Advanced Neuroimaging in Brain Tumors

Editor

SANGAM KANEKAR

RADIOLOGIC CLINICS OF NORTH AMERICA

www.radiologic.theclinics.com

Consulting Editor
FRANK H. MILLER

May 2021 • Volume 59 • Number 3

ELSEVIER

1600 John F. Kennedy Boulevard • Suite 1800 • Philadelphia, Pennsylvania, 19103-2899

http://www.theclinics.com

RADIOLOGIC CLINICS OF NORTH AMERICA Volume 59, Number 3
May 2021 ISSN 0033-8389, ISBN 13: 978-0-323-79421-3

Editor: John Vassallo (j.vassallo@elsevier.com)
Developmental Editor: Karen Solomon

Radiologic Clinics of North America (ISSN 0033-8389) is published bimonthly by Elsevier Inc., 360 Park Avenue South, New York, NY 10010-1710. Months of issue are January, March, May, July, September, and November. Periodicals postage paid at New York, NY and additional mailing offices. Subscription prices are USD 518 per year for US individuals, USD 1309 per year for US institutions, USD 100 per year for US students and residents, USD 611 per year for Canadian individuals, USD 1368 per year for Canadian institutions, USD 703 per year for international individuals, USD 1368 per year for international institutions, USD 100 per year for Canadian students/residents, and USD 315 per year for international students/residents. To receive student and resident rate, orders must be accompanied by name of affiliated institution, date of term and the signature of program/residency coordinatior on institution letterhead. Orders will be billed at individual rate until proof of status is received. Foreign air speed delivery is included in all *Clinics* subscription prices. All prices are subject to change without notice. **POSTMASTER:** Send address changes to *Radiologic Clinics of North America*, Elsevier Health Sciences Division, Subscription Customer Service, 3251 Riverport Lane, Maryland Heights, MO63043. **Customer Service: Telephone: 1-800-654-2452** (U.S. and Canada); **1-314-447-8871** (outside U.S. and Canada). **Fax: 1-314-447-8029. E-mail: journalscustomerservice-usa@elsevier.com (for print support); journalsonlinesupport-usa@elsevier.com (for online support)**.

Reprints. For copies of 100 or more of articles in this publication, please contact the Commercial Reprints Department, Elsevier Inc., 360 Park Avenue South, New York, New York 10010-1710. Tel.: +1-212-633-3874; Fax: +1-212-633-3820; E-mail: reprints@elsevier.com.

Radiologic Clinics of North America also published in Greek Paschalidis Medical Publications, Athens, Greece.

Radiologic Clinics of North America is covered in *MEDLINE/PubMed (Index Medicus), EMBASE/Excerpta Medica, Current Contents/Life Sciences, Current Contents/Clinical Medicine, RSNA Index to Imaging Literature, BIOSIS, Science Citation Index,* and *ISI/BIOMED*.

Printed in the United States of America.

Contributors

CONSULTING EDITOR

FRANK H. MILLER, MD, FACR
Lee F. Rogers MD Professor of Medical
Education, Chief, Body Imaging Section and
Fellowship Program, Medical Director, MRI,
Department of Radiology, Northwestern
Memorial Hospital, Northwestern University,
Feinberg School of Medicine, Chicago, Illinois

EDITOR

SANGAM KANEKAR, MD
Professor of Radiology and Neurology, Vice
Chair, Radiology Research, Chief, Division of
Neuroradiology, Penn State Milton Hershey
Medical Center, Penn State College of
Medicine, Hershey, Pennsylvania

AUTHORS

AMIT AGARWAL, MD
Associate Professor, Department of Radiology,
UT Southwestern Medical School and
Parkland Hospital, Dallas, Texas

SHRUTI AGARWAL, PhD
Division of Neuroradiology, The Russell H.
Morgan Department of Radiology and
Radiological Science, Johns Hopkins
School of Medicine, Baltimore, Maryland

CHAITRA BADVE, MBBS, MD
Assistant Professor, Department of Radiology,
Division of Neuroradiology, University
Hospitals Cleveland Medical Center,
Cleveland, Ohio

JAYAPALLI RAJIV BAPURAJ, MD
Division of Neuroradiology, Department of
Radiology, University of Michigan Medical
School, Michigan Medicine, Ann Arbor,
Michigan

PREM P. BATCHALA, MD
Assistant Professor of Nuclear Medicine and
Neuroradiology, Department of Radiology and
Medical Imaging, University of Virginia Health
System, Charlottesville, Virginia

ELHAM BEHESHTIAN, MD
Division of Neuroradiology, The Russell H.
Morgan Department of Radiology and
Radiological Science, Johns Hopkins School of
Medicine, Baltimore, Maryland

JOSEPH H. DONAHUE, MD
Assistant Professor of Neuroradiology,
Department of Radiology and Medical Imaging,
University of Virginia Health System,
Charlottesville, Virginia

**THOMAS J. ELUVATHINGAL MUTTIKKAL,
MD**
Assistant Professor of Neuroradiology,
Department of Radiology and Medical Imaging,
University of Virginia Health System,
Charlottesville, Virginia

CAMILO E. FADUL, MD
Professor of Neurology, Medicine, and
Neurological Surgery, Department of
Neurology, University of Virginia Health
System, Charlottesville, Virginia

DIANA GOMEZ-HASSAN, MD
Division of Neuroradiology, Department of Radiology, University of Michigan Medical School, Michigan Medicine, Ann Arbor, Michigan

SACHIN K. GUJAR, MBBS
Division of Neuroradiology, The Russell H. Morgan Department of Radiology and Radiological Science, Johns Hopkins School of Medicine, Baltimore, Maryland

MICHAEL J. HOCH, MD
Assistant Professor, Department of Radiology, University of Pennsylvania, Hospital of the University of Pennsylvania, Philadelphia, Pennsylvania

RANLIANG HU, MD
Assistant Professor, Department of Radiology and Imaging Sciences, Emory University, Emory University Hospital, Atlanta, Georgia

MICHAEL IV, MD
Clinical Associate Professor, Division of Neuroimaging and Neurointervention, Department of Radiology, Stanford University, Stanford, California

ROZITA JALILIANHASANPOUR, MD
Division of Neuroradiology, The Russell H. Morgan Department of Radiology and Radiological Science, Johns Hopkins School of Medicine, Baltimore, Maryland

SANGAM KANEKAR, MD
Professor of Radiology and Neurology, Vice Chair, Radiology Research, Chief, Division of Neuroradiology, Penn State Milton Hershey Medical Center, Penn State College of Medicine, Hershey, Pennsylvania

MANOHAR KURUVA, MD
Assistant Professor, Radiology and Imaging Sciences, Emory University, Atlanta, Georgia

LICIA P. LUNA, MD, PhD
Division of Neuroradiology, The Russell H. Morgan Department of Radiology and Radiological Science, Johns Hopkins School of Medicine, Baltimore, Maryland

SUGOTO MUKHERJEE, MD
Associate Professor of Neuroradiology, Department of Radiology and Medical Imaging, University of Virginia Health System, Charlottesville, Virginia

MARK E. MULLINS, MD, PhD
Professor, Radiology and Imaging Sciences, Emory University, Atlanta, Georgia

TAO OUYANG, MD
Assistant Professor, Department of Radiology, Penn State Health Milton Hershey Medical Center, Penn State College of Medicine, Hershey, Pennsylvania

SOHIL H. PATEL, MD
Associate Professor of Neuroradiology, Department of Radiology and Medical Imaging, University of Virginia Health System, Charlottesville, Virginia

KRISHNA PERNI, MD
Division of Neuroradiology, Department of Radiology, University of Michigan Medical School, Michigan Medicine, Ann Arbor, Michigan

JAY J. PILLAI, MD
Division of Neuroradiology, The Russell H. Morgan Department of Radiology and Radiological Science, Department of Neurosurgery, Johns Hopkins School of Medicine, Baltimore, Maryland

MARTIN G. POMPER, MD, PhD
Professor of Radiology and Radiological Science, The Russell H. Morgan Department of Radiology and Radiological Science, Johns Hopkins School of Medicine, Baltimore, Maryland

STEVEN P. ROWE, MD, PhD
Associate Professor, The Russell H. Morgan Department of Radiology and Radiological Science, Johns Hopkins School of Medicine, Baltimore, Maryland

DANIEL RYAN, MD
Division of Neuroradiology, The Russell H. Morgan Department of Radiology and Radiological Science, Johns Hopkins School of Medicine, Baltimore, Maryland

MOHAMMAD S. SADAGHIANI, MD, MPH
Resident Physician, The Russell H. Morgan Department of Radiology and Radiological

Science, Johns Hopkins School of Medicine, Baltimore, Maryland

HARIS I. SAIR, MD
Division of Neuroradiology, The Russell H. Morgan Department of Radiology and Radiological Science, Johns Hopkins School of Medicine, The Malone Center for Engineering in Healthcare, The Whiting School of Engineering, Johns Hopkins University, Baltimore, Maryland

SARA SHEIKHBAHAEI, MD, MPH
Resident Physician, The Russell H. Morgan Department of Radiology and Radiological Science, Johns Hopkins School of Medicine, Baltimore, Maryland

HYUNSUK SHIM, PhD
Professor, Radiation Oncology, Emory University, Atlanta, Georgia

LILJA B. SOLNES, MD, MBA
Associate Professor, The Russell H. Morgan Department of Radiology and Radiological Science, Johns Hopkins School of Medicine, Baltimore, Maryland

ASHOK SRINIVASAN, MD
Division of Neuroradiology, Department of Radiology, University of Michigan Medical School, Michigan Medicine, Ann Arbor, Michigan

AUSTIN TRINH, MD
Clinical Instructor, Division of Neuroimaging and Neurointervention, Department of Radiology, Stanford University, Stanford, California

BRENT D. WEINBERG, MD, PhD
Assistant Professor, Radiology and Imaging Sciences, Emory University, Atlanta, Georgia

MAX WINTERMARK, MD
Professor, Division of Neuroimaging and Neurointervention, Department of Radiology, Stanford University, Stanford, California

BRAD E. ZACHARIA, MD, MS
Associate Professor, Department of Neurosurgery and Otolaryngology, Penn State Health, Hershey, Pennsylvania

THOMAS ZACHARIA, MD
Professor, Department of Radiology, Penn State Health, Hershey, Pennsylvania

Contents

Molecular features are now essential in distinguishing between glioma histologic subtypes. Currently, isocitrate dehydrogenase mutation, 1p19q codeletion, and MGMT methylation status play significant roles in optimizing medical and surgical treatment. Noninvasive pretreatment and post-treatment determination of glioma subtype is of great interest. Although imaging cannot replace the genetic panel at present, image findings have shown promising signs to identify and diagnose the types and subtypes of gliomas. This article details key imaging findings in the most common molecular glioma subtypes and highlights recent advances in imaging technologies to differentiate these lesions noninvasively.

Neuroimaging plays an essential role in the initial diagnosis and continued surveillance of intracranial neoplasms. The advent of perfusion techniques with computed tomography and MR imaging have proven useful in neuro-oncology, offering enhanced approaches for tumor grading, guiding stereotactic biopsies, and monitoring treatment efficacy. Perfusion imaging can help to identify treatment-related processes, such as radiation necrosis, pseudoprogression, and pseudoregression, and can help to inform treatment-related decision making. Perfusion imaging is useful to differentiate between tumor types and between tumor and nonneoplastic conditions. This article reviews the clinical relevance and implications of perfusion imaging in neuro-oncology and highlights promising perfusion biomarkers.

Diffusion MR imaging exploits the diffusion properties of water to generate contrast between normal tissue and pathology. Diffusion is an essential component of nearly all brain tumor MR imaging examinations. This review covers the important clinical applications of diffusion weighted imaging in the pretreatment diagnosis and grading of brain tumors and assessment of treatment response. Diffusion imaging improves the accuracy of identifying treatment-related effects that may mimic tumor improvement or worsening. Fiber tractography models of eloquent white matter pathways are generated using diffusion tensor imaging. A practical and concise tractography guide is provided for anyone new to preoperative surgical mapping.

Neoplastic meningitis (NM) and paraneoplastic syndromes (PNSs) are a rare group of disorders present in patients with cancer. Clinical diagnosis of these conditions is challenging, and imaging and laboratory analysis play a significant role in diagnosing. Diagnosis of NM largely depends on documenting circulating tumor cells in the cerebrospinal fluid (CSF) and/or leptomeningeal and nodular enhancement on contrast-enhanced MR imaging of the brain or axial spine. PNSs encompass a variety of symptoms or syndromes. Paraneoplastic neuronal disorder diagnosis requires a multidimensional approach, high clinical suspicion, CSF and serum examination, and imaging. Neuroimaging is an integral part in the evaluation.

Neurologic injury arises from treatment of central nervous system malignancies as result of direct toxic effects or indirect vascular, autoimmune, or infectious effects. Multimodality treatment may potentiate both therapeutic and toxic effects. Symptoms range from mild to severe and permanent. Injuries can be immediate or delayed. Many early complications are nonspecific. Other early and delayed neurologic injuries, such as posterior reversible encephalopathy syndrome, dural sinus thrombosis, infarctions, myelopathy, leukoencephalopathy, and hypophysitis, have unique imaging features. This article reviews treatment options for neurologic malignancies and common and uncommon neurologic injuries that can result from treatment, focusing on radiologic features.

The 2016 World Health Organization brain tumor classification is based on genomic and molecular profile of tumor tissue. These characteristics have improved understanding of the brain tumor and played an important role in treatment planning and prognostication. There is an ongoing effort to develop noninvasive imaging techniques that provide insight into tissue characteristics at the cellular and molecular levels. This article focuses on the molecular characteristics of gliomas, transcriptomic subtypes, and radiogenomic studies using semantic and radiomic features. The limitations and future directions of radiogenomics as a standalone diagnostic tool also are discussed.

Nonneoplastic entities may closely resemble the imaging findings of primary or metastatic intracranial neoplasia, posing diagnostic challenges for the referring provider and radiologist. Prospective identification of brain tumor mimics is an opportunity for the radiologist to add value to patient care by decreasing time to diagnosis and avoiding unnecessary surgical procedures and medical therapies, but requires familiarity with mimic entities and a high degree of suspicion on the part of the interpreting radiologist. This article provides a framework for the radiologist to identify "brain tumor mimics," highlighting imaging and laboratory pearls and pitfalls, and illustrating unique and frequently encountered lesions.

Tumor predisposition syndromes represent a heterogeneous group of multiorgan disorders, with many having substantial central nervous system involvement. This article highlights the common and uncommon manifestations of these syndromic disorders, the underlying genetic pathways, and the imaging findings. Radiologists must be aware of the diagnostic criteria, optimal imaging techniques (both for diagnosis and surveillance), as well as the innumerable imaging manifestations of these syndromes. Multidisciplinary approach and teamwork are essential in managing these patients, with imaging having a central role as more of these patients get diagnosed earlier and survive longer.

PROGRAM OBJECTIVE
The objective of the *Radiologic Clinics of North America* is to keep practicing radiologists and radiology residents up to date with current clinical practice in radiology by providing timely articles reviewing the state of the art in patient care.

TARGET AUDIENCE
Practicing radiologists, radiology residents, and other healthcare professionals who provide patient care utilizing radiologic findings.

LEARNING OBJECTIVES
Upon completion of this activity, participants will be able to:
1. Describe the current state of imaging in brain cancer.
2. Discuss the imaging techniques employed for the diagnoses and for follow up of the brain tumors.
3. Recognize advances in imaging technologies to differentiate the most common molecular glioma subtypes.

ACCREDITATION
The Elsevier Office of Continuing Medical Education (EOCME) is accredited by the Accreditation Council for Continuing Medical Education (ACCME) to provide continuing medical education for physicians.

The EOCME designates this journal-based CME activity for a maximum of 12 *AMA PRA Category 1 Credit*(s)™. Physicians should claim only the credit commensurate with the extent of their participation in the activity.

All other healthcare professionals requesting continuing education credit for this enduring material will be issued a certificate of participation.

DISCLOSURE OF CONFLICTS OF INTEREST
The EOCME assesses conflict of interest with its instructors, faculty, planners, and other individuals who are in a position to control the content of CME activities. All relevant conflicts of interest that are identified are thoroughly vetted by EOCME for fair balance, scientific objectivity, and patient care recommendations. EOCME is committed to providing its learners with CME activities that promote improvements or quality in healthcare and not a specific proprietary business or a commercial interest.

The planning committee, staff, authors, and editors listed below have identified no financial relationships or relationships to products or devices they or their spouse/life partner have with commercial interest related to the content of this CME activity:
Amit Agarwal, MD; Shruti Agarwal, PhD; Chaitra Badve, MBBS, MD; Jayapalli Rajiv Bapuraj, MD; Prem P. Batchala, MD; Elham Beheshtian, MD; Regina Chavous-Gibson, MSN, RN; Joseph H. Donahue, MD; Thomas J. Eluvathingal Muttikkal, MD; Camilo E. Fadul, MD; Diana Gomez-Hassan, MD; Sachin K. Gujar, MBBS; Michael J. Hoch, MD; Ranliang Hu, MD; Michael Iv, MD; Rozita Jalilianhasanpour, MD; Sangam Kanekar, MD; Manohar Kuruva, MD; Pradeep Kuttysankaran; Licia P. Luna, MD, PhD; Sugoto Mukherjee, MD; Mark E. Mullins, MD, PhD; Tao Ouyang, MD; Sohil H. Patel, MD; Krishna Perni, MD; Jay J. Pillai, MD; Martin G. Pomper, MD, PhD; Steven P. Rowe, MD, PhD; Daniel Ryan, MD; Mohammad S. Sadaghiani, MD, MPH; Haris I. Sair, MD; Sara Sheikhbahaei, MD, MPH; Hyunsuk Shim, PhD; Ashok Srinivasan, MD; Austin Trinh, MD; John Vassallo; Brent D. Weinberg, MD, PhD; Max Wintermark, MD; Thomas Zacharia, MD.

The planning committee, staff, authors, and editors listed below have identified financial relationships or relationships to products or devices they or their spouse/life partner have with commercial interest related to the content of this CME activity:
Lilja B. Solnes, MD, MBA: consultant/advisor: Progenics Pharmaceuticals, Inc.

Brad E. Zacharia, MD, MS: speaker's bureau: Nico Corporation; consultant/advisor: Medtronic

UNAPPROVED/OFF-LABEL USE DISCLOSURE
The EOCME requires CME faculty to disclose to the participants:
1. When products or procedures being discussed are off-label, unlabelled, experimental, and/or investigational (not US Food and Drug Administration [FDA] approved); and
2. Any limitations on the information presented, such as data that are preliminary or that represent ongoing research, interim analyses, and/or unsupported opinions. Faculty may discuss information about pharmaceutical agents that is outside of FDA-approved labelling. This information is intended solely for CME and is not intended to promote off-label use of these medications. If you have any questions, contact the medical affairs department of the manufacturer for the most recent prescribing information.

TO ENROLL
To enroll in the *Radiologic Clinics of North America* Continuing Medical Education program, call customer service at 1-800-654-2452 or sign up online at http://www.theclinics.com/home/cme. The CME program is available to subscribers for an additional annual fee of USD 356.00.

METHOD OF PARTICIPATION

In order to claim credit, participants must complete the following:

1. Complete enrolment as indicated above.
2. Read the activity.
3. Complete the CME Test and Evaluation. Participants must achieve a score of 70% on the test. All CME Tests and Evaluations must be completed online.

CME INQUIRIES/SPECIAL NEEDS

For all CME inquiries or special needs, please contact elsevierCME@elsevier.com.

RADIOLOGIC CLINICS OF NORTH AMERICA

RELATED SERIES

Advances in Clinical Radiology
www.advancesinclinicalradiology.com
MRI Clinics
www.mri.theclinics.com
Neuroimaging Clinics
www.neuroimaging.theclinics.com
PET Clinics
www.pet.theclinics.com

Preface
Advanced Neuroimaging in Brain Tumors

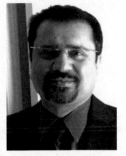

Sangam Kanekar, MD
Editor

The 2003 Human Genome Project and 2016 World Health Organization classification have made significant impacts on our understanding of brain tumors. Current research in brain tumors is focused on tumor genomics to identify novel therapeutic targets, devise personalized treatment options, and improve individual patient outcomes. In parallel, brain tumor imaging has also seen rapid growth with the development of advanced imaging techniques that provide insight into tissue characteristics at the cellular and molecular level. Molecular imaging techniques have made remarkable progress with the development of niche areas of texture analysis/radiomics and the applications of machine learning and artificial intelligence techniques.

Structural and molecular imaging plays a major role in diagnosis, treatment planning, and follow-up of the brain tumor. Preoperative imaging includes routine structural MR imaging along with various functional and molecular imaging techniques to aid the neurosurgeon in maximizing tumor excision. MR imaging, in particular, remains the basis for analyzing residual tumors, assessing treatment response, and guiding management. This *Radiologic Clinics of North America* issue strives to describe the current state of imaging in Brain Cancer, covering the imaging techniques employed for the diagnoses and for follow-up of the brain tumors.

I, along with my coauthors, present before you an issue of *Radiology Clinics of North America* dedicated to "Advanced Neuroimaging in Brain Tumors." This issue has 12 articles, predominately dedicated to the imaging approach in the preoperative and postoperative follow-up of the brain tumor. This subsequently plays a significant role in triage and treatment strategies.

I thank all the authors for their contributions that made this issue an outstanding and extensive review on "Advanced Neuroimaging in Brain Tumors." I take this opportunity to thank Dr Frank Miller, MD for graciously providing me a platform to present this topic to a wider audience. I wish to thank the departments of radiology, neurosurgery, and radiation oncology at the Penn State Milton S. Hershey Medical Center. Finally, I thank my wife, Revati, and my children, Samika and Rachita, for their continued support and love.

Sangam Kanekar, MD
Division of Neuroradiology
Penn State Milton Hershey Medical Center
Penn State College of Medicine
Mail Code H066, 500 University Drive
Hershey, PA 17033, USA

E-mail address:
skanekar@pennstatehealth.psu.edu

Radiol Clin N Am 59 (2021) xv
https://doi.org/10.1016/j.rcl.2021.02.004
0033-8389/21/© 2021 Published by Elsevier Inc.

Imaging Findings of New Entities and Patterns in Brain Tumor
Isocitrate Dehydrogenase Mutant, Isocitrate Dehydrogenase Wild-Type, Codeletion, and MGMT Methylation

Sangam Kanekar, MD[a],*, Brad E. Zacharia, MD, MS[b]

KEYWORDS

- Glioma molecular status • IDH • Codeletion • MGMT • Radiomics

KEY POINTS

- Molecular features are necessary for diagnosis of glioma subtype and greatly impact prognosis and treatment response.
- Increased contrast enhancement, sharp tumor margins, and homogenous signal intensity are characteristic of IDH-mutant gliomas, whereas degree of necrosis is not.
- T2-FLAIR mismatch is specific to IDH-mutant, 1p19q nondeleted gliomas (diffuse astrocytoma).
- Advanced MR imaging techniques, such as sodium MR imaging, deep learning, diffusion kurtosis imaging, and texture analysis, are used to predict molecular subtypes.

BACKGROUND

The 2016 World Health Organization (WHO) Classification of Tumors of the Central Nervous System set forth a revised classification system for brain tumors. This update included molecular aberrations in the definition of particular brain tumors and, to some extent, explained why some tumors of identical cell types appear similar on histology but respond differently to the same therapy and have different prognoses.[1] Today, this is thought to be caused by different genetic makeups of tumors, generating tremendous interest in the reclassification of cancers. Several molecular markers including isocitrate dehydrogenase (IDH), 1p/19q codeletion, O6-methylguanine-DNA methyltransferase methylation (MGMT), telomerase reverse transcriptase gene (TERT), α-thalassemia/mental retardation syndrome X-linked gene (ATRX), and p53, were identified as necessary for diagnoses of various gliomas (Fig. 1).[1–3]

There is parallel effort from an imaging perspective to be able to obtain molecular and genetic information from structural and molecular imaging techniques to match the new genotypic classifications. A major initiative to accomplish this was The Cancer Genome Atlas, undertaken by the National Institutes of Health.[4] This led to the Cancer Imaging Program, which obtains radiologic imaging data for The Cancer Genome Atlas patients and makes it available via The Cancer Imaging Archive.[4] The first large-scale imaging genomic study performed in glioblastomas (GBM) paved the way for the potential correlation between imaging features and histologic patterns and genetic profiles of the tumor, known collectively as

[a] Department of Radiology and Neurology, Penn State Health, Hershey Medical Center, Mail Code H066, 500 University Drive, Hershey, PA 17033, USA; [b] Department of Neurosurgery and Otolaryngology, Penn State Health, 30 Hope Drive, Hershey, PA 17033, USA
* Corresponding author. PO Box 850, 500 University Drive, Hershey, PA 17033.
E-mail address: skanekar@pennstatehealth.psu.edu

Radiol Clin N Am 59 (2021) 305–322
https://doi.org/10.1016/j.rcl.2021.01.001
0033-8389/21/© 2021 Elsevier Inc. All rights reserved.

"radiohistogenomic interpretation."[5] Radiomic-imaging features play an important role in accurate and early prediction of tumor genotype when genetic sequencing is not available.

GENETIC FACTORS

The 2016 central nervous system (CNS) WHO classification offered an attempt to standardize the terminology combining histopathologic and molecular features. Today CNS tumor naming includes histologic appearance (ie, astrocytoma or oligodendroglioma), WHO grade (II, III), and genetic features. Work on genotyping and identifying specific markers for brain tumors is ongoing. Histologic appearance is decided by routine staining techniques used in histopathology, which decides the cell lineage for the tumor. WHO grading (WHO I, II, III, and IV) of the diffuse glioma depends on cellularity, cortical infiltration, nuclear pleomorphism, hyperchromasia, and mitotic figures. The new classification posits grade I gliomas as virtually nonexistent in adults. Currently, the main molecular makers of diagnostic significance for gliomas include IDH, 1p19q deletion, MGMT, TERT, ATRX, and a tumor protein p53 gene (TP53).[2,3]

Diffuse gliomas based on gene expression and available molecular markers are classified as follows: grade II (diffuse astrocytoma, *IDH* mutant) and grade III astrocytic tumors (anaplastic astrocytoma, *IDH* mutant), grade II (oligodendroglioma *IDH* mutant and 1p/19q codeleted) and grade III oligodendrogliomas (anaplastic oligodendroglioma *IDH* mutant and 1p/19q codeleted), grade IV GBM (GBM *IDH* mutant and *IDH* wild-type), and diffuse gliomas of childhood (diffuse midline glioma, H3-K27M-mutant) (see **Fig. 1**).[2,3] Whenever molecular diagnostic testing is not available or genetic assay testing is inconclusive, the Not Otherwise Specified (NOS) category is used.

Neuro-oncology teams are of the opinion that much work still needs to be done to have a clear understanding of the genetic basis for many of the other brain tumors, including GBM. Following the 2016 classification, the Consortium to Inform Molecular and Practical Approaches to CNS Tumor Taxonomy (cIMPACT-NOW) was created in late 2016 under the sponsorship of the International Society of Neuropathology to provide a forum to evaluate and recommend proposed changes to future CNS tumor classifications.[6] cIMPACT-NOW updates are intended to provide guidance for diagnosticians and potentially inform future WHO classifications. This article focuses on correlating the phenotypic and genotypic features of gliomas, gliomagenesis of GBM, IDH mutation, other molecular markers and mutations in diffuse gliomas, and their imaging correlates on various MR imaging techniques.

Isocitrate Dehydrogenase Status

In humans, IDH exists in three isoforms (IDH1, IDH2, and IDH3). IDH1 and IDH2 are proteins in the cytosol and mitochondria, respectively, that

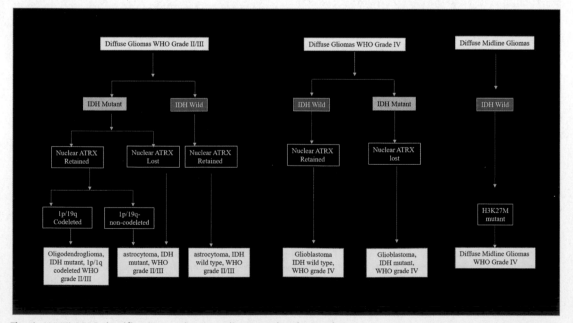

Fig. 1. WHO 2016 classification update on glioma molecular markers.

generate reduced nicotinamide adenine dinucleotide phosphate from NADP$^+$ by catalyzing the oxidative decarboxylation of isocitrate to α-ketoglutarate outside of the Krebs cycle (**Fig. 2**).[7–9] IDH3 functions to convert isocitrate to α-ketoglutarate and NAD$^+$ to NADH in the Krebs cycle. IDH plays an important role in cellular defense against oxidative stress. Cells with low levels of IDH become more sensitive to oxidative damage. IDH1 mutations involve an amino acid substitution (glycine to arginine) in the active site of the enzyme in codon 132 (R132H).[7–9] This mutation results in the abnormal production of 2-hydroxyglutarate (2HG), which causes histone and DNA methylation, thereby promoting tumorigenesis. IDH2 mutations occur in codon 172 and are associated with 2-hydroxyglutaric aciduria. These result in seizures, weak muscle tone (hypotonia), and progressive damage to the brain parenchyma.[7–9] Inhibition of these enzymes results in widespread histone and DNA methylation, which in turn leads to increased tumorigenesis.[4] Mutant IDH1 and IDH2 occur in more than 70% of WHO grade II and III astrocytomas, oligodendrogliomas, and in secondary GBM that developed from the previously mentioned lower-grade lesions.[10]

IDH1 and IDH2 are enzymes that function at the crossroads of cellular metabolism, epigenetic regulation, redox states, and DNA repair. The pro-oncogenic effect of *IDH* mutations is caused by the damage produced by high levels of reactive oxygen species to DNA and by 2HG, an oncometabolite that alters cell proliferation.[8,11] 2HG impairs the maturation of extracellular collagen in the brain capillary network basement membrane, which promotes cell migration to the extravascular space and intravascular fluid leakage into the extracellular space. This leakage is reflected as enhancement on contrast-enhanced MR imaging and permeability on MR perfusion imaging.

The Cancer Genome Atlas Research Network found an *IDH* mutation rate of 80% of grade II/III gliomas (diffuse astrocytomas, oligodendrogliomas, and oligoastrocytomas) and only 10% in GBM.[12,13] Based on these results, the WHO now recognizes the *IDH* mutation as a critical biomarker in glioma classification. Among the GBM, IDH1/IDH2 mutations are more commonly seen in secondary GBM originating from lower-grade diffuse gliomas than in primary GBM. When both IDH1/IDH2 mutant are negative, as in the primary GBM, it is labeled as IDH wild-type.[12–14] If IDH testing is not available, cannot be fully performed, or is inconclusive, the GBM is labeled IDH NOS. *IDH* status is considered an independent determinant of prognosis in patients

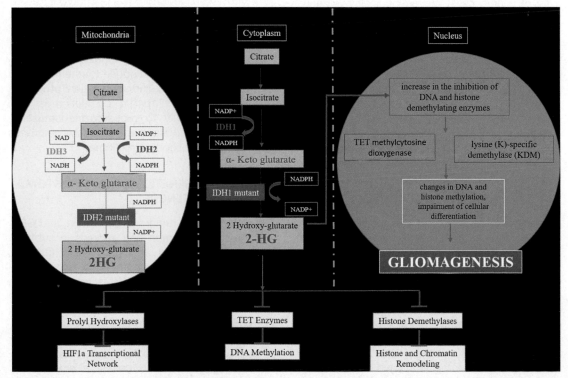

Fig. 2. Diagrammatic presentation of gliomagenesis.

with diffuse gliomas. Survival is higher in *IDH*-mutant patients than in *IDH* wild-type patients.

MGMT Methylation

MGMT is an apoptotic enzyme and DNA repair protein that inhibits the cross-linkage of double-stranded DNA, and repairs premutagenic, precarcinogenic, and pretoxic DNA damage.[15–17] Methylation within the MGMT gene promoter on chromosome 10q26.3 induces loss of function of the protein, ultimately leading to insufficient DNA repair and tumorigenesis.[16,17] For brain tumors, MGMT activity declines as glioma grade increases.

Alkylating chemotherapeutics (ie, methylating agents [procarbazine, dacarbazine streptozotocin, and temozolomide] and chloroethylating agents [carmustine, lomustine, nimustine, and fotemustine]) are commonly used in the treatment of brain tumors, malignant melanoma, and lymphoma because they are powerful inducers of apoptosis.[16–19] These alkylating agents cause mutations, sister chromatid exchanges, recombination and chromosomal aberrations, and DNA mismatch repair to DNA double-strand breaks that trigger cell death. However, their efficacy largely depends on MGMT expression. The loss of MGMT protein expression caused by MGMT promoter methylation reduces the DNA repair activity of glioma cells, preventing their resistance to alkylating agents. Patients with GBM and a methylated MGMT promoter are more sensitive to the killing effects of alkylating drugs because tumor cells with low MGMT expression are unable to repair such DNA lesions and are prone to apoptosis.[16–19] Cancer cells that overexpress MGMT are resistant to alkylating agents. Therefore, MGMT promoter methylation is the most relevant prognostic marker and is used to predict a therapeutic response to alkylating agents. Documentation of MGMT promoter methylation is important to decide the choice of chemotherapy or radiotherapy in patients with brain tumors.

Methylation of the promoter region of the MGMT gene is more frequently found in secondary GBMs compared with primary GBMs (75% vs 36%).[17,18] By knowing whether or not the MGMT promoter is methylated, response to temozolomide, a standard adjuvant chemotherapy treatment of GBMs, may be predicted.[16] Overall survival (OS) in methylated patients is better when temozolomide is given concurrently with radiation therapy. In unmethylated patients, radiotherapy alone is more effective.[16,18,19] In addition, GBM patients with MGMT promoter methylation have better OS and progression-free survival (PFS) than those without methylated MGMT promoters regardless of therapeutic intervention. MGMT promoter methylation is also a strong predictor of pseudoprogression and IDH mutation to the extent that almost all patients with an IDH mutation also exhibit MGMT promoter methylation.

1p/19q Codeletion

According to the 2016 WHO classification of CNS tumors, 1p19q codeletion is required for the diagnosis of oligodendroglioma.[20] A 1p/19q codeletion is the complete deletion of the short arm of chromosome 1 (1p) and the long arm of chromosome 19 (19q).[3,12] It is a definitive marker for grades II and III (anaplastic) oligodendroglioma. In contrast, a patient that is IDH positive and lacks a 1p19q codeletion carries a diagnosis of a diffuse astrocytoma (see **Fig. 1**).[20,21]

It is important to remember that oligodendroglial tumors have neither *ATRX* nor *TP53* gene mutations. An oligodendroglioma that is IDH-mutant but has not been analyzed for 1p/19q status is designated as oligodendroglioma NOS, whereas an oligodendroglioma that is IDH-mutant with a 1p deletion but an intact 19q is designated as diffuse glioma, IDH-mutant with 1p loss/19q retention, Not Elsewhere Classified (NEC).[3,12,22,23] Histopathologically diagnosed oligodendrogliomas without 1p19q codeletion is classified as a diffuse glioma of the oligodendroglial phenotype. Pediatric oligodendrogliomas are IDH negative, do not display 1p/19q codeletion, and are classified as NOS.

The presence of 1p/19q codeletion is associated with a favorable response to chemotherapy and radiotherapy and ultimately patient prognosis and survival.[20,21,24] 1p/19q codeletion is also linked to sensitivity to procarbazine-lomustine-vincristine chemotherapy and improved outcomes in patients with oligodendroglioma.[22,24]

MOLECULAR GENETICS OF GLIOBLASTOMA AND GLIOMAGENESIS

Gliomas are CNS tumors of glial origin, and GBM are the most common and aggressive subtype. On the phenotyping and genotyping features, GBM is classified into primary (95%) and secondary GBMs (5%). Primary GBMs are aggressive, highly invasive, and more commonly seen in the elderly.[2,3,25,26] Secondary GBMs are much less common, arise from low-grade gliomas, mostly seen younger than the age of 45, and have a better prognosis. GBMs are histologically indistinguishable but show distinctive genetic alterations that allows differentiation.

Genetic alterations occur in major key pathways to form GBMs. Gliomagenesis is a multifactorial process involving several genetic mutations. The introduction of genotyping has had a major impact on the classification, treatment, and understanding of outcome for GBMs. IDH status classifies GBMs into three types: IDH wild-type, IDH-mutant, and IDH NOS.[2,3,11,12]

1. IDH wild-type GBMs are also called primary or de novo GBMs. They form around 95% of the total GBMs and are primarily seen in patients older than 55. In contrast to the IDH-mutant, IDH wild-type follow an aggressive course and have poor prognosis. They are associated with various genetic alterations including epidermal growth factor receptor (EGFR), MGMT, the phosphatase and tensin homolog, TP53, platelet-derived growth factor receptor-α (PDGFRA), neurofibromin 1 (NF1), cyclin-dependent kinase inhibitor 2A and B (CDKN2A/B) genes, and telomerase reverse transcriptase (TERT) promoter.[27–29]

The most commonly pathway involved is receptor tyrosine kinases, which bind with growth factors inducing a conformational shift.[27–29] This shift activates the kinase function of the receptor tyrosine kinases allowing cross-phosphorylation of tyrosine residues in preparation for downstream signaling cascades. EGFR functions in the proliferation, migration, differentiation, and survival of all types of CNS cells.[28,29] In GBM cells, EGFR signaling gets activated either through overexpression of the receptor and its ligand amplifying the EGFR function. Amplification of the EGFR gene and activating mutations of its protein product are hallmarks of primary GBM and are associated with TP53 mutations.[3,13,28,29] PTEN amplification and loss of chromosome 10 are additional features of primary GBMs. Verhaak and colleagues[30] described a robust gene expression–based molecular classification of GBMs into proneural, neural, classical, and mesenchymal subtypes that integrate multidimensional genomic data to establish patterns of somatic mutations and DNA copy number. Primary GBMs represent the classical, mesenchymal, and neural subtypes. The mesenchymal and classical subtypes are typically associated with more aggressive, higher-grade gliomas. The classical subtype demonstrates a greater preponderance of EGFR amplification, decreased rates of TP53 mutation, and p16INK4A and p14ARF deletion.[30]

2. IDH-mutant GBMs, also called secondary GBMs, usually arise from diffuse WHO grade II or III gliomas. Genetic alterations common to secondary GBMs include TP53 mutations and IDH1/2 mutations.[27,28,31] TP53 mutations are detectable in the early stages of secondary GBM. IDH1/2 mutations rarely occur in primary GBMs and are therefore the most reliable indicator to differentiate between primary and secondary GBMs. Secondary GBMs are also associated ATRX (80%) and retinoblastoma protein 1 (Rb1) mutations, reflecting its origin from lower-grade gliomas.[27,28] It is primarily seen within the frontal lobe and corresponds to the proneural histologic subtype on the Verhaak and colleagues[30] classification. The proneural subtype is less aggressive; seen in younger patients; and has alterations in TP53, PDGFRA, PIK3C, and IDH1[30]

3. The NOS group includes tumors for which the IDH status cannot be determined.[3,6] Another recently introduced category is NEC, used when diagnostic testing has been successfully performed, but the results do not allow for a WHO categorization. In contrast, the NOS designation is used when a full molecular work-up has not been undertaken or was not successful. NEC diagnoses are descriptive diagnoses where the pathologist uses a non-WHO term to describe the tumor.

Tumor heterogeneity, one of the hallmarks of GBM, is the presence of multiple different cell subpopulations within a single tumor. It is caused by cancer stem cells that possess varying degrees of stemness, the ability to self-renew and differentiate into different tumor cell types, and clonal evolution that may enhance genetic diversity within the affected tissues.[32,33] This heterogeneity varies from different zones of the GBM, namely the core, interface, and peripheral brain zones. Because tumor fragments from the same patient may have different molecular subtypes in different zones, GBM grading is complex. GBM also shows epithelial to mesenchymal transitions, thought to be caused by signaling pathways of Wnt, transforming growth factor-β, and NOTCH.[32,33] This transition is partly responsible for the migration, diffusion invasion, and angiogenesis of GBM. By virtue of the inherent heterogeneity of these tumors, not all of the cells within a glioma respond to chemotherapy and radiation, resulting in tumor progression/recurrence.

IMAGING

Phenotyping and genotyping using tumor tissue remains the gold standard for characterizing the histologic type and genetic make of the tumor; it is thereby the predominant factor in deciding choice the treatment and prognosis. However, pathology and genotyping have their own limitations. One major downside of pathologic analysis is intratumoral heterogeneity, even across molecular subtypes. It is often not feasible to study every section of invasive tumor, and the availability of the newer diagnostic tools, such as immunohistochemistry, genotyping, and molecular markers, is limited and expensive. Another clinical limitation of genotyping is that the study of a tumor's genetic profile can only be done on tumor tissue samples processed in the primary institution or laboratory. Furthermore, the usefulness of these techniques is limited once the patient is on radiation or chemotherapy. Unfortunately, there is still no worldwide standard for processing and analyzing tissue samples. The quest for developing a noninvasive, cheaper, and specific technique to identify the molecular/genomic makeup of tumors is still ongoing.

ROLE OF MR IMAGING

At present, imaging modalities have limitations in locating the point mutation of a tumor's genetic material. However, the Cancer Imaging Program and The Cancer Imaging Archive have paved the way to correlate imaging features and histologic patterns with the genetic profile of the tumor; this is called "radiohistogenomic interpretation."[13,27,34] Thus, in the absence of genetic sequencing, imaging modalities play an important role.

Molecular imaging using MR imaging techniques, such as diffusion-weighted imaging/apparent diffusion coefficient (ADC), MR spectroscopy, MR perfusion, dynamic susceptibility contrast MR perfusion, and diffusion tensor imaging has shown promising results in understanding the genetic profile and biologic behavior of the tumor. Both structural and molecular imaging play an important role in the radiohistogenomic classification of the brain tumor. Markers that have been found useful in these classifications include location of the tumor, ADC values, FLAIR/T2 hyperintensities, chemical analysis of the tumor mass and surrounding brain using MR spectroscopy, and texture analysis using a combination of the previously mentioned techniques. These techniques are widely used to diagnose the IDH status; MGMT methylation; and, to a lesser extent, 1p/19q codeletion.[13,18,27,34] Extensive radiogenomic research is in progress to find imaging correlates of the other new molecular markers, such as TERT promoters, ATRX, TP53 mutations, TP53, diffuse midline gliomas, H3 K27M-mutant,

and wingless and sonic hedgehog activation.[13,18,27,30,34] A noninvasive prediction of IDH mutation is important because maximal surgical resection, including enhancing and nonenhancing tumors, may contribute to a better prognosis in IDH1-mutant gliomas. Although a survival benefit was noted in the complete resection of enhanced IDH1 wild-type gliomas, no survival benefit was observed in further resection of the nonenhanced portion.

KEY IMAGING FINDINGS
MGMT Methylation

Standard methods of imaging are limited in their ability to distinguish molecular subtypes of gliomas. These imaging modalities have not been able to clearly differentiate MGMT methylated from unmethylated tumors. Several investigations have evaluated the value of ADC for predicting MGMT promoter methylation, but the results are inconclusive.[35,36] However, a minimum ADC value may have some prognostic value in preoperatively estimating the status of MGMT promoter methylation (84% sensitive, 91% specific).[35] If a relationship were to be found between ADC and MGMT promoter methylation, this would be especially useful in noninvasively predicting methylation because accurate measurement of methylation is difficult because of small biopsy specimens and regional heterogeneity of GBM.

Knowing that MGMT promoter methylation has been used as a prognostic biomarker, researchers have also addressed the role of MGMT methylation via imaging in GBMs.[37] Using various MR imaging techniques, it was noted that the diagnostic performance of MR imaging for prediction of MGMT promoter methylation with recently diagnosed GBM patients was clinically viable.[37] This study found that MGMT promoter methylation in GBMs shows less edema, high ADC, and low perfusion on MR imaging, with a sensitivity at 79% (95% confidence interval, 72%–85%), a specificity of 78% (95% confidence interval, 71%–84%), and the area under the receiver operating curve (AUC) at 0.86 (95% confidence interval, 0.82–0.88).[37]

Another study evaluating MGMT promoter methylation in primary GBMs through imaging looked at the relationship between ADC and relative cerebral blood flow (rCBF) values in a manually drawn region of interest.[38] Using a combination of tumor location, necrosis, ADC, and rCBF, the highest AUC resulted in 0.914.[38] This suggests that ADC and rCBF, when used with other known factors of GBMs, are associated with the prediction of MGMT promoter methylation.[38]

Isocitrate Dehydrogenase Mutation

Determination of IDH mutation status is important and is usually determined via polymerase chain reaction, gene sequencing, and immunohistochemistry.[39] However, recent advances in imaging have afforded the potential to define the IDH status of diffuse gliomas (Table 1).[39,40] Radiogenomic texture analysis may show that a tumor's molecular differences and biologic behavior are mirrored in imaging features and that these parameters can be used for patient stratification to optimize glioma treatment.[39,40] This classification is clinically significant because IDH wild-type tumors have worse prognoses compared with secondary IDH-mutant tumors or others with more aggressive biologic behavior. The following is a compiled list of imaging findings correlated with IDH status:

- IDH-mutant tumors are primarily located in the frontal lobe or subventricular region of the frontal horns of the lateral ventricles and are less likely to invade eloquent areas of the brain.[18,21,41,42] IDH-mutant tumors are rare in the occipital lobe. IDH-mutant gliomas tend to be larger, exhibit slower growth, and have better defined contours than IDH wild-type gliomas.[18,42]
- Gliomas with IDH wild-type usually are multilobar; cross the midline; involve the corpus callosum; involve more than one lobe; and commonly affect eloquent areas and deeper structures, such as the diencephalon and brainstem.[18,42]
- IDH wild-type GBMs associated with unmethylated MGMT gene promoters are located predominantly in the right hemisphere and have poor prognoses. IDH-mutant MGMT methylated GBMs show better prognosis with temozolomide are located predominantly in the left hemisphere.[18,34]
- The presence of large portions of nonenhanced tumor in GBMs is strongly associated with the IDH1 mutation (Fig. 3). Large nonenhanced portions are caused by low VEGF levels in IDH-mutant tumors. IDH wild-type GBMs usually show smaller nonenhancing component.
- Yamashita and colleagues[43] suggested that percentage of cross-sectional necrosis area inside the enhancing lesion and necrosis area are significantly higher in patients with IDH1 wild-type than in those with IDH1 mutant GBMs (Fig. 4). The optimal cutoff for percentage of cross-sectional necrosis area inside the enhancing lesion was 22.5 with 72.7% sensitivity, 81.8% specificity, and 74.2%

accuracy. The optimal cutoff for necrosis area was 151 mm^2 with 72.7% sensitivity, 81.8% specificity, and 74.2% accuracy. The AUCs for percentage of cross-sectional necrosis area inside the enhancing lesion and necrosis area were 0.739 and 0.772, respectively.
- Zhou and colleagues[44] used textural analysis and found that according to the Visually Accessible Rembrandt Images (VASARI) annotations, increased proportion of necrosis and decreased lesion size were the most predictive for IDH-mutation status.
- ADC values correlate inversely with the cellularity of the tumor. Because of the lower cellularity of IDH-mutant tumors than IDH wild-type tumors, ADC values of IDH-mutant grade II and III astrocytomas are higher than those of wild-types (see Figs. 3C and 4B). An ADC mean of 1.2 can be used as a cutoff value to differentiate IDH wild-type and IDH-mutant gliomas. ADC means less than 1.08 have poor survival.[43] In addition, IDH-mutant tumors with codeletion 1p/19q, such as oligodendroglioma, have been shown to have greater ADC values and fractional anisotropy on diffusion tensor imaging imaging.
- Enhancement on postcontrast scans has historically been used to grade the aggressiveness of the tumor. However, the pattern of enhancement and perfusion largely depend on the chemical mediators that promote angiogenesis, such as EGFR, VEGF, and platelet-derived growth factors. Mutant GBMs show a more homogeneous, nodular, and less intense enhancement pattern compared with the wild-type tumors. IDH-mutant GBMs often have a greater proportion of nonenhanced tumor, whereas the ring enhancement with a central area of necrosis is a more common feature of IDH wild-type tumors.[18,45] It is found that a lower T2 abnormality to contrast enhancement volume ratio and central necrosis was predictive of the mesenchymal GBM subtype.
- MR imaging and computed tomography (CT) perfusion has been extensively studied to differentiate between the mutant and wild-type of GBMs. Because of low neovascularization, IDH-mutant GBMs have low relative cerebral blood volume value (1.09 ± 0.34 mL/100 g) compared with IDH wild-type GBMs (2.08 ± 0.54 mL/100 g) that show extensive angiogenesis.[46] Law and colleagues[47] demonstrated that the prognosis for patients with low-grade but highly perfused tumors was worse than that in

Table 1
Common genetic aberration and markers in the glioma

Genetic Aberration	CNS Tumor Association	Comments
IDH1/IDH2 mutation	Frequent in WHO grade II and III astrocytomas, oligodendrogliomas, secondary glioblastomas Required for diagnosis: Astrocytoma, IDH-mutant vs wild-type Anaplastic astrocytoma, IDH-mutant vs wild-type Glioblastoma, IDH-mutant vs wild-type Oligodendroglioma, IDH-mutant and lp/19q-codeleted Anaplastic oligodendroglioma, IDH-mutant and lp/19q-codeleted	IDH-mutant status signifies better prognosis compared with that of IDH wild-type even with the histologically same WHO grade
MGMT promoter hypermethylation	Reported as independent favorable prognostic factor in glioblastomas (irrespective of treatment)	Suggests improved prognosis in malignant glioma and predicts response to temozolomide chemotherapy and radiotherapy
EGFR amplification	Common in IDH wild-type glioblastomas (~40%)	Over expression of EGFR is responsible for proliferation and migration/infiltration in IDH wild-type
ATRX	Supportive for diagnosis of IDH-mutant diffuse astrocytoma/anaplastic astrocytoma/glioblastoma	ATRX mutations are almost always seen along with other mutations in the histone regulation, such as IDH, H3 K27M, and TP53
TP53 mutation	Supportive for diagnosis of IDH-mutant diffuse astrocytoma/anaplastic astrocytoma/glioblastoma	TP53 mutations also occur in IDH wild-type astrocytic tumors, but are rare in oligodendrogliomas
1p/19q codeletion	Required for diagnosis of: Oligodendroglioma, IDH-mutant, and 1p/19q codeleted Anaplastic oligodendroglioma, IDH-mutant, and 1p/19-codeleted	1p/19q codeletion is associated with sensitivity to procarbazine-lomustine-vincristine chemotherapy and improved outcome in patient with oligodendroglioma
H3 K27M mutation H3 Histone Family Member 3A (H3F3A) or Histone	Required for the diagnosis of diffuse midline glioma, H3 K27M-mutant	Signifies poor prognosis in diffuse midline glioma
TERT promoter mutation	Encountered in all grades of diffuse gliomas, ranging from WHO grade II to IV	TERT promoter mutations and long telomere length predict poor survival and radiotherapy resistance in gliomas

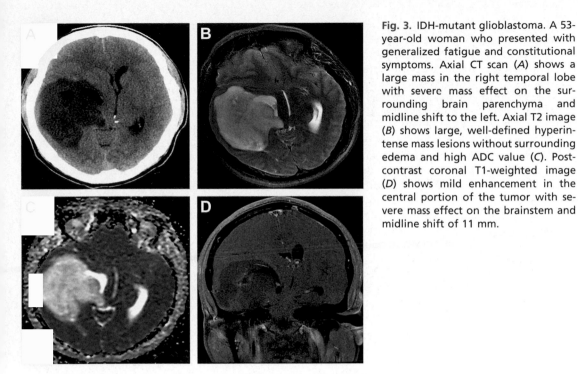

Fig. 3. IDH-mutant glioblastoma. A 53-year-old woman who presented with generalized fatigue and constitutional symptoms. Axial CT scan (*A*) shows a large mass in the right temporal lobe with severe mass effect on the surrounding brain parenchyma and midline shift to the left. Axial T2 image (*B*) shows large, well-defined hyperintense mass lesions without surrounding edema and high ADC value (*C*). Postcontrast coronal T1-weighted image (*D*) shows mild enhancement in the central portion of the tumor with severe mass effect on the brainstem and midline shift of 11 mm.

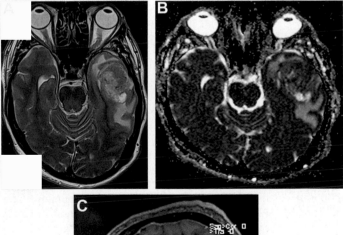

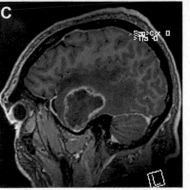

Fig. 4. IDH wild-type glioblastoma. A 62-year-old man presented to the emergency department with right-sided numbness and difficulties with fine motor skills. Axial T2-weighted image (*A*) shows heterointense mass in the left temporal lobe with large perilesional T2 hyperintensity. Axial ADC image (*B*) shows low ADC in the soft tissue component and few cystic areas. Sagittal postcontrast T1-weighted image (*C*) shows a necrotic mass with peripheral enhancement.

patients with high-grade, low-perfusion tumors. Yamashita and colleagues[43] using the arterial spin labeling technique, demonstrated that absolute tumor blood flow (aTBF) and relative tumor blood flow (rTBF) were significantly higher in patients with IDH wild-type GBMs than in patients with IDH-mutant GBMs. The optimal cutoff for aTBF was 70.0 mL/100 g/min with 76.5% sensitivity, 88.9% specificity, and 79.1% accuracy. The optimal cutoff for rTBF was 1.55 with 88.2% sensitivity, 77.8% specificity, and 86.0% accuracy, with the AUCs for aTBF and rTBF being 0.850 and 0.873, respectively.

- MR spectroscopy has shown encouraging results in differentiating types of glioma mutation. Mutations of the IDH1 and IDH2 genes result in an overreduction of the a-ketoglutarate to 2HG metabolite, leading to an accumulation of 2HG.[8,9,39,40] Using special proton MR spectroscopy point-resolved spectroscopy sequences, 2HG accumulation is analyzed qualitatively and quantitatively. Choi and colleagues[39] showed the existence of 2HG and glutamate multiplets in patients with IDH-mutated grade II-III tumors with 100% sensitivity and specificity. A maximum 2HG peak was identified at approximately 2.25 ppm, near the γ-aminobutyric acid peak (at 2.2–2.4 ppm) and located to the left of the N-acetylaspartate peak, at 2.0 ppm. Documentation of the 2HG peak is seen with IDH-mutation gliomas, and its absence is consistent with IDH wild-type tumors. MR spectroscopy has also been found useful in documenting the treatment response with DH1/2-mutant inhibitors.

Additionally, the VASARI, created by the Cancer Imaging Archive is a set of MR imaging features that are used to create uniform descriptions for gliomas. Researchers found that several of these features were significant predictors of IDH1-mutation status and 1p/19q codeletion status.[48] The following were considered to be independently associated with predicting IDH1 mutation based on the model generated (AUCs for predictive model, 0.859 and 0.778 for the discovery and validation sets, respectively)[48]: nonlobar tumor location, proportion of enhancing tumors of greater than 33%, multifocal/multicentric diffusion, and well-defined nonenhancing margin.

Determining IDH-mutation status is not only potentially useful in distinguishing gliomas from other lesions, it may help influence surgical decision-making, and help monitor treatment response or failure.[39,40] This method may also be useful in distinguishing between gliosis and lower-grade gliomas, possibly avoiding unnecessary biopsies or repeat surgical resections in ambiguous cases.[39,40]

1p/19q Codeletion on Imaging

1p/19q testing is not readily available in many locations. When formal 1p/19q testing is not possible, MR imaging features are likely to be more specific for determining 1p/19q status than histologic phenotype.[49–51] Genetically defined IDH-mutant codeletion oligodendrogliomas and IDH-mutant noncodeleted astrocytic gliomas differ in regards to tumor margins, heterogeneity, and ADC values.[49,51] Johnson and colleagues[49] found that 1p/19q codeleted oligodendrogliomas had poorly circumscribed borders in comparison with non-1p/19q codeleted astrocytic gliomas (**Fig. 5**). Even though there seem to be correlations between MR imaging findings and biomarkers in lower-grade gliomas, it is widely believed that conventional MR imaging findings are not sufficiently specific enough to predict histologic and/or molecular subtype of a low-grade glioma in an individual patient.

On MR imaging, more than 50% T2-FLAIR mismatch is strongly predictive of a noncodeleted astrocytic gliomas. The T2/FLAIR mismatch sign is represented as a homogeneous high signal on T2 sequence but as a bright rim and dark center on FLAIR images (**Fig. 6**). Patel and colleagues[50] showed that the substantial T2-FLAIR mismatch is specific to the IDH-mutant-noncodeleted molecular subtype of IDH-mutant gliomas, with 100% positive predictive value in the test and validation sets, with a high level of interrater agreement.[52] A T2-FLAIR mismatch on CT correlates with a markedly hypodense tumor. If a glioma were to be IDH-mutant, patients would significantly benefit from a gross total tumor resection compared with partial resection. Therefore, the T2-FLAIR mismatch sign may provide useful information to neurosurgeons before treatment planning stages of patient care encounters (see **Fig. 2**). Identification of this MR imaging biomarker may contribute to pretreatment planning and promote accurate and timely patient counseling.

The tumor is likely 1p/19q-codeleted if there are calcifications identified on CT or susceptibility weighted images. Johnson and colleagues[49] have also documented that noncircumscribed borders correlate with 1p/19q codeletion, but this appearance is also seen in 45% of noncodeleted tumors. Sharp borders are thought to be a better indicator for a noncodeleted tumor. Additionally, oligodendrogliomas are heterogenous on T1 and/or T2-weighted MR imaging and show ADC value less

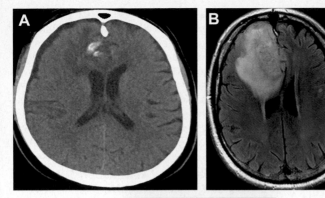

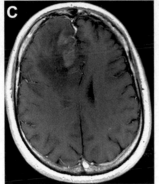

Fig. 5. Codeleted oligodendroglioma. A 39-year-old man with right frontal lobe oligodendroglioma, *IDH*-mutant, and 1p/19q codeleted, showing characteristic imaging features. Axial CT image (*A*) shows the right frontal lobe calcified mass with mild mass effect on the ventricular system. Axial FLAIR image (*B*) shows a hyperintense infiltrative mass in the right frontal lobe, which shows mild fluffy enhancement on its medial side on postcontrast T1 weighted images (*C*).

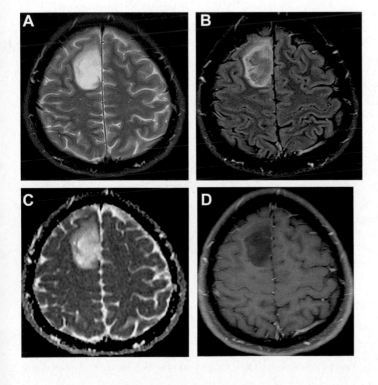

Fig. 6. Nondeleted astrocytoma. A 48-year-old man with a right frontal lobe diffuse astrocytoma, *IDH*-mutant, and 1p/19q noncodeleted, showing characteristic imaging features. Axial T2 image (*A*) shows a well-defined hyperintense mass in the right frontal lobe without much perilesional edema. Axial FLAIR image (*B*) shows hypointensity to isointensity in the central portion of the mass with surrounding hyperintensity. This is called T2-FLAIR mismatch sign. Mass shows high ADC and no enhancement on axial ADC (*C*) and postcontrast T1-weighted image (*D*).

than or equal to 1.41 mm^2/s with 73.7% sensitive and 74.1% specific for 1p/19q codeleted oligodendroglioma.[49,51] A single 1p19q codeleted tumor with immunohistochemistry negative for *IDH1* does not exhibit calcifications or greater than 50% T2-FLAIR mismatch. Simple MR imaging markers may be helpful in predicting the 1p/19q status, but an accuracy of 82% is insufficient to replace formal 1p/19q testing for all patients.[49–51]

OTHER MOLECULAR MARKERS AND MUTATIONS IN DIFFUSE GLIOMAS

Today, neuro-oncologic practice is increasingly dependent on molecular diagnostics of tumor tissue. Various mutations and molecular markers have been identified in brain tumors (**Table 2**). Depending on the genetic analysis of the tumor, tumor treatment has become personalized and identifying these mutations has become mandatory to select therapies promoting better OS and PFS. With the development of next-generation sequencing panels, multiple mutations are

detected in a single analysis. Next-generation sequencing panels also allow for the simultaneous detection of genome-wide methylation profiling and fusion and chromosomal copy aberrations. Mutations of the ATRX, TP53, and MGMT genes usually occur after the IDH mutation.[2,3,6] Currently, there is no specific imaging marker to diagnose these mutations; however, ancillary and indirect imaging findings may help in the search for a genetic mutation or molecular marker.

α-Thalassemia/Mental Retardation Syndrome X-Linked and TP53 Mutations

ATRX encodes a chromatin remodeling protein important in DNA replication, telomere stability, gene transcription, chromosome congression, and cohesion during cell division. ATRX mutation results in the abnormal lengthening of telomerase, an enzyme important for chromatin maintenance and remodeling.[3,6,53] ATRX mutations are rarely seen without other mutations in the genes for histone regulation proteins, such as IDH, H33 K27M,

Table 2
Distinguishing MR imaging features between IDH wild-type and IDH-mutant glioma

MR Parameters	IDH Wild-Type	IDH-Mutant
	Primary/de novo glioblastoma (90%)	Secondary glioblastomas (10%) (from diffuse or anaplastic astrocytoma)
Location/age	Supratentorial, >60 y	Frontal lobe, <45 y
Lobes	Multilobar, cross the midline	Single lobe, sparing of eloquent areas
Size and contours	Usually smaller, ill-defined, infiltrative margins	Larger and better defined contours
Growth	Faster growth, % NEC and NEC area significantly higher	Slow growth, limited necrosis
Enhancement	Heterogeneous, ring enhancement with central area of necrosis is a common feature	More homogeneous or nodular and less intense enhancement, large nonenhacing portion
DWI-ADC	ADC$_{mean}$ low, <1.2 and low FA	ADC$_{mean}$ higher FA: high
Promoter methylation	High relative CBV value (2.08 ± 0.54 mL/100 g), which shows extensive angiogenesis	Low relative CBV value (1.09 ± 0.34 mL/100 g),
MR spectroscopy	Absence of a 2HG peak	Maximum 2HG peak was identified at approximately 2.25 ppm
Median overall survival Surgery + RT Surgery + RT + CTX	9.9 mo 15 mo	24 mo 31 mo

Abbreviations: CBV, cerebral blood volume; CTX, chemotherapy; DWI, diffusion-weighted imaging; FA, fractional anisotropy; NEC, necrosis area; % NEC, percentage of cross-sectional necrosis area inside the enhancing lesion; RT, radiotherapy.

or TP53.[53,54] TP53 is a tumor suppressor gene located on the short arm of chromosome 17. TP53 is a cell-cycle regulatory protein that slows or prevents the passage from the G1 phase to the S phase of mitosis if the genetic material has undergone DNA damage. Loss of TP53 leads to DNA damage, hypoxia, oncogene activation, microtubule disruption, and oxidative damage, which contribute to CNS tumors pathogenesis including medulloblastoma, GBM, IDH-mutant astrocytomas, and hereditary syndromes.[53–55] IDH-mutant astrocytic tumors frequently carry an ATRX and a TP53 gene mutation. Loss of nuclear ATRX during immunohistochemical staining is a strong predictor an of ATRX mutation, whereas strong and extensive nuclear staining for TP53 signifies the presence of a TP53 mutation.

Pediatric Gliomas

Before the 2016 tumor classification, pediatric and adult gliomas were under one umbrella because of their histologic similarities. Now they are independent of one another because their varying genetic profiles. Unlike adult gliomas, pediatric diffuse gliomas do not have changes in the IDH or ATRX genes, nor do they exhibit the 1p/19q codeletion.[3] Some differences include that WHO grade I gliomas are almost exclusively in pediatric or young adult patients and that GB incidence is rarer in childhood. IDH and ATRX gene mutations commonly seen in adult diffuse gliomas are not found in pediatric GBMs; rather, more than 95% of pediatric GBM cases exhibit the H3-K27M gene mutation.[56]

Diffuse Midline Glioma and H3 K27M-Mutant

Diffuse intrinsic pontine gliomas are malignant brain tumors that account for 75% to 80% of brainstem tumors in children.[56,57] Histone H3 K27M is a mutation in the H3F3A gene that encodes histone H3.3, a protein that replaces lysine by methionine at position 27 (H3-K27M-mutant).[56] This leads to a global reduction of H3 K27 trimethylation and a lateration in the epigenetic setting of the cell including DNA methylation. This drives gene expression patterns thought to block glial differentiation and promote gliomagenesis. H3 K27M mutations are commonly seen with diffuse midline gliomas but are not exclusive to them. This mutation has been identified in a subset of posterior fossa ependymomas; anaplastic gangliogliomas; and, although rarely, pilocytic astrocytomas. Tumors with an H3 K27M mutation exhibit more aggressive behavior. Diffuse midline gliomas have a predilection for young adults and children but may also occur in adults. With an H3 K27M mutation diffuse midline gliomas carry a poor prognosis, with a 2-year survival rate less than 10%.

As the name suggests, diffuse midline gliomas are seen along the midline involving CNS structures, including the thalamus, hypothalamus, third ventricle, pineal region, cerebellum, brainstem (previously known as diffuse intrinsic pontine glioma), and spinal cord. The imaging features of histone H3 K27M mutant gliomas are heterogeneous. Thalamic gliomas (**Fig. 7**) demonstrate contrast enhancement and necrosis in 50% of patients, pontine gliomas demonstrate variable contrast enhancement in 67% of patients, and cervical spine gliomas demonstrate uniform enhancement.[58] Cervical spine gliomas with histone H3 K27M mutation demonstrate leptomenigeal metastatic spread, whereas thalamic and pontine gliomas demonstrate local spread and recurrence. The prognosis is dependent on multiple factors, such as patient age, symptom duration, treatment type, and radiologic presence of contrast ring enhancement within diffuse intrinsic pontine gliomas. The type and site of mutation play a vital role in survival. Correlating imaging findings with molecular/genetic analysis remains challenging because of the morbidity associated with biopsies. H3 K27M mutant diffuse intrinsic pontine gliomas have worse OS than the H3.1-mutated subgroup. On imaging, poor outcomes correlate with ring enhancement and lower baseline ADC values.[58]

TERT Promoter Mutations

TERT promoter mutations are encountered in all grades of diffuse gliomas ranging from grade II oligodendrogliomas, the best prognosis, to grade IV GBM, the worst prognosis. The prevalence of TERT mutations is most common in GBMs (IDH wild-type, 1p19q not codeleted) and oligodendrogliomas (IDH-mutant, 1p19q codeleted).[59–61] These genetic aberrations are valuable diagnostic markers. The interaction of TERT mutations, IDH mutations, and 1p19q codeletion status is complex and depends on other combinations to determine survival.[60] For example, IDH wild-type diffuse astrocytomas (not 1p19q codeleted) of all grades (II to IV) that have a TERT mutation exhibit significant reductions in survival rate, most strikingly in grade II and III tumors. TERT promoter mutations and long telomere length predict poor survival and radiotherapy resistance in gliomas.

TREATMENT, PROGNOSIS, AND ISOCITRATE DEHYDROGENASE MUTATIONS

A detailed discussion of glioma treatment is out of the scope of this article. We highlight the salient

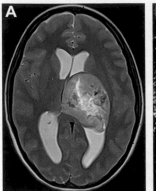
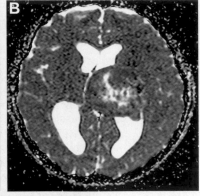
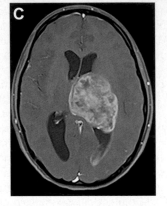

Fig. 7. Diffuse midline glioma with H3 K27M mutation. Axial T2-weighted image (A) demonstrates heterointense mass centered over the left thalamus with well-defined margins and without perilesional edema. On axial ADC image (B), mass shows low ADC except in the region of the necrosis. Contrast-enhanced T1-weighted image (C) shows intense enhancement of the thalamic mass with leptomeningeal enhancement along the left trigone and occipital horn.

genotyping and imaging features, which guide the oncology team in deciding an appropriate treatment. The main focus of glioma treatment has been to improve OS and have a PFS. By elevating the understanding of gliomagenesis and the phenotyping and genotyping classifications, the effort to develop therapeutic drugs, combined regimes, and minimally invasive surgeries to treat gliomas can continue.

IDH mutations are the initiating event in the oncogenesis of IDH-mutant gliomas. Noninvasive, preoperative identification of the IDH mutation is gaining ground, especially because genetic testing is not available across the globe. IDH1 mutation status is associated with a dramatic improvement in survival across the full spectrum of gliomas.[62] Therefore, pretreatment identification of IDH1 mutation in low-grade gliomas via radiographic characteristics may warrant early intervention as opposed to observation. Furthermore, IDH-mutant gliomas are found to be more susceptible to temozolomide as opposed to IDH wild-type lesions, which may be better targeted with alternative therapeutic interventions.[62,63] IDH-mutation status may also influence the extent of surgical resection.[62] High-grade IDH1-mutant may benefit

from resection of nonenhancing surrounding tissue, but similar results were not found for IDH1 wild-type high-grade gliomas. IDH status plays a significant role in surgical treatment plans, patient counseling, and adjuvant therapy.

Today, the treatment of GBM and diffuse glioma is largely decided by the mutation status and other available markers besides the tumor histology. This is also applicable when deciding the surgical approach and resection. There are emerging data that resection of the nonenhancing tumor component improves survival in patients with IDH-mutant but not IDH wild-type GBM, further strengthening the argument for noninvasive, preoperative classification of gliomas.[64,65]

In accordance with the Stupp protocol, a temozolomide and radiotherapy combination followed by temozolomide maintenance treatment is recommended on diagnosis of GBM in a patient younger than 70 years of age regardless of IDH status.[66] In patients diagnosed with IDH wild-type, however, radiotherapy alone is recommended for patients with a negative MGMT methylation status, whereas the GBM protocol is recommended for patients with a positive MGMT methylation status. There is ongoing effort to find the appropriate DH1/2-mutant inhibitors to improve IDH1/2-mutant glioma treatment. These inhibitors can quantitatively inhibit IDH1/2 mutants and reduce 2HG to normal levels.[67,68] They also partially reverse histone modification and DNA hypermethylation, thereby playing a protective role. IDH1/2-mutant enzyme inhibitors have shown great potential in clinical trials: ivosidenib (AG-120) and enasidenib (AG-221) are the preferred reversible selective inhibitors of IDH1- and IDH2-mutant enzymes, respectively.[67,68] Enasidenib was approved by the Food and Drug Administration as a first-in-class inhibitor for the treatment of relapsed or refractory IDH2-mutated acute myeloid leukemia.

PROGNOSIS

Patients with an IDH-mutant GBM generally show substantially longer OS than those with IDH wild-type GBM. This prognostic impact also applies to the diffuse grade II and anaplastic grade III astrocytomas with *IDH* mutants. An interesting finding is that the OS of patients with IDH wild-type anaplastic astrocytoma was worse than patients with IDH-mutant GBM (WHO grade IV). However, this rule may not hold true for all *IDH* mutants and IDH wild-type gliomas. cIMPACT Update 3 clarifies that besides IDH status, prognosis also depends on other factors including the microvascular proliferation and necrosis. Therefore, cIMPACTNOW Update 3 requires the detection of an EGFR amplification, a TERT promoter mutation, or a complete gain of chromosome 7 combined with a complete deletion of chromosome 10 in addition to the histologic and IDH status of the tumor to establish the correct genotypic diagnosis.

SUMMARY

The treatment of the brain tumors is more personalized and is moving toward targeted therapeutics because of a better understanding of tumor genetics and molecular markers. However, the increase in the number and importance of distinct genetic mutations has led to a search of noninvasive and less expensive biomarkers to identify and classify these tumors. *IDH* gene mutations reflect alterations in metabolism, cellularity, and angiogenesis, which may manifest characteristic features on FLAIR-T2, diffusion-weighted imaging/ADC, MR spectroscopy, and DSC-PWI. Although imaging cannot replace the genetic panel at present, image findings have shown promising signs to identify and diagnose the types and subtypes of gliomas.

CLINICS CARE POINTS

- Molecular aberrations in the particular brain tumors, explains why some tumors of identical cell types appear similar on histology but respond differently to the same therapy and have different prognoses.

- Several molecular markers including isocitrate dehydrogenase (IDH), 1p/19q codeletion, O6-methylguanine-DNA methyltransferase methylation (MGMT), telomerase reverse transcriptase gene (TERT), athalassemia/mental retardation syndrome X-linked gene (ATRX), and p53, have been identified as necessary for to classify and understand the behavior and progression of the tumor.

- The Cancer Imaging Program and The Cancer Imaging Archive have paved the way to correlate imaging features and histologic patterns with the genetic profile of the tumor; this is called "radiohistogenomic interpretation."

- At present, imaging modalities have limitations in locating the point mutation of a tumor's genetic material.

DISCLOSURE

B.E. Zacharia: NICO Corp, Speaker's Bureau; Medtronic Inc, consultant.

REFERENCES

1. Gupta A, Dwivedi T. A simplified overview of World Health Organization Classification Update of Central Nervous System Tumors 2016. J Neurosciences Rural Pract 2017;08(04):629–41.
2. Louis DN, Perry A, Burger P, et al. International Society of Neuropathology-Haarlem consensus guidelines for nervous system tumor classification and grading. Brain Pathol 2014;24:429–35.
3. Louis DN, Perry A, Reifenberger G, et al. The 2016 World Health Organization Classification of Tumors of the Central Nervous System: a summary. Acta Neuropathol (Berl) 2016;131:803–20.
4. Clark K, Vendt B, Smith K, et al. The Cancer Imaging Archive (TCIA): maintaining and operating a public information repository. J Digit Imaging 2013;26:1045–57.
5. Traylor J, Ravikumar V, Rao A, et al. COMP-07. machine learning predicts progression and survival in glioma using radiohistogenomic features. Neuro Oncol 2019;21(Supplement_6):vi62.
6. Louis DN, Ellison DW, Brat DJ, et al. cIMPACT-NOW: a practical summary of diagnostic points from Round 1 updates. Brain Pathol 2019;29(4):469–72.

7. Dang L, White DW, Gross S, et al. Cancer-associated IDH1 mutations produce 2-hydroxyglutarate. Nature 2009;462(7274):739–44.

8. Lee SM, Koh HJ, Park DC, et al. Cytosolic NADP(+)-dependent isocitrate dehydrogenase status modulates oxidative damage to cells. Free Radic Biol Med 2002;32(11):1185–96.

9. Corpas FJ, Barroso JB, Sandalio LM, et al. Peroxisomal NADP-dependent isocitrate dehydrogenase. Characterization and activity regulation during natural senescence. Plant Physiol 1999;121:921–8.

10. Cohen AL, Holmen SL, Colman H. IDH1 and IDH2 mutations in gliomas. Curr Neurol Neurosci Rep 2013; 13(5). https://doi.org/10.1007/s11910-013-0345-4.

11. Horbinski C. What do we know about IDH1/2 mutations so far, and how do we use it? Acta Neuropathol (Berl) 2013;125:621–36.

12. Yan H, Parsons DW, Jin G, et al. IDH1 and IDH2 mutations in gliomas. N Engl J Med 2009;360(8): 765–73.

13. The Cancer Genome Atlas (TCGA) Research Network. Comprehensive genomic characterization defines human glioblastoma genes and core pathways. Nature 2008;455:1061–8.

14. Phillips HS, Kharbanda S, Chen R, et al. Molecular subclasses of high-grade glioma predict prognosis, delineate a pattern of disease progression, and resemble stages in neurogenesis. Cancer Cell 2006;9(3):157–73.

15. Binabaj MM, Bahrami A, ShahidSales S, et al. The prognostic value of MGMT promoter methylation in glioblastoma: a meta-analysis of clinical trials. J Cell Physiol 2018;233(1):378–86.

16. Hegi ME, Diserens A-C, Gorlia T, et al. MGMT gene silencing and benefit from temozolomide in glioblastoma. N Engl J Med 2005;352:99701993.

17. Christmann M, Verbeek B, Roos WP, et al. O6-Methylguanine-DNA methyltransferase (MGMT) in normal tissues and tumors: enzyme activity, promoter methylation and immunohistochemistry. Biochim Biophys Acta 2011;1816(2):179–90.

18. Carrillo JA, Lai A, Nghiemphu PL, et al. Relationship between tumor enhancement, edema, IDH1 mutational status, MGMT promoter methylation, and survival in glioblastoma. AJNR Am J Neuroradiol 2012;33:1349–55.

19. Chen R, Ravindra VM, Cohen AL, et al. Molecular features assisting in diagnosis, surgery, and treatment decision making in low-grade gliomas. Neurosurg Focus 2015;38:E2.

20. Boots-Sprenger SHE, Sijben A, Rijntjes J, et al. Significance of complete 1p/19q co-deletion, IDH1 mutation and MGMT promoter methylation in gliomas: use with caution. Mod Pathol 2013;26(7):922–9.

21. Brat DJ, Verhaak RGW, Aldape KD, et al. Comprehensive, integrative genomic analysis of diffuse lower-grade gliomas. N Engl J Med 2015;372(26):2481–98.

22. Chamberlain MC, Born D. Prognostic significance of relative 1p/19q codeletion in oligodendroglial tumors. J Neurooncol 2015;125:249–2451.

23. Jenkinson MD, du Plessis DG, Smith TS, et al. Histological growth patterns and genotype in oligodendroglial tumours: correlation with MRI features. Brain 2006;129(Pt 7):1884–91.

24. Jenkins RB, Blair H, Ballman Kv, et al. A t(1;19)(q10; p10) mediates the combined deletions of 1p and 19q and predicts a better prognosis of patients with oligodendroglioma. Cancer Res 2006;66(20): 9852–61.

25. Ohgaki H, Dessen P, Jourde B, et al. Genetic pathways to glioblastoma: a population-based study. Cancer Res 2004;64:6892–9.

26. Arevalo OJ, Valenzuela R, Esquenazi Y, et al. The 2016 World Health Organization. Classification of tumors of the central nervous system: a practical approach for gliomas. Part 1: basic tumor genetics. Neurographics 2017;7(5):334–43.

27. Belden CJ, Valdes PA, Ran C, et al. Genetics of glioblastoma: a window into its imaging and histopathologic variability. Radiographics 2011;31:1717–40.

28. Liu Q, Liu Y, Li W, et al. Genetic, epigenetic, and molecular landscapes of multifocal and multicentric glioblastoma. Acta Neuropathol (Berl) 2015;130:587–97.

29. Nicholas MK, Lukas RV, Jafri NF, et al. Epidermal growth factor receptor-mediated signal transduction in the development and therapy of gliomas. Clin Cancer Res 2006;12:7261–70.

30. Verhaak RG, Hoadley KA, Purdom E, et al. Integrated genomic analysis identifies clinically relevant subtypes of glioblastoma characterized by abnormalities in PDGFRA, IDH1, EGFR, and NF1. Cancer Cell 2010;17(1):98–110.

31. Liu XY, Gerges N, Korshunov A, et al. Frequent ATRX mutations and loss of expression in adult diffuse astrocytic tumors carrying IDH1/IDH2 and TP53 mutations. Acta Neuropathol (Berl) 2012;124:615–25.

32. Gerlinger M, Rowan AJ, Horswell S, et al. Intratumor heterogeneity and branched evolution revealed by multiregion sequencing. N Engl J Med 2012;366: 883–92.

33. Stieber D, Golebiewska A, Evers L, et al. Glioblastomas are composed of genetically divergent clones with distinct tumourigenic potential and variable stem cell associated phenotypes. Acta Neuropathol 2014;127:203–19.

34. Gutman DA, Cooper LA, Hwang SN, et al. MR imaging predictors of molecular profile and survival: multi-institutional study of the TCGA glioblastoma data set. Radiology 2013;267:560–9.

35. Romano A, Calabria LF, Tavanti F, et al. Apparent diffusion coefficient obtained by magnetic resonance imaging as a prognostic marker in glioblastomas: correlation with MGMT promoter methylation status. Eur Radiol 2013;23(2):513–20.

36. Moon WJ, Choi JW, Roh HG, et al. Imaging parameters of high grade gliomas in relation to the MGMT promoter methylation status: the CT, diffusion tensor imaging, and perfusion MR imaging. Neuroradiology 2012;54(6):555–63.

37. Suh CH, Kim HS, Jung SC, et al. Clinically relevant imaging features for MGMT promoter methylation in multiple glioblastoma studies: a systematic review and meta-analysis. AJNR Am J Neuroradiol 2018; 39(8):1439–45.

38. Han Y, Yan L-F, Wang X-B, et al. Structural and advanced imaging in predicting MGMT promoter methylation of primary glioblastoma: a region of interest based analysis. BMC Cancer 2018;18(1):215.

39. Choi C, Ganji SK, DeBerardinis RJ, et al. 2-hydroxyglutarate detection by magnetic resonance spectroscopy in IDH-mutated glioma patients. Nat Med 2012;18(4):624–9.

40. Tietze A, Choi C, Mickey B, et al. Noninvasive assessment of isocitrate dehydrogenase mutation status in cerebral gliomas by magnetic resonance spectroscopy in a clinical setting. J Neurosurg 2018;128:391–8.

41. Ellingson BM, Lai A, Harris RJ, et al. Probabilistic radiographic atlas of glioblastoma phenotypes. AJNR Am J Neuroradiol 2013;34:533–40.

42. Wang YY, Zhang T, Li SW, et al. Mapping p53 mutations in low-grade glioma: a voxel-based neuroimaging analysis. AJNR Am J Neuroradiol 2015;36:70–6.

43. Yamashita K, Hiwatashi A, Togao O, et al. MR imaging based analysis of glioblastoma multiforme: estimation of IDH1 mutation status. AJNR Am J Neuroradiol 2016;37:58–65, 10.

44. Zhou H, Vallières M, Bai H, et al. MRI features predict survival and molecular markers in diffuse lower-grade gliomas. Neuro Oncol 2017;19(6):862–70.

45. Wang YY, Wang K, Li SW, et al. Patterns of tumor contrast enhancement predict the prognosis of anaplastic gliomas with IDH1 mutation. AJNR Am J Neuroradiol 2015;36:2023–9.

46. Kickingereder P, Sahm F, Radbruch A, et al. IDH mutation status is associated with a distinct hypoxia/angiogenesis transcriptome signature which is non-invasively predictable with rCBV imaging in human glioma. Sci Rep 2015;5:16238.

47. Law M, Young RJ, Babb JS, et al. Gliomas: predicting time to progression or survival with cerebral blood volume measurements at dynamic susceptibility-weighted contrast-enhanced perfusion MR imaging. Radiology 2008;247(2):490–8.

48. Park YW, Han K, Ahn SS, et al. Prediction of IDH1-mutation and 1p/19q-codeletion status using preoperative MR imaging phenotypes in lower grade gliomas. AJNR Am J Neuroradiol 2018;39(1):37–42.

49. Johnson DR, Diehn FE, Giannini C, et al. Genetically defined oligodendroglioma is characterized by indistinct tumor borders at MRI. AJNR Am J Neuroradiol 2017;38(4):678–84.

50. Patel SH, Poisson LM, Brat DJ, et al. T2–FLAIR mismatch, an imaging biomarker for IDH and 1p/19q status in lower-grade gliomas: a TCGA/TCIA project. Clin Cancer Res 2017;23(20):6078–86.

51. Sherman JH, Prevedello DM, Shah L, et al. MR imaging characteristics of oligodendroglial tumors with assessment of 1p/19q deletion status. Acta Neurochir (Wien) 2010;152:182–1834.

52. Lai A, Kharbanda S, Pope WB, et al. Evidence for sequenced molecular evolution of IDH1 mutant glioblastoma from a distinct cell of origin. J Clin Oncol 2011;29(34):4482–90.

53. Kannan K, Inagaki A, Silber J, et al. Whole-exome sequencing identifies ATRX mutation as a key molecular determinant in lower-grade glioma. Oncotarget 2012;3:1194–203.

54. Ham SW, Jeon HY, Jin X, et al. TP53 gain-of-function mutation promotes inflammation in glioblastoma. Cell Death Differ 2019;26(3):409–25.

55. Zhukova N, Ramaswamy V, Remke M, et al. Subgroup-specific prognostic implications of TP53 mutation in medulloblastoma. J Clin Oncol 2013; 31(23):2927–35.

56. Solomon DA, Wood MD, Tihan T, et al. Diffuse midline gliomas with histone H3–K27M mutation: a series of 47 cases assessing the spectrum of morphologic variation and associated genetic alterations. Brain Pathol 2016;26:569–80.

57. Appin CL, Brat DJ. Biomarker-driven diagnosis of diffuse gliomas. Mol Aspects Med 2015;45:87–96.

58. Aboian MS, Solomon DA, Felton E, et al. Imaging characteristics of pediatric diffuse midline gliomas with histone H3 K27M mutation. AJNR Am J Neuroradiol 2017;38(4):795–800.

59. Chen R, Smith-Cohn M, Cohen AL, et al. Glioma subclassifications and their clinical significance. Neurotherapeutics 2017;14(2):284–97.

60. Eckel-Passow JE, Lachance DH, Molinaro AM, et al. Glioma groups based on 1p/19q, IDH, and TERT promoter mutations in tumors. N Engl J Med 2015; 372(26):2499–508.

61. Vuong HG, Altibi AMA, Duong UNP, et al. TERT promoter mutation and its interaction with IDH mutations in glioma: combined TERT promoter and IDH mutations stratifies lower-grade glioma into distinct survival subgroups. A meta-analysis of aggregate data. Crit Rev Oncol Hematol 2017;120:1–9.

62. SongTao Q, Lei Y, Si G, et al. IDH mutations predict longer survival and response to temozolomide in secondary glioblastoma. Cancer Sci 2012;103(2): 269–73.

63. Okita Y, Narita Y, Miyakita Y, et al. IDH1/2 mutation is a prognostic marker for survival and predicts response to chemotherapy for grade II gliomas

concomitantly treated with radiation therapy. Int J Oncol 2012;41(4):1325–36.

64. Patel SH, Bansal AG, Young EB, et al. Lopes MB extent of surgical resection in lower-grade gliomas: differential impact based on molecular subtype. AJNR Am J Neuroradiol 2019;40(7):1149–55.

65. Delev D, Heiland DH, Franco P, et al. Surgical management of lower-grade glioma in the spotlight of the 2016 WHO classification system. J Neurooncol 2019;141(1):223–33.

66. Stupp R, Mason WP, van den Bent MJ, et al. Radiotherapy plus concomitant and adjuvant temozolomide for glioblastoma. N Engl J Med 2005;352(10): 987–96.

67. Rohle D, Popovici-Muller J, Palaskas N, et al. An inhibitor of mutant IDH1 delays growth and promotes differentiation of glioma cells. Science 2013;340: 626–30.

68. Huang J, Yu J, Tu L, et al. Isocitrate dehydrogenase mutations in glioma: from basic discovery to therapeutics development. Front Oncol 2019;9:506.

Clinical Review of Computed Tomography and MR Perfusion Imaging in Neuro-Oncology

Austin Trinh, MD[a], Max Wintermark, MD[b], Michael Iv, MD[c],*

KEYWORDS

• Perfusion • Neuro-oncology • Glioblastoma • Fractional tumor burden

KEY POINTS

• Advanced perfusion imaging can offer enhanced evaluation of tumoral physiology to guide the diagnosis, intraoperative sampling, and grading of brain tumors.
• Perfusion imaging is useful when differentiating between tumor types and neoplastic and nonneoplastic conditions.
• Hemodynamic parameters obtained from perfusion imaging can guide clinical decision making for treatment-related processes, such as radiation necrosis.

INTRODUCTION

Neuroimaging plays an essential role in the initial diagnosis and continued surveillance of intracranial neoplasms, with multiple studies showing the utility of perfusion imaging in assessing tumor physiology and hemodynamics.[1] Although conventional MR imaging techniques are useful in evaluating the anatomy and structure of the brain, advanced imaging approaches can provide useful information about physiology and function not visible on the anatomic images.[2] Specifically, perfusion imaging can estimate cerebral blood flow (CBF) and cerebral blood volume (CBV) as markers of angiogenesis within intracranial tumors, can generate transfer constant (k-trans) as a permeability marker in tumors before and after treatment, and can help to distinguish between tumor and treatment effect in previously treated tumors. To date, the most useful perfusion parameters in the clinical neuro-oncology setting are CBF and CBV, which are acquired with exogenous contrast agents (eg, dynamic susceptibility contrast [DSC] MR imaging[3] and iodinated contrast-enhanced computed tomography [CT] perfusion imaging)[4] or without contrast agents (eg, arterial spin labeling [ASL] imaging).[2] In this article, we review the clinical relevance and implications of perfusion imaging in neuro-oncology and highlight promising perfusion biomarkers.

COMPUTED TOMOGRAPHY PERFUSION

CT perfusion provides information on brain hemodynamics by analyzing the first passage of an intravenous contrast bolus through the cerebral vessels. Raw images are acquired on a multislice CT scanner and are subsequently post-processed by software to generate hemodynamic perfusion maps. This permits quantitative and

[a] Division of Neuroimaging and Neurointervention, Department of Radiology, Stanford University, 300 Pasteur Drive, Grant Building, Room S031, Stanford, CA 94305-5105, USA; [b] Division of Neuroimaging and Neurointervention, Department of Radiology, Stanford University, 300 Pasteur Drive, Grant Building, Room S047, Stanford, CA 94305-5105, USA; [c] Division of Neuroimaging and Neurointervention, Department of Radiology, Stanford University, 300 Pasteur Drive, Grant Building, Room S031E, Stanford, CA 94305-5105, USA
* Corresponding author.
E-mail address: miv@stanford.edu
Twitter: @mwNRAD (M.W.); @Michael_Iv_MD (M.I.)

Radiol Clin N Am 59 (2021) 323–334
https://doi.org/10.1016/j.rcl.2021.01.002
0033-8389/21/© 2021 Elsevier Inc. All rights reserved.

qualitative assessment of CBV and CBF (**Fig. 1**). CBV refers to the volume of blood within a given region of brain tissue and is measured in milliliters per 100 g of brain tissue. A closely associated and often interchangeably used term is relative cerebral blood volume (rCBV). This accounts for capillary permeability by measuring CBV relative to an internal control (such as the contralateral normal-appearing white matter) and is expressed as an overall ratio. CBF refers to the amount of blood per unit time passing through a given region of brain tissue and is measured in milliliters per 100 g per minute of brain tissue.[5] Fractional tumor burden (FTB) is a newer perfusion-derived metric and is defined as the volume fraction of tumor voxels higher or lower than a specified CBV threshold.[6]

An advantage of using CT perfusion over perfusion MR imaging is the linear relationship between iodine concentration and attenuation on CT, providing a more absolute measurement of vascular parameters.[5] CT also has the benefit of wider availability, faster scanning times, and lower cost compared with MR imaging.[4] CT can also be used in patients with contraindications to MR imaging, such as in those with medical implants. However, CT does require radiation exposure to the patient, which may be additive if serial imaging is needed. In addition, soft tissue resolution on CT is inferior to MR imaging.[4]

PERFUSION MR IMAGING

Perfusion MR imaging techniques take advantage of endogenous or exogenous tracers. With regards to exogenous agents, perfusion MR imaging is based on the concept of following an injected bolus of contrast agent over time, which is then used to investigate the perfusion characteristics of brain tumors. Contrast-enhanced perfusion imaging is accomplished with DSC and dynamic contrast-enhanced (DCE) imaging. With regards to endogenous agents, ASL imaging can be used; this technique magnetically labels spins using protons within arterial blood to estimate CBF.[7] In the next paragraphs, we briefly review the techniques of DSC, DCE, and ASL and highlight the clinically relevant parameters acquired from each technique for brain tumor imaging (**Fig. 2**).

Dynamic Susceptibility Contrast

DSC MR imaging uses a bolus tracking technique that is most frequently based on T2 (spin echo) or T2* (gradient echo imaging) effects before, during, and after administration of a gadolinium-based contrast agent.[8] In DSC imaging, injection of a contrast agent causes a transient drop in signal intensity reflective of the effects of the paramagnetic contrast agent. The spin echo technique has the advantage of minimizing brain, bone, and air interfaces and is more sensitive to signal changes from contrast material passage through small vessels. The main disadvantage of spin echo imaging is the requirement of a higher dose of contrast, which is needed to produce signal changes comparable with gradient echo imaging.[9] Gradient echo DSC is faster in terms of image acquisition and takes advantage of first-pass imaging and magnification

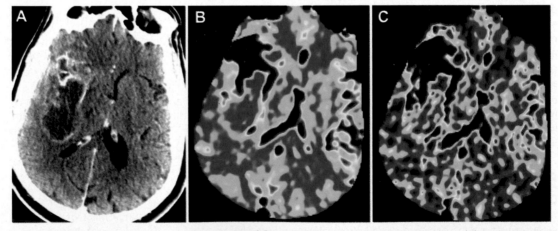

Fig. 1. CT perfusion in a 67-year-old man acquired for evaluation of stroke-like symptoms. (*A*) Postcontrast CT image shows a large peripherally enhancing necrotic mass in the right temporal lobe. (*B*) Post-processed cerebral blood flow and (*C*) cerebral blood volume images acquired from perfusion imaging show significantly elevated (*red color*) perfusion within the anterior and peripheral aspects of the mass. Histopathology following surgical resection revealed glioblastoma.

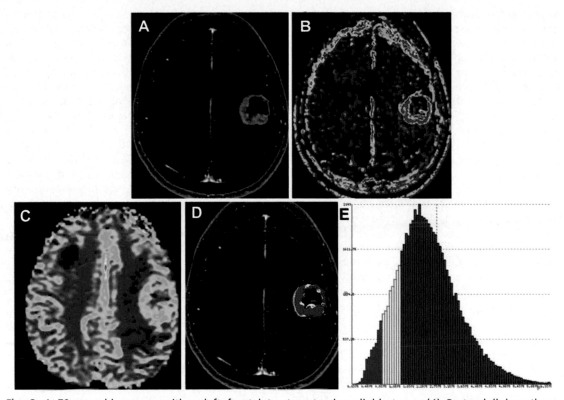

Fig. 2. A 70-year-old woman with a left frontal treatment-naive glioblastoma. (*A*) Postgadolinium three-dimensional (3D) T1-weighted MR image shows a large necrotic mass in the left frontal lobe. (*B*) K-trans map acquired from dynamic contrast-enhanced perfusion imaging shows elevated k-trans (*red color*) throughout much of the lesion. (*C*) CBV and (*D*) FTB images acquired from dynamic susceptibility contrast-enhanced perfusion imaging also show elevated CBV and FTB$_{high}$, respectively. (*E*) FTB histogram shows the distribution of contrast-enhancing voxels with low FTB (*blue*), intermediate FTB (*yellow*), and high FTB (*red*), with the greatest proportion of contrast-enhancing lesion voxels having high FTB.

of contrast-induced signal loss through susceptibility-weighted images. A disadvantage of this technique, however, is related to inherent susceptibility artifacts produced by blood, calcification, or larger vessels. Nonetheless, with either approach, contrast preloading, gamma variate curve fitting, or other leakage correction methods are commonly used to reduce T1 relaxation effects and to account for residual T2/T2* effects.[10,11] Much like CT perfusion, DSC allows for the calculation of multiple perfusion parameters, such as CBF, CBV, and FTB.[6]

Dynamic Contrast Enhancement

DCE MR imaging uses bolus tracking on T1-weighted imaging, where permeability characteristics of brain tumors are assessed. Advantages of DCE include acquisition with a lower contrast dose and better temporal resolution compared with that of T2- or T2*-weighted DSC imaging. This is because T1-weighted imaging-based DCE

measures the relaxivity effects rather than the susceptibility effects of the injected dose of a paramagnetic contrast agent. The relaxivity effect refers to the generated signal of T1 shortening related to relaxation time, which is inherently stronger than susceptibility. Also, shorter injection times may result in better quantitation of CBV and CBF provided that the temporal resolution of the pulse sequence can allow for dynamic tracking of the injected contrast bolus over multiple time points to extract and estimate T1 signal and concentration.[9] However, DCE suffers from the necessity of advanced and complex pharmacokinetic modeling to account for the nonlinear relationship between the acquired signal intensity and contrast concentration. Nonpharmacokinetic model-based analyses with DCE have attempted to avoid this problem but have unclear physiologic and clinical basis and utility.[11]

Despite several choices for modeling, the Extended Tofts Model, which is a two-compartment model of the vascular and extracellular-extravascular spaces, is frequently used in brain tumor imaging. In this model, the leakage of contrast is measured quantitatively and a triexponential enhancement curve is fitted to a theoretic model based on compartmental analysis.[12] This allows for many parameters to be obtained, such as the k-trans, volume of the extravascular extracellular space, and blood plasma volume.[5] Of these, k-trans has been the most widely used and investigated in clinical neuro-oncology. It is important to know that although k-trans is thought to be a marker of permeability, it is more reflective of blood flow in certain conditions. For example, in situations where there is high permeability, the flux of gadolinium-based contrast agent is primarily limited by flow and, therefore, k-trans primarily reflects blood flow. In situations where there is low permeability, the contrast leakage is limited in its ability to flow into the extravascular-extracellular space and, therefore, k-trans primarily reflects permeability.[13]

Arterial Spin Labeling

ASL imaging is a noncontrast technique that takes advantage of an endogenous tracer by magnetically labeling spins using protons within arterial blood.[7,14] The MR imaging sequence acquisition is built in such way that a delay allows the labeled water molecules to flow into the brain tissue and exchange with the brain tissue water, which results in small changes in the magnetization of the tissue water. When evaluated in conjunction with control (unlabeled) images, CBF images are generated after subtraction from the labeled images.[2] Although not yet widely used or established in clinical practice, this technique for acquiring cerebral perfusion offers several advantages over DSC and DCE, primarily because it does not require injection of a gadolinium-based contrast agent. Therefore, ASL is a promising technique for assessing perfusion in patients who have renal dysfunction or severe allergic reactions to gadolinium or who require frequent follow-up contrast-enhanced examinations.[3] However, widespread clinical applications of this method have been limited, in part because of longer acquisition times and sensitivity of the technique to patient motion.[9]

CLINICAL USE OF PERFUSION IMAGING IN NEURO-ONCOLOGY

Although conventional MR imaging is essential for the diagnosis and evaluation of brain tumors, it does not confer much information about tumor vascularity and physiology. Perfusion imaging is valuable because it is used to help grade tumors; differentiate between tumor types; differentiate

tumors from nonneoplastic lesions; guide intraoperative sampling; and, most importantly, determine efficacy of treatment.[15] The initial differentiation between neoplastic and nonneoplastic lesions is difficult with conventional MR imaging, often requiring direct tissue sampling for diagnostic confirmation.[8] Perfusion imaging can help to distinguish between infectious and neoplastic lesions, as CBV of infection tends to be significantly lower than CBV of metastases or glioblastomas, likely reflective of their respective vascular densities.[16] However, there is potential for overlap between low-grade tumors and non-neoplastic lesions.[15] Thus, systematic incorporation of perfusion imaging as part of a multiparametric approach, potentially with MR spectroscopy, can aid in improving diagnostic confidence.[8,17]

Grading of Tumors

MR and CT perfusion imaging have shown to be helpful in determining the initial grade of gliomas based on increased or decreased tumor perfusion,[5] with studies showing that specific perfusion metrics correlate strongly with overall histopathologic grade.[18] These perfusion metrics can predict tumor behavior, because tumor aggressiveness and growth are associated with endothelial hyperplasia and endothelial neovascularization.[19] As such, it is not surprising that higher CBV correlates with lesion vascularity and higher tumor grade.[16] However, there is a substantial overlap of perfusion markers in tumors of varying grades and histology, which somewhat limits the discriminatory ability of perfusion imaging in certain tumor types and in differentiating between higher grades of tumors (eg, grade III and IV gliomas).[8] K-trans has shown promise in differentiating between low-grade (grade I) and higher-grade (grade II, III, or IV) tumors, although larger multicenter studies are still needed to validate its use in the clinic.[19]

Differentiation Between Tumor Types

An important and often difficult diagnostic dilemma exists when differentiating between glioblastoma, solitary brain metastasis, and primary central nervous system lymphoma. This is because of their similar and often times overlapping appearance on conventional MR imaging, presenting as solitary and avidly enhancing lesions with peripheral T2 hyperintensity.[20] It is important to distinguish between these entities, because management (surgery and/or chemotherapy) is different.[20,21] A study by Neska-Matuszewska and colleagues[20] found that maximum CBV within the tumor core enabled discrimination of less perfused primary central nervous system lymphomas from that of the more hyperperfused glioblastomas and metastases. When discriminating between glioblastoma and metastasis, maximum CBV within the perilesional zone was found to be most helpful. Increased CBV was observed within the peritumoral zones, reflecting the infiltrative and highly vascular nature of glioblastomas. Alternatively, decreased CBV was observed within the perilesional zone of metastases, reflecting regional vasogenic edema rather than nonenhancing infiltrative tumor.[20]

Differentiation Between Tumor and Nonneoplastic Conditions

On conventional imaging, aggressive neoplasms, such as a necrotic glioblastoma, may mimic and may be difficult to differentiate from other entities, such as a cerebral abscess, because these entities can appear as rim-enhancing lesions with regional edema.[22] Perfusion imaging is helpful in these cases, because higher-grade neoplasms tend to have increased neovascularity and capillary density and, therefore, higher CBV, whereas abscesses tend to have significantly lower CBV.[23] Other studies have found that neoplastic lesions also demonstrate higher CBV when compared with infectious lesions. For example, Floriano and colleagues[24] found that a rCBV value less than 1.3 yielded a 92.6% specificity for identifying infectious lesions, adding support for the use of perfusion imaging in distinguishing between infectious and neoplastic brain lesions.

Tumefactive demyelinating lesions can also mimic higher-grade neoplasms, given their aggressive appearance on structural MR imaging. However, it has been demonstrated that tumefactive demyelinating lesions have lower CBV than high-grade gliomas because of the absence of neoangiogenesis, a prominent feature of high-grade tumors.[5,8]

Tumor Sampling

Although the optimal management of low-grade gliomas is surgical resection, watchful waiting is reasonable in certain patients. With watchful waiting, imaging is used to ensure tumor stability over time. If tumor progresses on imaging or shows changes indicative of transformation to a higher-grade lesion (eg, new or increasing enhancement or perfusion), then intervention may be necessary. However, some higher-grade tumors may lack enhancement altogether.[25] In addition, the presence of contrast enhancement may not always indicate a higher-grade tumor because its presence is only reflective of a disrupted blood-brain barrier.[8] Furthermore, although nonenhancing tumors are more likely to be of higher grade in older patients, diagnosis of lower-grade tumors cannot be reliably made without a proper biopsy.[25]

Stereotactic guided biopsy is commonly used for sampling of tumor tissue (Fig. 3). However, because of the internal heterogeneity of brain tumors, sampling error remains a problem. Studies have shown that regions of increased CBV on perfusion imaging can help to guide biopsies in patients with gliomas. CBF and CBV maps are used to identify areas of maximum hyperperfusion within a lesion to guide intraoperative sampling, because these areas are most likely to yield diagnostic tissue representative of the highest grade component of tumor.[8,26] Beyond CBV, the use of FTB has shown the highest correlation with actual tumor content, further supporting that perfusion MR imaging can potentially reduce sampling error in histopathologic diagnosis and improve target selection for stereotactic biopsy.[27,28]

Distinguishing Between Tumor and Treatment Response

Perfusion imaging may serve as an early response marker of treatment efficacy. For example, CBV values may be more useful after initiation of cytotoxic therapy than enhancing tumor volume alone.[8] Bag and colleagues[29] found that higher post-treatment peritumoral CBV and CBF values in patients with newly diagnosed glioblastomas were associated with poor prognosis. Also, a greater than 5% increase in CBV correlated with poor overall survival when acquired 4 weeks after treatment was initiated.[29] Iv and colleagues[6] showed that FTB_{high} (defined as all contrast-enhancing lesion voxels with normalized rCBV >1.75) performed better than mean normalized rCBV, FTB_{low} (defined as all contrast-enhancing lesion voxels with normalized rCBV <1), and FTB_{mid} (defined as all contrast-enhancing lesion voxels with normalized rCBV between 1 and 1.75) in differentiating tumor from treatment effect in the recurrent glioblastoma setting and also impacted clinical decision-making.[6] These findings are likely related to the heterogeneity of tumor, which can have areas of high and low blood volume because of varying areas of angiogenesis and necrosis, whereas treated tissue typically has low blood volume.

Post-treatment Follow-up

In 1990, Macdonald and colleagues[30] published outlined criteria to evaluate malignant glioma response to treatment. The criteria consisted of two-dimensional measurements of enhancing

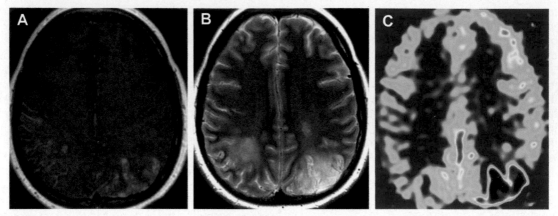

Fig. 3. A 29-year-old woman with history of an undifferentiated uterine sarcoma. (*A*) Postgadolinium 3D T1-weighted black blood image shows parenchymal and leptomeningeal enhancement within the parietal lobes bilaterally. (*B*) Extensive T2 signal is present in these areas. (*C*) Cerebral blood flow image acquired from arterial spin labeling perfusion imaging shows an area of high blood flow only in the left parietal lobe. Because the exact nature of these imaging findings was unclear in the context of progressive disease on serial imaging (not shown), persistent seizures, and unremarkable cerebrospinal fluid studies, intraoperative sampling was performed for tissue diagnosis. The biopsy was performed in the area of greatest perfusion. Histopathology revealed sarcoma metastases.

tumors using cross-sectional images, while incorporating neurologic status and corticosteroid use. With the development and growing use of antiangiogenic agents that drastically affected imaging findings, newer criteria have been made available for use when evaluating post-treatment response (Response Assessment in Neuro-Oncology [RANO] criteria). This construct is primarily used in the context of a clinical trial and in clinical research. The response assessment consists of measurements of contrast enhancement, progression or decrease (response) in size, durability of response, measurability, number of target lesions (up to five), and consideration and incorporation of corticosteroids, clinical status, and pseudoprogression. There are similar but different criteria for high-grade gliomas (RANO-HGG), low-grade gliomas (RANO-LGG), patients undergoing immunotherapy (iRANO), and brain metastases (RANO-BM), with multiple working RANO groups in progress.[31] A shortcoming of these criteria is the reliance on gadolinium enhancement, which is sensitive for tumoral changes but overall nonspecific when compared with other more advanced MR imaging sequences.[32] In addition to incorporating clinical findings with response criteria, clinicians today face the additional challenge of managing patients that have either new or established lesions seen on follow-up MR imaging.[33]

Pseudoprogression

A well-known phenomenon observed during the imaging surveillance of treated glioma patients is

the increase in size of the contrast-enhancing lesion, or contrast-enhancing volume, followed by subsequent improvement or eventual stabilization. This initial increase in size and enhancement is termed pseudoprogression.[34] Pseudoprogression often appears several weeks or months after the initial treatment.[33] It reflects transiently increased contrast enhancement, which can often mimic tumor progression and can complicate evaluation using radiologic criteria for progression, because it represents an exaggerated response to therapy.[8,34] The cause of pseudoprogression is believed to be the result of transient interruption of myelin synthesis secondary to injury to primary oligodendrocytes, with studies suggesting an overall transient course with spontaneous recovery.[33] Although pseudoprogression is commonly seen after concomitant radiotherapy-temozolomide, it can also be seen after radiotherapy alone or in combination with chemotherapy. Pseudoprogression is seen in approximately 20% of patients treated with concomitant radiotherapy-temozolomide and is often seen in the 2- to 6-month period after chemoradiotherapy, with a median of approximately 3 months.[34]

Differentiation from progressive disease is a hallmark for avoiding premature trial failures in the setting of pseudoprogression and selecting timely alternate therapies.[8] The challenge in differentiating between pseudoprogression and progressive disease using conventional T1-weighted postcontrast MR imaging is because contrast enhancement is nonspecific and only a marker of blood-brain barrier disruption.[35,36] The inflammatory response in pseudoprogression and angiogenic response in active tumor can demonstrate increased vascular permeability and contrast enhancement on MR imaging; therefore, it is often difficult to differentiate between these entities using conventional MR imaging alone. Perfusion MR imaging provides the advantage of quantifying blood volume, in addition to physiologic blow flow and permeability, which can provide a more discriminating diagnostic tool (**Figs. 4** and **5**).[35] For example, studies have found that an enhancing lesion with a normalized relative CBV ratio higher than 2.6 is suggestive of tumor recurrence, and a relative CBV value lower than 0.6 suggests nontumoral contrast-enhancing tissue. Overall, studies demonstrate that an increase in the relative CBV value favors tumor recurrence and a decrease favors pseudoprogression.[34] Another study by Young and colleagues[35] found that perfusion MR imaging estimates of blood volume and permeability can successfully identify pseudoprogression within a subgroup of patients that initially presented with radiographic worsening. This was characterized by lower perfusion parameters and overall higher permeability. This suggests that despite nearly identical appearances on conventional MR imaging, the addition of perfusion imaging may play an important role in the early diagnosis of treatment effects versus treatment failure.[35] Based on a recent 2017 meta-analysis of perfusion-weighted imaging in distinguishing treatment effect from tumor, perfusion imaging demonstrated promising accuracy.[11] A caveat is the heterogeneity of imaging techniques and highly variable proposed cutoff CBV values, which are potentially useful as a general guide. A particular threshold value that is optimized at a single institution might be more sufficient if applied consistently to a patient and subsequently followed over time.[11] Mean CBV may also be inadequate early in lesion evolution for observing the overall dominant or predicted behavior of tumor. As such, CBV trends or histograms identifying temporal and spatial variations may be more predictive.[8]

Radiation Necrosis

Radiation necrosis and pseudoprogression are distinct entities on a spectrum of post-treatment enhancement.[8] In contrast to pseudoprogression, radiation necrosis typically appears months to several years after the initial treatment. Although its mechanism is not fully understood, it is thought to be characterized by increased vascular permeability with proinflammatory mediators and cytokines, mixed with quiescent tumor and necrosis, which results in edema and contrast enhancement that is difficult to distinguish from progressive disease on conventional MR imaging.[34] The area of necrosis results in a space-occupying lesion with mass effect and can result in neurologic dysfunction or sequelae,[33] which makes delineation between radiation necrosis and tumor progression a diagnostic challenge. Both entities often manifest as a mass-like lesion with regional edema and progressive enhancement on serial studies.[18] Often, conventional imaging is inconclusive and advanced MR imaging techniques are necessary.[2] This imaging dilemma is not uncommon, with a recent meta-analysis revealing that 36% of patients with an enhancing lesion on post-treatment MR have treatment-related changes, whereas true progression only occurred in 60% of the patients.[37,38]

In these cases, perfusion imaging has shown to be helpful (**Fig. 6**).[18] CBV measurements using

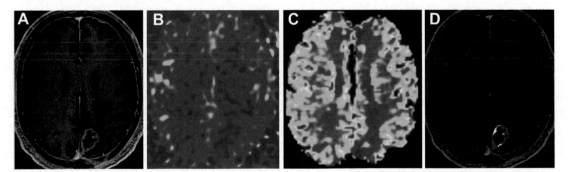

Fig. 4. A 65-year-old man with history of left posterior parietal glioblastoma previously treated with surgical resection and chemoradiation, presenting for follow-up 3 months after therapy. (*A*) Postgadolinium 3D T1-weighted image shows a heterogeneously enhancing lesion in the left posterior parietal lobe, at the site of previously treated glioblastoma. (*B*) Cerebral blood flow image from arterial spin labeling and (*C*) cerebral blood volume image from DSC imaging show low blood flow and volume, respectively, within the lesion. (*D*) Fractional tumor burden image from DSC shows primarily low fractional tumor burden (*blue*) within the lesion. Perfusion characteristics are suggestive of pseudoprogression (treatment effect). Nonetheless, the patient underwent surgical resection, and histopathology confirmed necrosis and reactive changes without tumor cells.

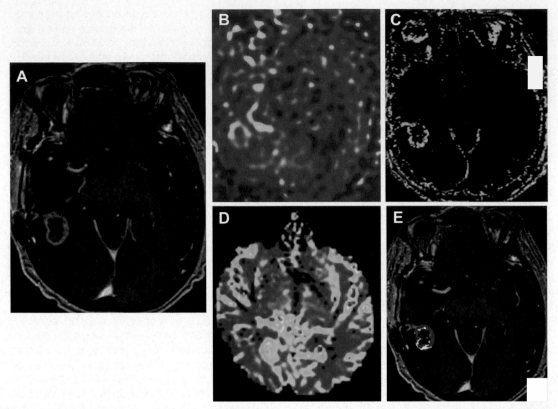

Fig. 5. A 70-year-old woman with history of right temporal glioblastoma, previously treated with surgical resection and chemoradiation, presenting for follow-up 2 months after therapy. (*A*) Postgadolinium 3D T1-weighted image shows a heterogeneously enhancing lesion in the right temporal lobe, at the site of the previously treated glioma. (*B*) CBF image from arterial spin labeling, (*C*) k-trans image from dynamic contrast enhancement, and (*D*) CBV image from dynamic susceptibility contrast-enhanced imaging show mild-to-moderately elevated CBF, k-trans, and CBV, respectively, within the lesion. (*E*) Fractional tumor burden image from DSC shows primarily high fractional tumor burden (*red*). Perfusion characteristics are suggestive of residual/recurrent tumor. The patient underwent surgical resection, and histopathology confirmed the diagnosis of residual/recurrent glioblastoma.

perfusion MR imaging may predict the status of contrast enhancing lesions and provide results similar to fluorodeoxyglucose (FDG)-PET with regards to differentiation between tumor recurrence and radiation necrosis.[39] In a study by Larsen and colleagues,[39] measurements of CBV were performed on patients with contrast enhancing lesions on MR imaging, which correlated well with FDG-PET examination findings. The lesions that regressed demonstrated lower CBV and generally corresponded to regions of decreased metabolism on FDG-PET (radiation necrosis). Lesions that progressed demonstrated higher CBV and corresponded to regions of higher metabolic activity on FDG-PET (tumor recurrence).[33] However, this is partially limited by the use of different CBV thresholds, which is dependent on the specific perfusion MR imaging protocol at a certain institution.[8] In a study by Barajas

and colleagues,[40] perfusion MR imaging was retrospectively studied to determine whether a progressively enhancing lesion represented recurrent glioblastoma or radiation necrosis. The authors found that CBV tended to be significantly higher in tumor, and that significantly lower parameters were found in patients with radiation necrosis. As indicated by the findings of these studies, the ability of perfusion values to distinguish between radiation necrosis and tumor is caused by inherent differences in their hemodynamic characteristics, which is further supported by histologic studies that demonstrated that tumor vasculature was significantly elevated in tissue specimens obtained from the contrast-enhancing portions of glioblastoma.[18] Besides perfusion-weighted imaging, the addition of MR spectroscopy is helpful to differentiate between tumor progression and radiation necrosis, the latter of which demonstrates a

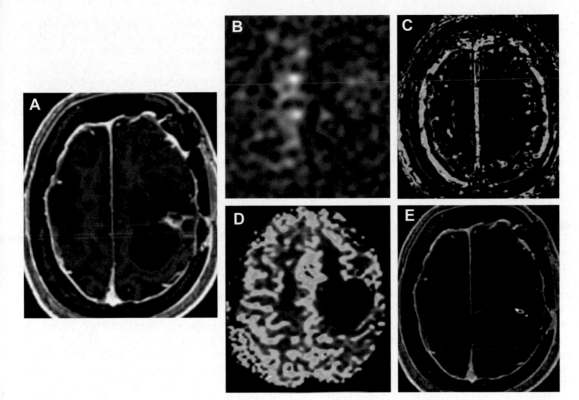

Fig. 6. A 72-year-old man with history of brain metastases from non–small cell lung cancer and previous treatment of a dominant left frontal metastasis with surgical resection and stereotactic radiosurgery, more than 4 years prior. (A) Postgadolinium 3D T1-weighted image shows a heterogeneously enhancing lesion in the left frontal lobe, at the site of the previously treated metastasis. (B) Arterial spin labeling images were suboptimal because of poor labeling. (C) K-trans image acquired from dynamic contrast-enhanced imaging and (D) CBV image acquired from dynamic susceptibility contrast-enhanced imaging show no increase in k-trans and CBV, respectively, within the lesion. (E) Fractional tumor burden image from DSC shows primarily low fractional tumor burden (blue) within the lesion. Perfusion features are suggestive of radiation necrosis (treatment effect). Nonetheless, the patient underwent a surgical resection, and histopathology revealed radiation necrosis and extensive gliosis without neoplasm.

high lipid/lactate peak, low N-acetylaspartate (NAA) peak, and a low choline peak as compared with normal brain parenchyma and pretreatment brain tumor.[2]

Pseudoregression (Pseudoresponse)

The advent of antiangiogenic therapy has led to often deceptive improvements in imaging findings, termed pseudoregression or pseudoresponse. This consists of relative decreases in contrast enhancement and peritumoral edema and is noted in up to 25% to 60% of the patients.[41,42] The most common agents used in these treatments are bevacizumab, which is a recombinant antibody, and cediranib, a receptor tyrosine kinase inhibitor. Additionally, pseudoregression may be associated with several other immunotherapeutic treatment agents, which are currently being studied.[31]

It is thought that the rapid radiographic response related to pseudoregression represents a direct action on blood vessel permeability rather than a true antitumor effect.[2] Typically, these findings are evident after several days, and can coincide with a transient improvement of clinical symptoms. However, the decrease in contrast enhancement in cases of pseudoregression is not associated with a decrease in tumor or overall survival.[43] Despite the shortcomings of conventional techniques, perfusion MR imaging can demonstrate areas of persistent increased perfusion values within the responsive lesion.[41]

Furthermore, studies have shown that the information provided by perfusion imaging can provide valuable information about changes in vascular function during therapy, which may aid in the identification of patients who are more likely to respond to prior therapies, or as an early indicator of patient response to antiangiogenic therapy. A study by Essock-Burns and colleagues[44] emphasized two parameters derived from perfusion maps: peak height, defined as the maximum increase in relaxivity of the greatest gadolinium influx, which is used as an estimate of vascular density; and percent signal recovery defined as the relative return to baseline of the signal intensity-time curve reflective of the bolus through a voxel, which is used as an estimate of leakage. These parameters were chosen in lieu of relative CBV because they did not require extensive curve fitting.[44] The study found that those with true response demonstrated a decrease in peak height and an increase in percent signal recovery which was attributed to an improvement in vessel permeability caused by antiangiogenic treatment. However, other studies demonstrate conflicting results, with a study by Stadlbaeur and colleagues demonstrating that changes in CBV were not significant enough to be suitable for differentiation between a true response and pseudoresponse.[41,45] A further confounder in the assessment of response is the tendency for antiangiogenic agents to promote progression of nonenhancing disease, thought be secondary to selection of a more invasive tumor subtype that does not require angiogenesis.[2]

SUMMARY

Through the years, there has been increased clinical utility of perfusion techniques using CT and MR imaging. These techniques have the potential to overcome the shortcomings of conventional MR imaging and can offer better approaches to tumor grading and provide physiologic information to aid advanced biopsy techniques. Furthermore, perfusion MR imaging is helpful to distinguish tumor from treatment-related processes, such as radiation necrosis, pseudoprogression, and pseudoregression.[41] Although the heterogeneity of image acquisition and processing techniques across sites remains a significant hurdle, the use of perfusion imaging in neuro-oncology has thus far proven to be promising.

CLINICS CARE POINTS

- Advanced perfusion imaging can offer enhanced evaluation of tumor physiology and hemodynamics to establish diagnosis, grade tumors, guide intraoperative sampling, and monitor therapeutic efficacy.

- Perfusion imaging is useful to differentiate between tumor types and between tumor and nonneoplastic conditions, such as infection or demyelination.

- Physiologic parameters obtained from perfusion imaging can help to identify treatment-related processes, such as radiation necrosis, pseudoprogression, and pseudoregression, and can help to guide clinical decision-making.

DISCLOSURE

The authors have nothing to disclose.

REFERENCES

1. De Simone M, Muccio CF, Pagnotta SM, et al. Comparison between CT and MR in perfusion imaging assessment of high-grade gliomas. Radiol Med 2013;118(1):140–51.
2. Lequin M, Hendrikse J. Advanced MR imaging in pediatric brain tumors, clinical applications. Neuroimaging Clin N Am 2017;27(1):167–90.
3. Järnum H, Steffensen EG, Knutsson L, et al. Perfusion MRI of brain tumours: a comparative study of pseudo-continuous arterial spin labelling and dynamic susceptibility contrast imaging. Neuroradiology 2010;52(4):307–17.
4. Jain R. Perfusion CT imaging of brain tumors: an overview. AJNR Am J Neuroradiol 2011;32(9):1570–7.
5. Griffith B, Jain R. Perfusion imaging in neuro-oncology: basic techniques and clinical applications. Magn Reson Imaging Clin N Am 2016;24(4):765–79.
6. Iv M, Liu X, Lavezo J, et al. Perfusion MRI-based fractional tumor burden differentiates between tumor and treatment effect in recurrent glioblastomas and informs clinical decision-making. AJNR Am J Neuroradiol 2019;40(10):1649–57.
7. Detre JA, Alsop DC. Perfusion magnetic resonance imaging with continuous arterial spin labeling: methods and clinical applications in the central nervous system. Eur J Radiol 1999;30(2):115–24.
8. Boxerman JL, Shiroishi MS, Ellingson BM, et al. Dynamic susceptibility contrast MR imaging in glioma: review of current clinical practice. Magn Reson Imaging Clin N Am 2016;24(4):649–70.
9. Petrella JR, Provenzale JM. MR perfusion imaging of the brain: techniques and applications. AJR Am J Roentgenol 2000;175(1):207–19.
10. Gharzeddine K, Hatzoglou V, Holodny AI, et al. MR perfusion and MR spectroscopy of brain neoplasms. Radiol Clin North Am 2019;57(6):1177–88.

11. Patel P, Baradaran H, Delgado D, et al. MR perfusion-weighted imaging in the evaluation of high-grade gliomas after treatment: a systematic review and meta-analysis. Neuro Oncol 2017;19(1): 118–27.

12. Tofts PS, Kermode AG. Measurement of the blood-brain barrier permeability and leakage space using dynamic MR imaging. 1. Fundamental concepts. Magn Reson Med 1991;17(2):357–67.

13. Essig M, Shiroishi MS, Nguyen TB, et al. Perfusion MRI: the five most frequently asked technical questions. AJR Am J Roentgenol 2013;200(1):24–34.

14. Khashbat Md D, Abe Md T, Ganbold Md M, et al. Correlation of 3D arterial spin labeling and multiparametric dynamic susceptibility contrast perfusion MRI in brain tumors. J Med Invest 2016;63(3–4): 175–81.

15. Hourani R, Brant LJ, Rizk T, et al. Can proton MR spectroscopic and perfusion imaging differentiate between neoplastic and nonneoplastic brain lesions in adults? AJNR Am J Neuroradiol 2008;29(2): 366–72.

16. Hakyemez B, Erdogan C, Bolca N, et al. Evaluation of different cerebral mass lesions by perfusion-weighted MR imaging. J Magn Reson Imaging 2006;24(4):817–24.

17. Al-Okaili RN, Krejza J, Woo JH, et al. Intraaxial brain masses: MR imaging-based diagnostic strategy–initial experience. Radiology 2007;243(2):539–50.

18. Yoon RG, Kim HS, Koh MJ, et al. Differentiation of recurrent glioblastoma from delayed radiation necrosis by using voxel-based multiparametric analysis of MR imaging data. Radiology 2017;285(1): 206–13.

19. Law M, Yang S, Babb JS, et al. Comparison of cerebral blood volume and vascular permeability from dynamic susceptibility contrast-enhanced perfusion MR imaging with glioma grade. AJNR Am J Neuroradiol 2004;25(5):746–55.

20. Neska-Matuszewska M, Bladowska J, Sąsiadek M, et al. Differentiation of glioblastoma multiforme, metastases and primary central nervous system lymphomas using multiparametric perfusion and diffusion MR imaging of a tumor core and a peritumoral zone: searching for a practical approach. PLoS One 2018;13(1):e0191341.

21. Sperduto PW, Chao ST, Sneed PK, et al. Diagnosis-specific prognostic factors, indexes, and treatment outcomes for patients with newly diagnosed brain metastases: a multi-institutional analysis of 4,259 patients. Int J Radiat Oncol Biol Phys 2010;77(3): 655–61.

22. Toh CH, Wei KC, Chang CN, et al. Differentiation of brain abscesses from glioblastomas and metastatic brain tumors: comparisons of diagnostic performance of dynamic susceptibility contrast-enhanced perfusion MR imaging before and after

23. mathematic contrast leakage correction. PLoS One 2014;9(10):e109172.

23. Holmes TM, Petrella JR, Provenzale JM. Distinction between cerebral abscesses and high-grade neoplasms by dynamic susceptibility contrast perfusion MRI. AJR Am J Roentgenol 2004;183(5):1247–52.

24. Floriano VH, Torres US, Spotti AR, et al. The role of dynamic susceptibility contrast-enhanced perfusion MR imaging in differentiating between infectious and neoplastic focal brain lesions: results from a cohort of 100 consecutive patients. PLoS One 2013;8(12): e81509.

25. Barker FG, Chang SM, Huhn SL, et al. Age and the risk of anaplasia in magnetic resonance-nonenhancing supratentorial cerebral tumors. Cancer 1997;80(5):936–41.

26. Prah MA, Al-Gizawiy MM, Mueller WM, et al. Spatial discrimination of glioblastoma and treatment effect with histologically-validated perfusion and diffusion magnetic resonance imaging metrics. J Neurooncol 2018;136(1):13–21.

27. Maia AC, Malheiros SM, da Rocha AJ, et al. Stereotactic biopsy guidance in adults with supratentorial nonenhancing gliomas: role of perfusion-weighted magnetic resonance imaging. J Neurosurg 2004; 101(6):970–6.

28. Hoxworth JM, Eschbacher JM, Gonzales AC, et al. Performance of Standardized relative CBV for quantifying regional histologic tumor burden in recurrent high-grade glioma: comparison against normalized relative CBV using image-localized stereotactic biopsies. AJNR Am J Neuroradiol 2020; 41(3):408–15.

29. Bag AK, Cezayirli PC, Davenport JJ, et al. Survival analysis in patients with newly diagnosed primary glioblastoma multiforme using pre- and post-treatment peritumoral perfusion imaging parameters. J Neurooncol 2014;120(2):361–70.

30. Macdonald DR, Cascino TL, Schold SC, et al. Response criteria for phase II studies of supratentorial malignant glioma. J Clin Oncol 1990;8(7): 1277–80. https://doi.org/10.1200/JCO.1990.8.7.1277.

31. Okada H, Weller M, Huang R, et al. Immunotherapy response assessment in neuro-oncology: a report of the RANO working group. Lancet Oncol 2015; 16(15):e534–42.

32. Falk Delgado A, Van Westen D, Nilsson M, et al. Diagnostic value of alternative techniques to gadolinium-based contrast agents in MR neuroimaging-a comprehensive overview. Insights Imaging 2019;10(1):84.

33. Parvez K, Parvez A, Zadeh G. The diagnosis and treatment of pseudoprogression, radiation necrosis and brain tumor recurrence. Int J Mol Sci 2014; 15(7):11832–46.

34. Fatterpekar GM, Galheigo D, Narayana A, et al. Treatment-related change versus tumor recurrence

in high-grade gliomas: a diagnostic conundrum–use of dynamic susceptibility contrast-enhanced (DSC) perfusion MRI. AJR Am J Roentgenol 2012;198(1): 19–26.

35. Young RJ, Gupta A, Shah AD, et al. MRI perfusion in determining pseudoprogression in patients with glioblastoma. Clin Imaging 2013;37(1):41–9.

36. Omuro AM, Leite CC, Mokhtari K, et al. Pitfalls in the diagnosis of brain tumours. Lancet Neurol 2006; 5(11):937–48.

37. Abbasi AW, Westerlaan HE, Holtman GA, et al. Incidence of tumour progression and pseudoprogression in high-grade gliomas: a systematic review and meta-analysis. Clin Neuroradiol 2018;28(3):401–11.

38. Zakhari N, Taccone MS, Torres CH, et al. Prospective comparative diagnostic accuracy evaluation of dynamic contrast-enhanced (DCE) vs. dynamic susceptibility contrast (DSC) MR perfusion in differentiating tumor recurrence from radiation necrosis in treated high-grade gliomas. J Magn Reson Imaging 2019;50(2):573–82.

39. Larsen VA, Simonsen HJ, Law I, et al. Evaluation of dynamic contrast-enhanced T1-weighted perfusion MRI in the differentiation of tumor recurrence from radiation necrosis. Neuroradiology 2013;55(3):361–9.

40. Barajas RF, Chang JS, Sneed PK, et al. Distinguishing recurrent intra-axial metastatic tumor from radiation necrosis following gamma knife radiosurgery using dynamic susceptibility-weighted contrast-enhanced perfusion MR imaging. AJNR Am J Neuroradiol 2009;30(2):367–72. https://doi.org/10.3174/ajnr.A1362.

41. van Dijken BRJ, van Laar PJ, Smits M, et al. Perfusion MRI in treatment evaluation of glioblastomas: clinical relevance of current and future techniques. J Magn Reson Imaging 2019;49(1):11–22.

42. Wen PY, Macdonald DR, Reardon DA, et al. Updated response assessment criteria for high-grade gliomas: response assessment in neuro-oncology working group. J Clin Oncol 2010;28(11):1963–72.

43. Brandsma D, van den Bent MJ. Pseudoprogression and pseudoresponse in the treatment of gliomas. Curr Opin Neurol 2009;22(6):633–8.

44. Essock-Burns E, Lupo JM, Cha S, et al. Assessment of perfusion MRI-derived parameters in evaluating and predicting response to antiangiogenic therapy in patients with newly diagnosed glioblastoma. Neuro Oncol 2011;13(1):119–31.

45. Stadlbauer A, Pichler P, Karl M, et al. Quantification of serial changes in cerebral blood volume and metabolism in patients with recurrent glioblastoma undergoing antiangiogenic therapy. Eur J Radiol 2015;84(6):1128–36.

Application of Diffusion Weighted Imaging and Diffusion Tensor Imaging in the Pretreatment and Post-treatment of Brain Tumor

Ranliang Hu, MD[a], Michael J. Hoch, MD[b],*

KEYWORDS

• ADC • Anisotropy • Brain mapping • Glioma • Neurosurgery • Tractography

KEY POINTS

- Clinical diffusion weighted imaging exploits the random motion of water molecules to generate contrast between normal tissue and disease.
- Diffusion is a valuable sequence in the initial evaluation of intracranial tumors, which can narrow the differential diagnosis and increase diagnostic confidence.
- Noninvasive presurgical mapping of eloquent white matter by diffusion tractography can reduce operative complication rates.
- Interpreting radiologists should understand the common causes of nonvisualized fibers by clinical tractography to better guide surgery.

INTRODUCTION

Diffusion MR imaging is a powerful technique that exploits the diffusion properties of water to generate contrast between normal tissue and pathology. The relative restriction of random water movement (diffusion) in vivo is measured using paired diffusion sensitizing gradients, which causes greater signal loss in diffusing relative to stationary spins. Since its introduction 30 years ago, diffusion MR imaging has transformed the practice of radiology by demonstrating high sensitivity and specificity for ischemic, infectious, toxic-metabolic, and neoplastic conditions.[1] In brain tumor imaging, diffusion MR imaging has been used to assess tumor type and grade, treatment response, and guide surgical intervention.[2–4]

Diffusion weighted imaging (DWI) is the most basic implementation of diffusion MR imaging and assumes a simple but clinically useful model of isotropic gaussian diffusion. DWI is "diffusion weighted" because it is not a true map of diffusion but also contains T2 and other contrasts; therefore, at least one additional set of images with no or little diffusion weighting is also required to calculate the apparent diffusion coefficient (ADC), a semiquantitative measure that relates to the actual diffusion coefficient and removes the contribution of "T2 shine-through."

Diffusion tensor imaging (DTI) expands on DWI by fitting a tensor model of diffusion, taking into account anisotropic diffusion in different directions and enabling calculation of metrics, such as fractional anisotropy (FA) (**Table 1**). Furthermore, DTI has been used to produce models of white matter bundles in the brain, or fiber tractography (FT), which is useful for neurosurgical planning and

[a] Department of Radiology & Imaging Sciences, Emory University, Emory University Hospital, 1364 Clifton Road, BG 20, Atlanta, GA 30322, USA; [b] Department of Radiology, University of Pennsylvania, Hospital of the University of Pennsylvania, 3400 Spruce Street, Suite 130, Philadelphia, PA 19104, USA
* Corresponding author.
E-mail address: Michael.Hoch@pennmedicine.upenn.edu

Radiol Clin N Am 59 (2021) 335–347
https://doi.org/10.1016/j.rcl.2021.01.003
0033-8389/21/© 2021 Elsevier Inc. All rights reserved.

Table 1
Description of diffusion tensor–derived metrics

Metric	Definition	Notes
Axial diffusivity	Diffusion magnitude along the primary orientation of axonal fiber bundles	Largest or principal eigenvalue
Radial diffusivity	Diffusion magnitude perpendicular to the axonal fiber bundles	Average of the two minor eigenvalues
Mean diffusivity	Directionally averaged diffusivity of water in a voxel	Average of all 3 eigenvalues; equals ADC
Fractional anisotropy	Degree of coherent directionality of intravoxel diffusivity	Values from 0 to 1 0 = unrestricted 1 = linear

intraoperative navigation. Although there is much exciting research in this area, a detailed physics review of advanced diffusion methods is beyond the scope of this article. The current clinical applications of diffusion imaging for evaluation of brain tumors is our focus.

DIFFUSION WEIGHTED IMAGING
Pretreatment

DWI is a useful sequence in the initial evaluation of intracranial tumors and tumor-like lesions. Restricted diffusion, as demonstrated by increased DWI signal and correspondingly reduced ADC, is caused by decreased free motion of water molecules, either because of high cellular density (eg, lymphoma and medulloblastoma) or high protein content (eg, epidermoid cyst). When used in conjunction with clinical history and other imaging features, DWI can help narrow the differential diagnosis and increase diagnostic confidence.

Extra-axial masses

Meningiomas are the most commonly encountered extra-axial lesion in clinical practice and can have a variable appearance on DWI. Qualitatively, some meningiomas can have slightly increased signal on DWI compared with the adjacent brain parenchymal. Lower ADC values have been reported to be associated with high-grade (atypical or malignant) meningiomas.[5] Similarly, there are also preliminary reports of using ADC to differentiate between hemangiopericytomas from meningiomas (higher ADC in the former), but further study is needed to confirm these findings.[6]

Dermoid and epidermoid cysts are along the histologic spectrum of ectodermal inclusion cysts and are classified depending on the presence of only epidermal component (epidermoid) or epidermal and dermal appendages (dermoid). Desquamated keratin in epidermoid cysts gives them the characteristic high DWI signal, enabling it to be readily differentiated from similar cystic lesions, such as arachnoid cyst.[7] Dermoid cysts can have variable high DWI signal depending on amount of desquamated keratin, but they also have high T1 signal because of their lipid content. Practically, clear distinction between dermoid and epidermoid at imaging is not crucial, because it does not alter management of these related benign entities.

Intra-axial masses

Diffusion imaging is helpful in the evaluation of pediatric and adult intra-axial tumors. In children, medulloblastomas and other embryonal tumors typically demonstrate high DWI signal and reduced ADC because of their high cellularity and nuclear-to-cytoplasmic ratio. This enables reliable distinction from other posterior fossa masses, such as ependymoma (**Fig. 1**) and pilocytic astrocytoma, which tend to have intermediate or facilitated diffusion.[8] Atypical teratoid/rhabdoid tumor is an aggressive embryonal tumor that also demonstrates restricted diffusion, but typically presents in a younger age group than medulloblastomas (<2 years vs mid to later childhood).

DWI plays a key role in the differentiation of gliomas and lymphomas, two of the most commonly encountered adult brain tumors. Central nervous system lymphoma are usually homogeneously hyperintense on DWI and has significantly lower ADC than glioblastoma, $0.630 \pm 0.155 \times 10^{-3}$ mm^2/s versus $0.963 \pm 0.119 \times 10^{-3}$ mm^2/s.[9] Diffusion within glioma varies from intermediate to high and correlates with histologic grade, with higher-grade tumors, such as anaplastic astrocytomas and glioblastoma, demonstrating lower ADC than

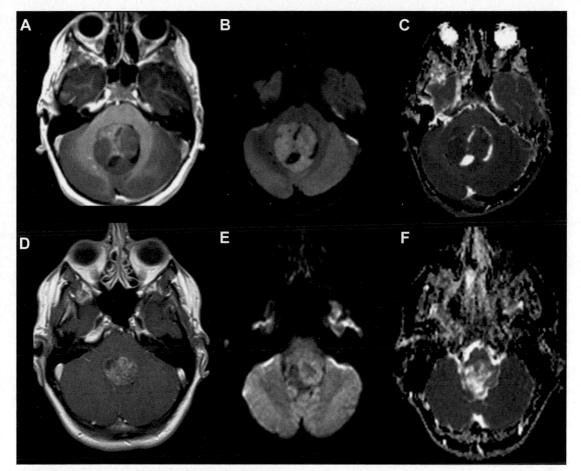

Fig. 1. Two different fourth ventricle tumors demonstrating heterogeneous enhancement on T1 postcontrast images. Medulloblastoma (*A*) demonstrating high signal intensity on DWI (*B*) and lower ADC than adjacent cerebellum (*C*). Ependymoma (*D*) demonstrating intermediate signal on DWI (*E*) but high ADC compared with the cerebellum (*F*).

low-grade gliomas (World Health Organization I and II).[10] Glioblastomas, in particular, are more heterogeneous than untreated lymphoma, with solid enhancing component demonstrating mild hyperintensity on DWI because of a combination of T2 shine-through and intermediate diffusion, and necrotic components demonstrating facilitated diffusion. Intratumoral hemorrhage is also more common in glioblastoma, and its associated susceptibility artifact can produce erroneous high DWI signal that must be recognized to avoid misinterpretation.

Other central nervous system tumors, especially those in the category of "small-blue-round-cell" tumors, such as primitive neuroectodermal tumor, germ cell tumor, and retinoblastoma, can demonstrate restricted diffusion. These are rarer and their characteristic locations can often provide helpful clues. Metastatic brain tumors can have variable appearance on DWI, depending on their primary source. Some have reported that the peritumoral edema of metastatic lesions have higher ADC than the nonenhancing component of gliomas, presumably because of higher cellularity of the latter.[11]

Nonneoplastic processes, such intracranial abscess and tumefactive demyelination, can often mimic tumor and demonstrate restricted diffusion. In contrast to lymphoma and other tumors, however, it is the central necrotic component of the abscess that demonstrates intense restricted diffusion rather than the solid cellular portion. Intracranial abscesses also tend to have relevant history and laboratory findings that aid in diagnosis. However, tumefactive demyelination can pose a diagnostic dilemma and appear similar to brain tumors, but its diffusion restriction is often along a "front" of active demyelination, occurring in a characteristic incomplete rim rather than a solid mass (**Fig. 2**).

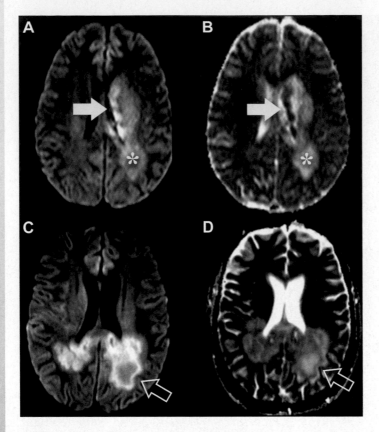

Fig. 2. Central nervous system lymphoma with foci of restricted diffusion (*arrows*) as shown on DWI (*A*) and ADC (*B*) along the left caudate and splenium, and extensive surrounding edema that demonstrates T2 shine-through (*asterisks*). (*C, D*) Tumefactive demyelination involving the splenium and periventricular white matter, with a thin rim of restricted diffusion along a front of active demyelination (*arrows*). Note the relative paucity of surrounding edema and mass effect despite a larger lesion in the case of tumefactive demyelination.

Post-treatment

A challenge in post-treatment imaging of brain tumors is the differentiation of treatment effects, from true tumor progression. Diffusion imaging can play a helpful role in this task when interpreted with detailed knowledge of tumor type and treatment history. In the immediate postsurgical setting, devitalized tissue along the resection cavity is expected to demonstrate restricted diffusion. Sometimes, however, the extent of restricted diffusion can extend beyond the surgical cavity and may involve large vascular territories, raising concern for perioperative infarction. This is more common when the mass is close to or encases vital vascular structures. Susceptibility artifact associated with postsurgical blood products can produce apparent hyperintensity on DWI and must be differentiated from true restricted diffusion.

Radiation therapy induces complex changes to the tumor and surrounding brain, which is dependent on tumor genetics, radiation dose, concurrent chemotherapy, and time. Paradoxic worsening of conventional image findings (enhancement and FLAIR) can occur within the first 3 months of completion of chemoradiation of high-grade gliomas, especially among tumors with IDH-1 mutation and methylation of the MGMT promoter.[12] This phenomenon is termed pseudoprogression and reflects an inflammatory response to tumor necrosis and connotes improved survival. A retrospective series evaluated the role of ADC ratio (minimal ADC in lesion/contralateral normal-appearing white matter) in differentiation between pseudoprogression and true progression, and found diagnostic accuracy of 86.7% when using ADC ratio alone, and 93.3% when used in a multiparametric model combined with dynamic susceptibility contrast perfusion and MR spectroscopy.[13] Interval increase in ADC after stereotactic radiosurgery of brain metastases has also been shown to be predictive of pseudoprogression, with accuracy of 77% according to one report.[14]

Radiation necrosis commonly occurs 3 months to a year following radiation and may be delayed for up to multiple years. Differentiation of radiation necrosis and tumor progression is difficult based on conventional imaging appearance, and addition of DWI has been shown to improve diagnostic accuracy. A recent study showed that addition of ADC cutoff of 1×10^{-3} mm^2/s to Brain Tumor Reporting and Data System improved its diagnostic performance either alone (area under the curve, 0.76–0.88), or in combination with dynamic susceptibility contrast (area under the curve, 0.92).[15] Complex techniques that consider heterogeneity within a lesion, such as volume-weighted voxel-based multiparametric clustering of diffusion and perfusion features, improved diagnostic accuracy over single imaging parameters.[16] With the growth of machine learning and radiomics, there will undoubtedly be newer algorithms that incorporate conventional and advanced imaging features to classify tumor outcome. However, heterogeneity within treated tumor itself, where radiation necrosis often coexists with viable tumor, poses a challenge to the development and implementation of automated techniques.

The vascular endothelial growth factor inhibitor bevacizumab is commonly used in recurrent glioblastoma. This medication has antiangiogenic effects and reduces blood-brain barrier permeability, thereby masking the enhancement of viable tumor (pseudoresponse). Restricted diffusion can occur in either the tumor bed or elsewhere in the brain, presumably caused by ischemic necrosis (**Fig. 3**). Restricted diffusion in malignant gliomas treated with bevacizumab that is persistent over time is usually associated with good outcomes.[17] However, pathologic studies have shown that progressive bevacizumab-induced restricted diffusion is associated with coagulative necrosis surrounded by viable tumor and associated with poor outcomes.[18] Thus, it is important to evaluate serial changes in diffusion restriction on follow-up imaging and to incorporate all clinical and imaging data available to make the most accurate assessment.

DIFFUSION TENSOR IMAGING
Pretreatment

To preserve functional tissue, state-of-the-art MR imaging preoperative mapping of brain tumor patients has become the standard of care across the country. Neuroradiology-generated preoperative mapping of eloquent white matter tracts helps the neurosurgeon balance morbidity with resecting as much tumor as possible, which correlates with improved patient survival.[19] The emergence of DTI with FT has allowed neurosurgeons to resect tumors with decreased complication rates[20,21] and increased median survival rates.[22]

Knowledge of the technical basis of DTI combined with white matter anatomy is essential in the application of preoperative FT. DTI uses the

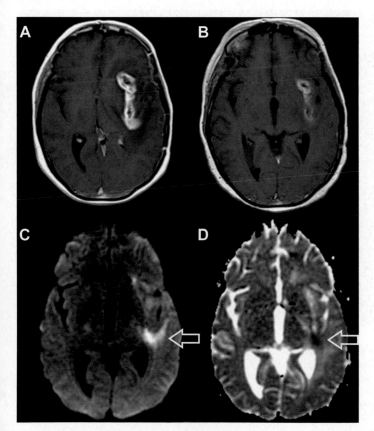

Fig. 3. Glioblastoma treated with bevacizumab demonstrating reduction of enhancement on pretreatment (*A*) and follow-up (*B*) T1 postcontrast images. Follow-up DWI (*C*) and ADC (*D*) shows diffusion restriction in the left temporal stem in the region of previous enhancement (*arrows*), corresponding to ischemic necrosis. Attention to this area on follow-up diffusion imaging is needed to assess for continued tumor response.

anisotropic diffusion of water along coherently organized white matter tracts. FA value of 1 means that diffusion happens along one axis and is restricted in other directions (ie, axonal bundle). Most clinical DTI protocols use at least 30 diffusion-encoded image sets at $b = 1000$ s/mm^2 along noncollinear directions in addition to $b = 0$ s/mm^2 image set with 2- to 3-mm isotropic voxels to create the diffusion tensor. Deterministic FT generates streamlines, originating from user-defined seed points, along the dominant diffusion direction of the tract in three-dimension (3D) from voxel to voxel. Tracking parameters can then be manipulated to constrain the streamlines to anatomically represent eloquent white matter pathways. Various technical aspects of FT have been discussed previously and are an essential review for anyone new to brain mapping.[23–26]

FT data are coregistered with volumetric structural sequences using various Food and Drug Administration–approved post-processing software for surgical navigation. The "buttonology" of these platforms varies, but the concepts of seed placement and tract titration are consistent. For nonenhancing tumors, it is paramount to fuse the tensor data with a 3D-FLAIR or T2 sequence. For enhancing lesions, postcontrast 3D-T1 images should be included. Seeds are placed in the plane perpendicular to the known trajectory of the desired tract to obtain as many streamlines as possible. A seed point can be drawn on several adjacent slices as another method to capture more streamlines. Our review focuses on two white matter tracts most frequently requested by our neurosurgical colleagues (corticospinal tract [CST] and arcuate fasciculus [AF]). Using real examples, we describe relevant anatomy, seed placement, and appropriate tract titration. A brief discussion on the limitations of clinical deterministic FT is included.

Motor: corticospinal tract

The CST or pyramidal tract is responsible for controlling movement in the contralateral torso, upper and lower extremities. It descends from the precentral gyrus and converges through the posterior limb internal capsule before traversing the brainstem.[26] It decussates at the caudal medulla and connects with spinal motor neurons. Using the direction-encoded color FA maps as a guide, the first seed is drawn in the axial plane to cover the cerebral peduncle (Fig. 4A). Cover as much of the peduncle as possible to ensure obtaining the CST fibers. The purpose of the second seed

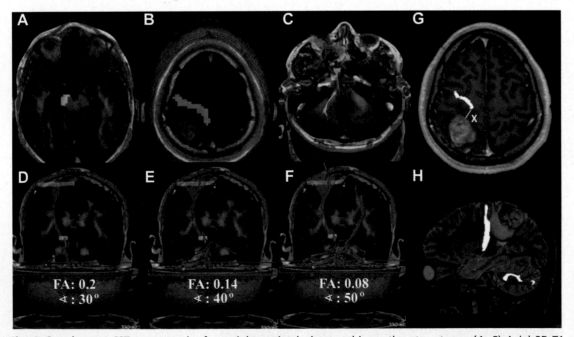

Fig. 4. Step-by-step CST tractography for a right parietal pleomorphic xanthoastrocytoma. (A, B) Axial 3D-T1 postcontrast images fused with direction-encoded color FA maps show the locations for seed placement: cerebral peduncle (blue) and precentral gyrus (pink). (C) Oblique axial image shows inclusion of streamlines only within both seed points. (D–F) Coronal images with different titration thresholds show sparse, appropriate, and excessive streamlines, respectively. (G) Axial 3D-T1 postcontrast and (H) sagittal 3D-T2 surgical navigation images show the 3D "burned-in" tract volume X mm from the enhancing tumor margin and along the nonenhancing signal abnormality.

point is to constrain the tract to match known anatomy.[27] The second seed is placed on axial images to cover the precentral gyrus subcortical white matter just inferior to the level of the hand knob (**Fig.** 4B). In the case of the CST the second seed point excludes the frontal pontine and parietal pontine fibers (**Fig.** 4C).

After the initial tract is generated, we then titrate our tract parameters to enhance the tract density while at the same time minimizing spurious fibers. An excellent review of CST parameter titration by Parizel and colleagues[28] provides suggested values. **Fig.** 4D–F shows examples of sparse, sufficient and excessive streamlines. A summary of parameters altering fiber tracking is found in **Table 2**. We report the smallest distance from the lesion's enhancing and nonenhancing margins relative to the visualized tract (**Fig.** 4G, H). Although this is not a universally accepted DTI practice because of the deterministic tractography limitations that are discussed later,[29] acknowledgment by surgeons that the tracts are estimated representations of white matter makes this a nonissue.

Language: arcuate fasciculus

The AF has been classically represented as the connection between the putative Broca and Wernicke language areas. Recent models of language connectivity in human cadaver[30] and DTI studies[31,32] favor the AF consisting of multiple complex components including indirect semantic and direct phonetic pathways. The AF extends from the caudal aspect of the superior and middle temporal gyri around the sylvian fissure and to the ipsilateral dorsal prefrontal cortex. To virtually dissect the AF, we place an initial seed on the direction-encoded color FA maps in the proximal frontal projections in the coronal plane at the level of the isthmus of the corpus callosum (**Fig.** 5A).

The second seed is placed in the genu of the AF in the axial plane at the level of the internal capsule (**Fig.** 5B). When titrating, a higher angle threshold (60°–80°) should be used to overcome the curved portion of the tract.

Most humans have left language lateralization and the left AF is typically larger (**Fig.** 5D, E).[33,34] It has been theorized that the left AF may play an additional role in acoustic processing and will be larger even in right language lateralized subjects.[35] However, the right or nondominant AF should not be regarded as trivial because it contributes to prosody.[36] In left-handed and ambidextrous patients that tend to have bilateral hemisphere contributions to speech, use caution if relying on tractography of the AF without functional MR imaging task data to predict language lateralization, because there can be less AF asymmetry.[34,37] Correlating the bilateral AF tractography pattern with the Edinburgh Handedness Inventory score[38] is essential for right-sided lesion cases for best representation of the tracts.[34] The putative Wernicke area has a greater variability in location compared with Broca area.[39] In cases of suspected atypical language center localization, fusing the FT data to the functional MR imaging task data can increase reporting confidence if the data sets have common areas of involvement (**Fig.** 6).

Challenges and limitations

Neuroradiologists need to understand the limitations of tractography, such as patient motion, signal noise, magnetic field geometric distortions, and eddy-current artifacts. Neurosurgeons need to know that once the craniotomy is performed and debulking occurs, the brain shifts and the 3D tracts loaded to the navigation software may no longer align with the patient.[40] Another major limitation to the deterministic tensor model is the

Table 2
Summary of post-processing fiber tracking parameters and suggested starting values for tract titration

Parameter[a]	Increasing Parameter Effect on Fiber Density	Suggested Starting Value	
		CST	AF
FA threshold	Decreases	0.16	0.12
Angle threshold	Increases	40°	60°
Step length	Decreases	1.5 mm	1.5 mm
Samples per voxel length	Increases	2	3

FA threshold: fiber tracking will stop if FA is smaller than this value. Angle threshold: fiber tracking will stop if turning angle is larger than this value. Step length: for the streamline marching algorithm; should be about one-quarter of the voxel size. If too small will cause much longer tracking time with little increase in accuracy. Samples per voxel length: sample rate for user-defined seed region. Values larger than 4 may cause errors.

[a] Not all parameters are available to manually adjust on different software platforms.

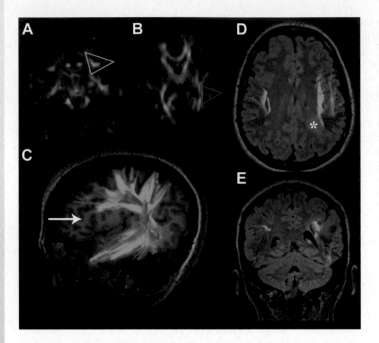

Fig. 5. (A, B) Coronal and axial direction-encoded color FA maps show the typical locations for seed placement for generating the left AF in a volunteer: periventricular *green triangle* and genu *purple triangle*. (C) Sagittal 3D-T1 image shows only streamlines included in both seed points. Note the lack of frontal fibers to the Broca area (*arrow*). (D, E) Axial and coronal 3D-FLAIR images with fused bilateral AF tracts show expected asymmetry in a right-handed (Edinburgh Handedness +100) individual with an infiltrative left parietal lesion (*asterisk*).

inability to resolve multiple fiber orientations within the imaging voxel.[41,42] This is known as the "crossing fiber problem." The estimate of tensor orientation is an average of the orientations of all the axons contained within the voxel. When the axons are coherently organized the tensor orientation reflects the underlying fibers. When the axons are not highly coherent, the voxel-averaged estimate of tensor orientation is not accurate and the tract stops prematurely or can continue spuriously. Although this issue is improved with higher angular resolution diffusion acquisitions[43] and

probabilistic tractography,[44] voxels containing multiple-fiber orientations are likely whenever the imaging resolution (2–3 mm) is larger than the axon dimensions (several microns).

The lateral projections of the CST and the corticobulbar tracts (movement of the face and tongue) are notoriously nonvisualized because of crossing the lateral aspect of the AF while entering the corona radiata (**Fig. 7**).[44,45] Routinely when generating the AF, the anterior component to Broca area is truncated for unknown reasons (**Fig. 5**C). This may be caused by crossing short frontal tracts

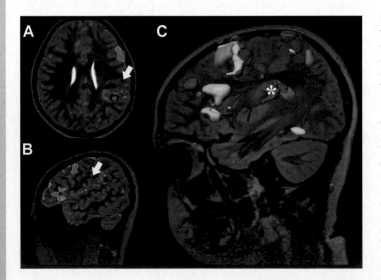

Fig. 6. Superimposing the DTI data to the functional MR imaging task data can increase confidence in mapping atypical language centers. (A, B) Axial and sagittal 3D-T2 images with coregistered verb generation (*blue*) and semantic decision (*red*) tasks for a left parietal extraventricular neurocytoma. There is a dominant receptive language center (*arrows*) in an atypical location in the supramarginal gyrus. Activity was not seen in the classic Wernicke location of posterior superior temporal gyrus. (C) 3D-FLAIR fused with left AF volume (*purple*) shows the streamlines involving the receptive language center (*asterisk*) increasing confidence. There was impairment of phonologic retrieval during intraoperative cortical stimulation of this center.

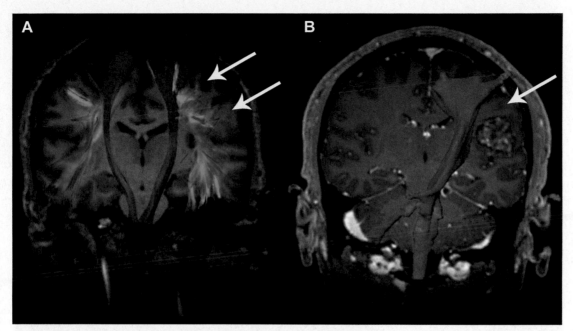

Fig. 7. (*A*) Coronal 3D-T1 fused with bilateral CST (*blue*) and AF (*green*) tracts in a volunteer shows the location of missing lateral CST and corticobulbar streamlines (*arrows*) from crossing fibers. (*B*) Coronal 3D-T1 postcontrast of a patient with a cavernoma shows missing lateral streamlines of the CST (*purple*) over the superior aspect of the lesion (*arrow*). It is important to report expected locations of nonvisualized fibers before surgery.

including the frontal aslant pathway.[46] An electrocorticography study combined with DTI of the AF found that language-related sites in the temporal lobe were far more likely to directly connect to the inferior precentral gyrus rather than Broca area.[47] This may suggest the AF plays a supporting role and interacts with other language tracts that have a direct connection to Broca area. Using knowledge of white matter anatomy one can anticipate where these classically "missing" fiber components would be relative to the lesion and inform the neurosurgeon in their report.

Absence of fibers may also occur when there is extensive edema, tumor infiltration, or frank destruction. Delineation of the two latter scenarios is problematic because both may occur with the same lesion. New research tractography approaches are able to overcome the "edema problem."[48] Until they are ready for widespread clinical implementation, reducing the FA threshold to increase visualization of absent fibers remains an alternative, albeit not always successful. Tumor imaging patterns with tractography have been previously described.[26] In the case of frank destruction by tumor, a near zero anisotropy is seen and the tract is not visualized no matter the decrease in FA threshold. With tract infiltration by tumor, the tract is deviated into an abnormal orientation with an abnormally low FA. In cases of peritumoral edema there is an abnormally low FA but no

deviation in tract orientation. These three patterns can each reduce FA, therefore one should not confuse FA values with white matter integrity. Observation of function during functional MR imaging training by the neuroradiologist or cortical activation with relevant tasks is superior to absence of DTI fibers (**Fig. 8**).

Post-treatment

Previous works have evaluated DTI as a means to predict functional recovery after surgery. They have evaluated distances and indirectly estimated axonal health via DTI metrics, such as FA and diffusivity. Lower FA averages and higher mean diffusivity in the ipsilateral CST have been linked to postoperative motor deficits.[49] FA values of interhemispheric connectivity were associated with postoperative aphasia in left-sided perisylvian brain tumors.[50] A tumor distance of 1 cm or less from the CST or AF most significantly predicts the occurrence of new deficits with current surgical techniques.[51] Furthermore, an intraoperative subcortical motor stimulation study showed a 1-cm gap of uncertainty between the bipolar electrode tip and generated DTI tracts.[52] Therefore we favor clearly describing "impression worthy" tracts that are 1 cm or less from the tumor margins in our functional MR imaging reports. The DTI tractography plans can improve safety of surgery by

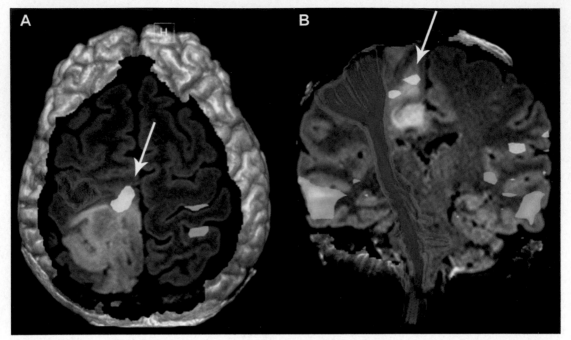

Fig. 8. (*A*) Axial and (*B*) coronal 3D-FLAIR images of a right parietal IDH-mutated glioma. The CST (*pink*) medial fibers to the leg/foot area of the right precentral gyrus are not visualized because of decreased FA from tumor infiltration. Foot motion was intact during patient training and superimposed functional MR imaging ankle flexion task data (*yellow*) show activity (*arrows*). Reporting the medial CST fibers are functioning even though not recognized by the tractography algorithm is crucial for surgical planning.

identifying challenging resection margins and informing the surgeons when to brace for a possible challenging postoperative recovery.

Diffusion tensor–derived quantitative measures can act as biomarkers for worsening disease in the absence of appreciable change on conventional MR imaging sequences. Restriction on DTI maps can detect low-grade glioma malignant transformation (axial diffusivity having highest sensitivity and specificity) at the same time point or earlier compared with contrast-enhanced images.[53] Significantly decreased FA at baseline in the glioma peritumoral nonenhancing signal abnormality is a predictor of local enhancing tumor recurrence.[54] These findings may be important for surgery or radiation planning. The toxic effects of chemoradiation therapy on cerebral white matter linked to cognitive changes are assessed with DTI. Connor and colleagues[55] showed mean, axial, and radial diffusivity significantly increased with radiation time course and dose and corresponding decrease in FA in white matter of high-grade glioma patients. They postulated the radiation-induced vascular permeability and neuroinflammation contributed to neurocognitive decline. The structural integrity of white matter is susceptible to the effects of chemotherapy. Medulloblastoma patients treated with chemotherapy

had decreased FA values in white matter structures compared with healthy age-matched control subjects. Reductions in FA values were associated with poor performance at school.[56]

CLINICS CARE POINTS

- Reduced ADC values are seen in highly cellular brain tumors, such as lymphoma, medulloblastoma, and atypical meningioma.

- Progressive reduced diffusion over time is associated with poor outcomes in malignant gliomas treated with bevacizumab.

- The arcuate fasciculi typically have greater hemispheric asymmetry than the corticospinal tracts and should be correlated with Edinburgh Handedness score.

- Tumor infiltration and edema can reduce FA values to the point that functioning fiber tracts are not recognized by deterministic tractography.

- Document eloquent fiber tracts that are 1 cm or less from the tumor margin in the functional MR imaging report impression.

DISCLOSURES

The authors have nothing to disclose.

REFERENCES

1. Schaefer PW, Grant PE, Gonzalez RG. Diffusion-weighted MR imaging of the brain. Radiology 2000;217(2):331–45.
2. Kono K, Inoue Y, Nakayama K, et al. The role of diffusion-weighted imaging in patients with brain tumors. AJNR Am J Neuroradiol 2001;22(6):1081–8.
3. Holodny AI, Ollenschlager M. Diffusion imaging in brain tumors. Neuroimaging Clin N Am 2002;12(1):107–24.
4. Hygino da Cruz LC Jr, Vieira IG, Domingues RC. Diffusion MR imaging: an important tool in the assessment of brain tumors. Neuroimaging Clin N Am 2011;21(1):27–49.
5. Filippi CG, Edgar MA, Uluğ AM, et al. Appearance of meningiomas on diffusion-weighted images: correlating diffusion constants with histopathologic findings. AJNR Am J Neuroradiol 2001;22(1):65–72.
6. Shankar JJS, Hodgson L, Sinha N. Diffusion weighted imaging may help differentiate intracranial hemangiopericytoma from meningioma. J Neuroradiol 2019;46(4):263–7.
7. Tsuruda JS, Chew WM, Moseley ME, et al. Diffusion-weighted MR imaging of the brain: value of differentiating between extraaxial cysts and epidermoid tumors. AJNR Am J Neuroradiol 1990;11(5):925–31 [discussion: 932–4].
8. Rumboldt Z, Camacho DLA, Lake D, et al. Apparent diffusion coefficients for differentiation of cerebellar tumors in children. AJNR Am J Neuroradiol 2006;27(6):1362–9.
9. Toh C-H, Castillo M, Wong AM-C, et al. Primary cerebral lymphoma and glioblastoma multiforme: differences in diffusion characteristics evaluated with diffusion tensor imaging. AJNR Am J Neuroradiol 2007;29(3):471–5.
10. Hilario A, Ramos A, Perez-Nuñez A, et al. The added value of apparent diffusion coefficient to cerebral blood volume in the preoperative grading of diffuse gliomas. AJNR Am J Neuroradiol 2011;33(4):701–7.
11. Lee EJ, terBrugge K, Mikulis D, et al. Diagnostic value of peritumoral minimum apparent diffusion coefficient for differentiation of glioblastoma multiforme from solitary metastatic lesions. AJR Am J Roentgenol 2011;196:71–6.
12. Li H, Li J, Cheng G, et al. IDH mutation and MGMT promoter methylation are associated with the pseudoprogression and improved prognosis of glioblastoma multiforme patients who have undergone concurrent and adjuvant temozolomide-based chemoradiotherapy. Clin Neurol Neurosurg 2016;151:31–6.
13. Matsusue E, Fink JR, Rockhill JK, et al. Distinction between glioma progression and post-radiation change by combined physiologic MR imaging. Neuroradiology 2010;52(4):297–306.
14. Knitter JR, Erly WK, Stea BD, et al. Interval change in diffusion and perfusion MRI parameters for the assessment of pseudoprogression in cerebral metastases treated with stereotactic radiation. Am J Roentgenol 2018;211(1):168–75.
15. Yang Y, Yang Y, Wu X, et al. Adding DSC PWI and DWI to BT-RADS can help identify postoperative recurrence in patients with high-grade gliomas. J Neurooncol 2020;146(2):363–71.
16. Yoon RG, Kim HS, Koh MJ, et al. Differentiation of recurrent glioblastoma from delayed radiation necrosis by using voxel-based multiparametric analysis of MR imaging data. Radiology 2017;285(1):206–13.
17. Mong S, Ellingson BM, Nghiemphu PL, et al. Persistent diffusion-restricted lesions in bevacizumab-treated malignant gliomas are associated with improved survival compared with matched controls. AJNR Am J Neuroradiol 2012;33(9):1763–70.
18. Nguyen HS, Milbach N, Hurrell SL, et al. Progressing bevacizumab-induced diffusion restriction is associated with coagulative necrosis surrounded by viable tumor and decreased overall survival in patients with recurrent glioblastoma. AJNR Am J Neuroradiol 2016;37(12):2201–8.
19. Claus EB, Horlacher A, Hsu L, et al. Survival rates in patients with low-grade glioma after intraoperative magnetic resonance image guidance. Cancer 2005;103:1227–33.
20. Ulmer JL, Berman JI, Meuller WN, et al. Issues in translating imaging technology and presurgical diffusion tensor imaging. In: Faro SH, Mohamed FB, Law M, et al, editors. Functional neuroradiology: principles and clinical applications. 1st edition. Boston (MA): Springer; 2011. p. 731–65.
21. Bello L, Castellano A, Fava E, et al. Intraoperative use of diffusion tensor imaging fiber tractography and subcortical mapping for resection of gliomas: technical considerations. Neurosurg Focus 2010;28(2):E6.
22. Wu JS, Zhou LF, Tang WJ, et al. Clinical evaluation and follow-up outcome of diffusion tensor imaging-based functional neuronavigation: a prospective, controlled study in patients with gliomas involving pyramidal tracts. Neurosurgery 2007;61(5):935–48 [discussion: 948–9].
23. Mukherjee P, Berman JI, Chung SW, et al. Diffusion tensor MR imaging and fiber tractography: theoretic underpinnings. AJNR Am J Neuroradiol 2008;29:632–41.
24. Mukherjee P, Chung SW, Berman JI, et al. Diffusion tensor MR imaging and fiber tractography: technical

considerations. AJNR Am J Neuroradiol 2008;29: 843–52.

25. Catani M, Howard RJ, Pajevic S, et al. Virtual in vivo interactive dissection of white matter fasciculi in the human brain. Neuroimage 2002;17:77–94.

26. Jellison BJ, Field AS, Medow J, et al. Diffusion tensor imaging of cerebral white matter: a pictorial review of physics, fiber tract anatomy, and tumor imaging patterns. AJNR Am J Neuroradiol 2004; 25:356–69.

27. Carpenter MB, Strong OS, Truex RC. Human neuro-anatomy: (formerly Strong and Elwyn's human neuroanatomy). 7th edition. Baltimore (MD): Lippincott Williams & Wilkins; 1976.

28. Parizel PM, Van Rompaey V, Van Loock R, et al. Influence of user-defined parameters on diffusion tensor tractography of the corticospinal tract. Neuroradiology J 2007;20:139–47.

29. Field A, Filippi C, Kalnin A, et al. ASFNR guidelines for clinical application of diffusion tensor imaging. 2012. Available at: www.asfnr.org/clinical-standards. Accessed April 21, 2020.

30. Dick AS, Tremblay P. Beyond the arcuate fasciculus: consensus and controversy in the connectional anatomy of language. Brain 2012;135:3529–50.

31. Catani M, Mesulam M. The arcuate fasciculus and the disconnection theme in language and aphasia: history and current state. Cortex 2008;44:953–61.

32. Glasser MF, Rilling JK. DTI tractography of the human brain's language pathways. Cereb Cortex 2008;18:2471–82.

33. Vernooij MW, Smits M, Wielopolski PA, et al. Fiber density asymmetry of the arcuate fasciculus in relation to functional hemispheric language lateralization in both right- and left-handed healthy subjects: a combined fMRI and DTI study. Neuroimage 2007;35(3):1064–76.

34. Propper RE, O'Donnell LJ, Whalen S, et al. A combined fMRI and DTI examination of functional language lateralization and arcuate fasciculus structure: effects of degree versus direction of hand preference. Brain Cogn 2010;73:85–92.

35. Hutsler J, Galuske RA. Hemispheric asymmetries in cerebral cortical networks. Trends Neurosci 2003;8: 429–35.

36. Ethofer T, Anders S, Erb M, et al. Cerebral pathways in processing of affective prosody: a dynamic causal modeling study. Neuroimage 2006;30:580–7.

37. Szaflarski JP, Binder JR, Possing ET, et al. Language lateralization in left-handed and ambidextrous people: fMRI data. Neurology 2002;2:238–44.

38. Oldfield RC. The assessment and analysis of handedness: the Edinburgh inventory. Neuropsychologia 1971;9(1):97–113.

39. Chang EF, Raygor KP, Berger MS. Contemporary model of language organization: an overview for neurosurgeons. J Neurosurg 2015;122:250–61.

40. Nimsky C, Ganslandt O, Hastreiter P, et al. Preoperative and intraoperative diffusion tensor imaging-based fiber tracking in glioma surgery. Neurosurgery 2005;56(1):130–7 [discussion: 138].

41. Basser PJ, Mattiello J, Le Bihan D. Estimation of the effective self-diffusion tensor from the NMR spin echo. J Magn Reson 1994;103:247–54.

42. Pierpaoli C, Basser PJ. Toward a quantitative assessment of diffusion anisotropy. Magn Reson Med 1996;36:893–906.

43. Caverzasi E, Hervey-Jumper SL, Jordan KM, et al. Identifying preoperative language tracts and predicting postoperative functional recovery using HARDI q-ball fiber tractography in patients with gliomas. J Neurosurg 2015;125:33–45.

44. Behrens TEJ, Berg HJ, Jbabdi S, et al. Probabilistic diffusion tractography with multiple fibre orientations: what can we gain? Neuroimage 2007;34: 144–55.

45. Holodny AI, Watts R, Korneinko VN, et al. Diffusion tensor tractography of the motor white matter tracts in man: current controversies and future directions. Ann N Y Acad Sci 2005;1064:88–97.

46. Catani M, Dell'Acqua F, Vergani F, et al. Short frontal lobe connections of the human brain. Cortex 2012; 48:273–91.

47. Brown EC, Jeong JW, Muzik O, et al. Evaluating the arcuate fasciculus with combined diffusion weighted MRI tractography and electrocorticography. Hum Brain Mapp 2014;35(5):2333–47.

48. Zhang H, Wang Y, Lu T, et al. Differences between generalized q-sampling imaging and diffusion tensor imaging in the preoperative visualization of the nerve fiber tracts within peritumoral edema in brain. Neurosurgery 2013;73:1044–53 [discussion: 1053].

49. Rosenstock T, Giampiccolo D, Schneider H, et al. Specific DTI seeding and diffusivity-analysis improve the quality and prognostic value of TMS-based deterministic DTI of the pyramidal tract. Neuroimage Clin 2017;16:276–85.

50. Sollmann N, Negwer C, Tussis L, et al. Interhemispheric connectivity revealed by diffusion tensor imaging fiber tracking derived from navigated transcranial magnetic stimulation maps as a sign of language function at risk in patients with brain tumors. J Neurosurg 2016;126:222–33.

51. Meyer EJ, Gaggl W, Gilloon B, et al. The impact of intracranial tumor proximity to white matter tracts on morbidity and mortality: a retrospective diffusion tensor imaging study. Neurosurgery 2017;80: 193–200.

52. Berman JI, Berger MS, Chung SW, et al. Accuracy of diffusion tensor magnetic resonance imaging tractography assessed using intraoperative subcortical stimulation mapping and magnetic source imaging. J Neurosurg 2007;107(3):488–94.

53. Freitag MT, Maier-Hein KH, Binczyk F, et al. Early detection of malignant transformation in resected WHO II low-grade glioma using diffusion tensor-derived quantitative measures. PLoS One 2016; 11(10):e0164679.

54. Bette S, Huber T, Gempt J, et al. Local fractional anisotropy is reduced in areas with tumor recurrence in glioblastoma. Radiology 2017;283(2):499–507.

55. Connor M, Karunamuni R, McDonald C, et al. Dose-dependent white matter damage after brain radio-therapy. Radiother Oncol 2016;121(2):209–16.

56. Khong PL, Kwong DLW, Chan GCF, et al. Diffusion-tensor imaging for the detection and quantification of treatment-induced white matter injury in children with medulloblastoma: a pilot study. AJNR Am J Neuroradiol 2003;24(4):734–40.

Clinical Applications of Magnetic Resonance Spectroscopy in Brain Tumors
From Diagnosis to Treatment

Brent D. Weinberg, MD, PhD[a],*, Manohar Kuruva, MD[a],
Hyunsuk Shim, PhD[b], Mark E. Mullins, MD, PhD[a]

KEYWORDS

- Brain tumor • Glioblastoma • Magnetic resonance spectroscopy • Pseudoprogression
- Radiation necrosis • Tumor progression

KEY POINTS

- Magnetic resonance spectroscopy (MRS) is an advanced MR imaging technique that allows noninvasive evaluation of tissue molecular composition.
- High-grade neoplasms, including brain tumors, have elevation of choline, a marker of cell membrane turnover, with decrease in N-acetyl aspartate, a marker of neuronal integrity.
- The most frequent applications of MRS in brain tumor care are differentiating tumor from other nonneoplastic pathology, estimating tumor grade, and differentiating tumor recurrence from radiation effects.
- Many pathologies overlap in spectroscopic appearance, and MRS is best interpreted in conjunction with other imaging findings and clinical considerations.
- Future developments may make whole-brain spectroscopic imaging a useful tool for prognostication and treatment planning.

INTRODUCTION

Magnetic resonance spectroscopy (MRS) is a technique that combines the ability of nuclear magnetic resonance (NMR) to differentiate molecules with the imaging features of localization unique to MR imaging. This provides a "molecular window" into the component chemistry of a given tissue, allowing for unique insight into physiologic or disease (pathophysiologic) processes. MRS requires no injected contrast agent and no ionizing radiation is involved, which are obvious safety benefits.

There are many applications of MRS to imaging of brain tumors that have been explored, some of which have already reached clinical practice and others that have been confined predominantly to research applications (**Table 1**). In clinical application, MRS can potentially differentiate primary brain tumors from other potential mimics, such as demyelinating disease, lymphoma, or infection. In addition, the "molecular signatures" of high-grade and low-grade tumors often differ, allowing prediction of how aggressive a tumor may be. After treatment, MRS can provide insight into whether treated tissue consists predominantly of radiation necrosis or tumor, a considerable diagnostic dilemma. More research-oriented applications include surveying a tumor to locate the most aggressive area to target for biopsy and

[a] Radiology and Imaging Sciences, Emory University, 1364 Clifton Road Northeast BG20, Atlanta, GA 30322, USA; [b] Radiation Oncology, Emory University, 1365 Clifton Road Northeast, Atlanta, GA 30322, USA
* Corresponding author.
E-mail address: brent.d.weinberg@emory.edu
Twitter: @brentweinberg (B.D.W.)

Radiol Clin N Am 59 (2021) 349–362
https://doi.org/10.1016/j.rcl.2021.01.004

Table 1	
Potential uses of magnetic resonance spectroscopy in brain tumor imaging	
Clinical Applications	**Research Applications**
Differentiating tumor from potential mimics	Three-dimensional evaluation of tumor heterogeneity
Metastatic disease	Detection of molecular/genetic features
Demyelinating disease	Isocitrate dehydrogenase mutation
Lymphoma	Treatment planning
Infection	Surgical resection/biopsy
Evaluation of treated tumor to differentiate	Radiation therapy
Recurrent tumor	
Pseudoprogression/radiation necrosis	

radiation therapy by using high-resolution whole brain spectroscopic MR imaging.

MRS has several limitations that have prevented it from reaching its full potential in brain tumor imaging. Despite the theoretic ability to differentiate tissues of different types, there is substantial overlap between the spectroscopic appearances of different diseases. MRS can be time-consuming and highly variable between different imaging locations; moreover, artifacts often limit evaluation.

This work provides an overview of the use of MR spectroscopy in brain tumor imaging, including general imaging principles and technique, key imaged metabolites, the typical appearance of overlapping disease processes, and practical limitations on MRS. The second section discusses ongoing development of new applications likely to have an impact on clinical care in coming years.

IMAGING TECHNIQUE

Early in the development of NMR, it was discovered that nuclei in different molecular environments resonated at slightly different frequencies.[1] In simplest terms, when subjected to an applied magnetic field, molecules precess at a resonant frequency that varies with the surrounding molecular environment. This effect, known as chemical shift, allows nuclei in different chemical environments to be distinguished based on their resonant frequencies. A shielding parameter, defined in parts per million (ppm), describes the relative change compared with a reference compound. The shielding parameter is a constant, whereas the chemical shift measured in Hz increases linearly with field strength. As a result, the resolution of spectroscopy increases with increasing field strength.

Most imaging spectroscopy applications image the hydrogen nucleus (^{1}H) because it is the most prevalent nucleus in tissue. Spectroscopy of other elements is possible,[2] although not used widely in

practice. For in vitro proton (^{1}H) spectroscopy, chemical shift values (δ) are reported in ppm relative to a tetramethylsilane (TMS). In vivo, compounds such as TMS are not available, so usually one of the indigenous spectral signals is used as a reference (eg, for the brain, the N-acetyl resonance of N-acetyl aspartate (NAA), set at 2.02 ppm, is often used).

Virtually all MRS studies are performed by collecting time domain data after application of either a 90° pulse, or an echo-type of sequence. The time domain signal is then converted to the frequency domain through Fourier transformation, which allows the viewing of the signal intensity as a function of frequency (ie, in the frequency domain). To accumulate sufficient signal to noise ratio (SNR), the scan can be repeated many (N) times and averaged together to improve SNR, which is proportional to the $\sqrt{N}$. Choosing an appropriate N and scan repetition time (TR) is required to balance image acquisition time and optimize SNR.[3,4] Successful ^{1}H MRS also requires water and lipid suppression techniques, because water and lipids are present at concentrations many-fold higher than target metabolites, which are usually present in the millimolar range. Magnetic field homogeneity and field strengths must be sufficient to allow resolution of the relatively small chemical shift range of protons ($\sim$10 ppm). Large and/or membrane-associated molecules are not usually well-seen, although their broad resonances contribute to the baseline of the spectrum.[5]

The information from a brain MR spectrum depends on several factors, such as the field strength, echo time, and type of pulse sequence. On a 1.5 T scanner with long echo times (TE) (eg, 140 or 280 ms), only choline (Cho), creatine (Cr), and NAA are typically observable in healthy adult brain, whereas compounds such as lactate, alanine, or others may be detectable if their concentrations are elevated above normal levels due to abnormal metabolic processes.[6–8] At short TE

($\leq$ 35 ms), additional compounds, including gluta-mate, glutamine, myo-inositol, lipids, and other macromolecules may become detectable.

Spatial localization allows signals to be recorded from well-defined structures or lesions within the brain.[9–12] In the 1980s, a wide range of spatial localization techniques were developed for in vivo spectroscopy[13]; however, many were either difficult to implement, involved too many radiofrequency pulses, or were inefficient. Out of this plethora of sequences, 2 emerged as simple and robust enough for wider use, each based on 3 slice-selective pulses applied in orthogonal directions. The STEAM sequence (Stimulated Echo Acquisition Mode)[14–17] uses three 90° pulses and detects the resulting stimulated echo from the volume intersected by all 3 pulses, whereas the PRESS sequence (Point REsolved Spectroscopy Sequence)[18,19] uses one 90° pulse and two 180° pulses to detect a spin echo from the localized volume. The sequence is designed so that signals from other regions outside the desired voxel are eliminated (usually by using crusher gradients).[14,20] Typical voxel sizes for brain ^{1}H MRS are approximately 8 cm.[3] Multi-voxel (2-dimensional [2D], or 3-dimensional [3D]) PRESS magnetic resonance spectroscopic imaging (MRSI) sequences are available on commer-cial MR scanners from most scanner vendors and are the most commonly applied MRS technique.[21]

METABOLITES

The most described metabolites in brain tumor spectroscopy are choline, NAA, creatine, lipids, myo-inositol, and lactate (summarized in **Table 2**). A representative normal spectrum from the cere-bral hemisphere is shown in **Fig. 1**. The area under each curve represents the number of spins identi-fied; however, this result is only quantitative if an external reference (of known concentration) is used. As such, the areas under the curve are usu-ally evaluated in a relative fashion. Some systems automatically produce relative area under the curve numbers. In the absence of these numbers, peak height is often used as a surrogate marker. Although alterations in the concentrations of each of these metabolites can be seen with various pathologies, a combination of the relative changes of these various metabolites in conjunc-tion with other imaging features can be useful in distinguishing primary brain tumors from metasta-ses, grading gliomas, and distinguishing recur-rence from radiation necrosis. Sometimes, ratios of metabolites (such as Cho/Cr, or Cho/NAA) can be used to increase the sensitivity of a particular

measure. In practice, this is one of the most commonly used approaches.

Cho (3.2 ppm) is a precursor of acetylcholine, a component of cell membranes. Elevated Cho is a marker of increased cell turnover, which can be seen with tumors and other proliferative pro-cesses. In combination with other imaging fea-tures, elevated Cho can identify high cellular turnover pathologies like gliomas and lymphoma compared with other pathologies with lower cellu-larity, such as radiation necrosis or infarction.[22,23]

NAA (2.0 ppm) is synthesized from acetylation of the amino acid aspartate in the neuronal mito-chondria and is a marker of neuronal viability. Reduction of NAA is seen in many pathologies, such as glioma and radiation necrosis, which involve destruction or replacement of neurons. Lymphoma or metastases tend to show low or absent NAA levels due to lack of neurons in the tumor component.[24]

Cr (3.0 ppm) has a role in storage and transfer of energy in neurons that have high metabolism. Cr is relatively maintained across a number of disease processes and serves as an internal control which can be used for ratio calculations, such as Cho/Cr.

Lactate (Lac, 1.3 ppm) is a marker of anerobic metabolism and is not seen in normal adult brain spectra due to exclusive aerobic metabolism in brain. Lactate is visualized in necrotic tissues with anaerobic metabolism which include abscesses and high-grade tumors.[25,26] Lactate overlaps with lipids at short TE, shows inversion at intermediate TE, and has a characteristic double peak at longer TE.[27]

Lipids (Lip, 1.3 ppm) are components of cell membrane and are increased in diseases with high cell turnover rates such as high-grade gliomas (HGGs). However this is not a specific feature and can be see with other pathologies with high cell turnover/destruction such as abscesses, infarc-tion, and metastases.[28]

Myo-Inositol (MI, 3.5 ppm) is a precursor of phos-phatidylinositol (a phospholipid) and of phosphati-dylinositol 4,5-bisphosphate. Elevations of MI are seen in low-grade gliomas; in contradistinction, reduction seen in World Health Organization grade IV gliomas and can be a useful marker in grading gli-omas.[29] Elevation of MI can also be seen with other pathologies like dementia of Alzheimer type and progressive multifocal leukoencephalopathy.

2-Hydroxyglutarate (2-HG, 2.25 ppm) is an onco-metabolite of increasing interest in recent times. Tumors with isocitrate dehydrogenase (IDH-1) mu-tations accumulate higher levels of 2-HG, and as a result detection of 2-HG can be used with reason-able accuracy for noninvasive detection of IDH-1 mutant gliomas.[30]

Table 2
Frequently encountered metabolites and their characteristics and clinical role in evaluating brain tumors

Metabolite	ppm	Elevated in	Decreased in	Clinical Significance in Brain Tumor Imaging
Choline	3.2 ppm	Neoplasms Inflammation Gliosis	Necrosis	Grading gliomas Distinguishing glioblastomas for metastases Radiation planning in gliomas Differentiating tumor progression vs pseudoprogression/ Radionecrosis
N-acetyl aspartate	2.0 ppm		Gliomas and more so in high-grade gliomas Radiation necrosis Metastases Lymphoma	Grading of gliomas Distinguishing gliomas from metastases
Creatine	3.0 ppm		High-grade gliomas Necrosis	Grading of gliomas Distinguishing metastases from glioblastoma
Lactate	1.3 ppm	Glioblastoma Abscesses	Not present in normal spectra	Grading of gliomas
Lipids	1.3 ppm with inversion at intermediate echo time	Glioblastoma Abscess Lymphoma Metastases		Grading of gliomas
Myo-Inositol	3.5 ppm	Low-grade gliomas Progressive multifocal encephalopathy	High-grade gliomas	Grading of gliomas
2-Hydroxyglutarate	2.5 ppm	Isocitrate dehydrogenase (IDH)-1 positive tumors		Detection of IDH-1 positive tumors

Other metabolites have been described in the research setting, including metabolites of other nuclei.[31,32] However, these have demonstrated little clinical importance.

CLINICAL RELEVANCE: DIAGNOSIS

Years ago, brain tumor workups commonly involved a 2-step process including an initial needle biopsy followed by a more definitive surgical resection. The transition to what is usually a single (initial) surgery has been ushered along by developments in neuroimaging, including advanced techniques. MRS is one of those techniques and, along with other methods, this constellation of imaging tools essentially serves as a sort of "virtual biopsy." In complex cases, such an approach can be used to differentiate gliomas from other diagnoses such as metastases, lymphoma, demyelination, edema, necrosis, and infection. Unfortunately, the spectroscopic profile of HGGs overlaps that of other brain tumors and even non-neoplastic diagnoses on many occasions. It is important to use advanced neuroimaging such as MRS in the context of conventional imaging, including MR imaging.

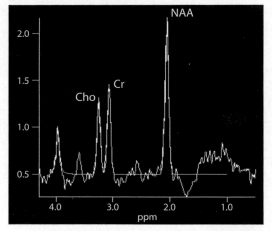

Fig. 1. MRS spectrum from an area of normal brain. Cho, Cr, and NAA are the dominant peaks, with NAA higher than both Cho and Cr.

Brain metastases, particularly when solitary, can have considerable overlap with the appearance of primary brain tumors on MR imaging. Both are characterized by enhancing masses with surrounding T2/fluid attenuated inversion recovery (FLAIR) hyperintense edema. Both metastases and gliomas are known to have elevated Cho and decreased NAA compared with adjacent normal white matter. However, lipids and macromolecules are higher in metastases than glioblastoma.[33] Evaluating spectroscopic results for the edema next to an enhancing mass may help with diagnosis, as the edema in gliomas more often contains infiltrating tumor cells and as a result has higher Cho/NAA and Cho/Cr.[24,33–35] As an example of this approach, please see **Fig. 2**. Placement of voxels within the enhancing abnormality is suggestive of a high-grade tumor (either glioma or metastasis), but elevated Cho in the nonenhancing abnormality is more consistent with a high-grade tumor.

Primary central nervous system lymphoma (PCNSL) also can mimic primary brain tumors in many cases; however, there remains some hope for the utility of MRS in these instances. For example, Nagashima and colleagues[36] recently reported that MI was significantly increased in HGGs compared with PCNSL. In addition to absolute value measurements, peak ratios have also been used to assist with differentiation. High-grade tumors such as lymphoma and HGG have higher elevation of Cho/NAA compared with nonneoplastic diagnoses, such as demyelination.[37] Although both lymphoma and HGG have Cho/NAA elevation, lymphoma is reported to have lower Cho/NAA than primary brain tumors.[38] **Fig. 3** shows an example of a patient with periventricular abnormality on brain MR imaging that is, most consistent with primary central nervous lymphoma on conventional imaging. MR spectroscopy in this setting was consistent with high-grade tumor (**Fig. 3**). Spectroscopy does rule out other

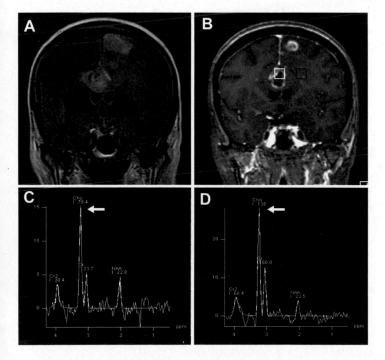

Fig. 2. Glioblastoma. An 86 year-old woman with new neurologic symptoms. Coronal FLAIR (A) and contrast-enhanced T1-weighted images (B) demonstrate a mass in the corpus callosum and left superior frontal gyrus with multiple areas of enhancement. Spectroscopy (TE 144 ms) from the corpus callosum (C, region of white box in B) shows markedly elevated Cho (white arrow) and relatively low NAA. Spectroscopy from the area of nonenhancing tumor in the left centrum semiovale (D, black box in B) shows similar findings in the nonenhancing areas, confirming infiltrative tumor.

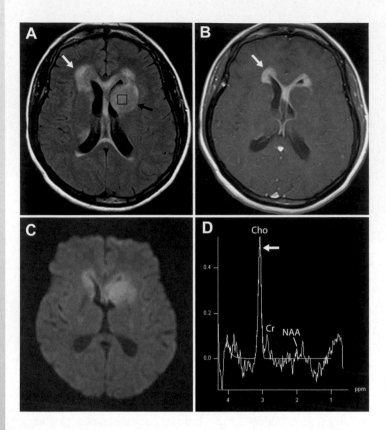

Fig. 3. Lymphoma. A 40 year-old woman with human immunodeficiency virus presented with altered mental status. FLAIR (*A*) though the basal ganglia showed masslike FLAIR hyperintensity and expansion of the left caudate (*black arrow*) with multiple periventricular masses that enhance on postcontrast T1-weighted images (*B, white arrows*). DWI (*C*) demonstrates associated hyperintensity. Spectroscopy (TE 140 ms) (*D*) from the caudate (*black box, A*) shows markedly elevated Cho (*white arrow*) with very low Cr and NAA.

possibilities such as infection in this case, although this appearance could easily be confused with glioblastoma, highlighting the importance of interpreting MRS alongside conventional imaging. For further review of intracranial lymphoma including MRS see an article by Brandao and Castillo.[39]

Tumefactive demyelinating lesions (TDLs) have an overlapping appearance with primary brain tumors. Results have been conflicting regarding the value of MRS in these cases. Ikeguchi and colleagues[40] found that a Cho/NAA ratio greater than 1.72 favors HGG over TDL. These results contrast with those of Saindane and colleagues[41] who found no difference Cho/Cr ratios in contrast-enhancing, central, or perilesional areas of TDLs and gliomas. TDL are most associated with loss of normal neuronal peaks including Cr and NAA. **Fig. 4** shows an example of tumefactive demyelination that has a typical appearance on conventional imaging. The MR spectroscopic results are most notable for the presence of prominent lactate and absence of peak ratios suggestive of high-grade tumor (**Fig. 4**). In our experience, prominent lactate is rarely associated with untreated brain tumors.

Another type of brain mass that can occasionally be misinterpreted as primary brain tumor is pyogenic brain abscess. The conventional imaging, especially diffusion-weighted imaging (DWI) and

apparent diffusion coefficient evaluation of the central nonenhancing material is traditionally quite helpful. As one might imagine, identification of lactate commonly overlaps both entities.[42] The classic MRS description of abscess includes presence of amino acid peaks such as valine, alanine, leucine, acetate, and succinate.[42] However, Pal and colleagues[43] found that amino acids, although found in 80% of abscesses, had a sensitivity and specificity of 0.72 and 0.30, respectively. The clinical utility of numbers like these is unclear at best.

To summarize, a Venn diagram of MRS for astrocytoma/glioma, lymphoma, TDL, and brain abscess would not have distinct circles. An individual patient may have an MRS pattern that suggests one of these diagnoses, but this result is best interpreted in the setting of the conventional MR imaging results and the clinical presentation. A combination of peak presence (especially combinations), peak height, area under the (peak) curve, and peak ratio may be helpful, whereas individual values are challenging to interpret. Future work using MRS as a multiparametric biomarker, including incorporation of machine learning techniques, may increase its ability to differentiate these diagnoses and predict patient prognosis.[34] In reviewing the literature, it is clear that the consensus is that there is no consensus.

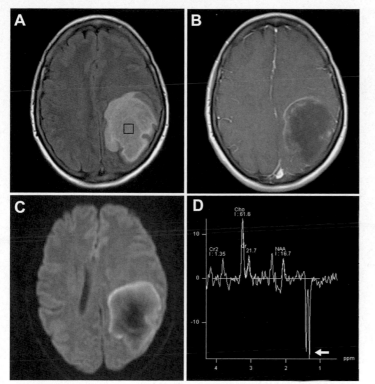

Fig. 4. Tumefactive demyelination. A 50-year-old woman with right-sided weakness. FLAIR (*A*) images show an expansile, FLAIR hyperintense mass in the left parietal lobe with a peripheral incomplete rim of enhancement on T1-weighted imaging (*B*). DWI (*C*) similarly shows a peripheral rim of abnormally hyperintense DWI. Spectroscopy (TE 135 ms) (*D*) from the central portion of the lesion (*black box, A*) shows elevated Cho, near complete loss of NAA, and a characteristic inverted doublet lactate peak at 1.3 ppm.

CLINICAL RELEVANCE: TUMOR GRADING

MRS has a clinical role in grading gliomas. In conjunction with other imaging features like hemorrhage, necrosis, and enhancement it can be useful to support a diagnosis of HGG versus low-grade glioma. Typical abnormal spectroscopic features of low-grade gliomas include modest Cho elevation, NAA reduction, and Cho/Cr ratio elevation (**Fig. 5**). MI and MI/Cr ratio can also be elevated. Low-grade gliomas typically lack Lac and Lip peaks. In some cases, low-grade gliomas may have only mild changes in Cho or NAA with some changes in MI. Therefore, it should be noted that short TE spectroscopy with more detectable metabolites is helpful in low-grade gliomas.

HGGs tend to have more dramatic MRS changes compared with low-grade tumors. Typical MRS features of grade III and IV gliomas include increased Cho and decreased Cr, NAA, and MI (**Fig. 2**). NAA is seen in higher concentrations in low-grade gliomas relative to HGGs and can be used as a marker of prognosis and grading gliomas.[44] Reductions in Cr can be seen and in combination with increased Cho results in higher Cho/Cr ratios in HGGs compared with low-grade gliomas.[44] There can be variations in spectroscopy abnormalities in glioblastoma depending on the area sampled, and sampling of necrotic regions may show only lipid and lactate peaks with reduced/absent Cho peak. Presence of lactate and lipid peaks suggests a grade IV tumor and is not commonly seen with grade III gliomas.

As there is considerable overlap in spectroscopy patterns of low-grade versus HGGs, semiquantitative analysis using ratios of various metabolites is used to better predict the grade. Commonly used ratios are Cho/Cr, Cho/NAA, and NAA/Cr. Typical pattern in HGGs is elevated Cho/Cr, Cho/NAA ratios and reduced NAA/Cr ratio. Cho/Cr is the most commonly used in clinical practice and in research studies. Wang and colleagues,[45] in a large meta-analysis, looked at 30 articles comprising 1228 patients and analyzed utility of various metabolite ratios in predicting grade of gliomas and distinguishing low-grade gliomas from HGGs. Quantitative synthesis of studies showed that the pooled sensitivity/specificity of Cho/Cr, Cho/NAA and NAA/Cr ratios was 0.75/0.60, 0.80/0.76 and 0.71/0.70, respectively. The area under the curve values for these metabolites were 0.83, 0.87, and 0.78, respectively. In this analysis, all 3 ratios had comparable performance and Cho/NAA ratio showed the highest accuracy. However, it should be noted that there was wide variation in the ratio cutoffs used in these studies.

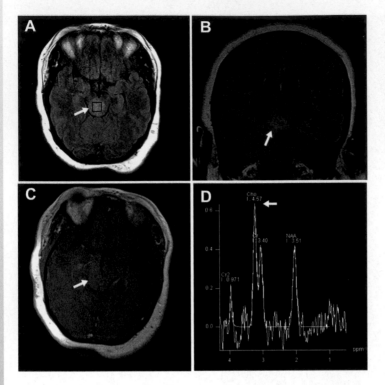

Fig. 5. Low-grade glioma. A 34-year-old woman with neurofibromatosis type 1. Axial (*A*) and coronal (*B*) FLAIR images show an expansile mass within the midbrain with no enhancement on postcontrast T1-weighted images (*C*) (*arrows*). Spectroscopy (TE 135 ms) (*D*) within the midbrain shows modest elevation of Cho (*arrow*) and depression of NAA. Spectroscopy is particularly important in this difficult to biopsy location.

CLINICAL RELEVANCE: FOLLOW-UP

MRS can be useful in the longitudinal follow-up of patients with brain tumor, particularly for troubleshooting cases in which there may be significant overlap between tumor progression and radiation effects. Worsening in both post–contrast enhancement on T1-weighted imaging and surrounding FLAIR hyperintense edema can both occur because of radiation injury to the tumor and surrounding normal tissue.[46] Pseudoprogression is the phenomenon of acute imaging worsening in the early phase after radiation, usually within the first 3 to 6 months after completing chemoradiation.[47] Pseudoprogression can occur in as many as 20% to 30% of primary brain tumors and is more common in patients with O6-methylguanine–DNA methyltransferase methylation.[48] Furthermore, pseudoprogression is associated with improved patient outcomes. It is important to differentiate pseudoprogression from true tumor progression, as tumor progression in this early period would indicate a failure of initial therapy, which would necessitate a change in therapy, often taking a patient off the well-tolerated and often effective temozolomide to begin another therapy such as lomustine. Interpretation guidelines such as the Response Assessment in Neuro-Oncology advise conservative interpretation of cases in the first 3 months after completing radiation, assuming imaging worsening is pseudoprogression as long

as they occur in the radiation treatment field.[49] Pseudoprogression is usually self-limited,[47] and when imaging does not improve on subsequent follow-up, interpretation is more nuanced and determining if worsening represents tumor progression is more challenging. Radiation necrosis can also occur in a delayed fashion any time from months to years after completing radiation therapy. It can have progressive worsening of enhancement, edema, and mass effect along with worsening patient symptoms. Later, radiation necrosis poses a considerable diagnostic dilemma because of its highly variable timing.

Advanced imaging, including MRS, can be a useful tool in differentiating treatment effects from tumor progression, and the imaging appearance of pseudoprogression and delayed radiation necrosis are similar. Radiation results in decreased NAA, Cho, and Cr compared with patients with tumor recurrence.[46] Using ratios including Cho/Cr can further improve performance of spectroscopy, with higher Cho/Cr in cases of tumor progression. In a meta-analysis of 477 lesions, MRS had moderate performance in differentiating radiation necrosis from glioma recurrence, with Cho/Cr ratio having a sensitivity, specificity, and areas under the curve of 0.83, 0.83, and 0.91, respectively.[50] Compared with progressive tumor, radiation necrosis is also more likely to show elevation in Lip and Lac (**Fig. 6**).[51]

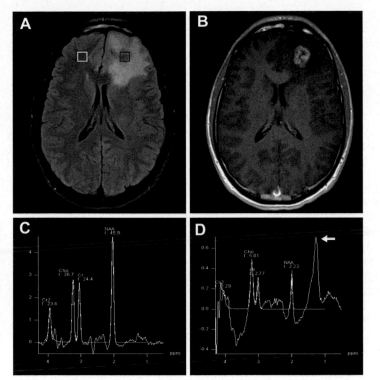

Fig. 6. Radiation necrosis. A 21-year-old with Ewing sarcoma metastasis to the left frontal lobe previously treated with radiation. Expansile mass in the left frontal lobe with surrounding abnormal FLAIR (*A*) and central enhancement on postcontrast T1 (*B*). Spectroscopy (TE 135 ms) of the contralateral normal white matter (*C*, from *white box* in *A*) shows relatively normal spectrum. Spectroscopy of the abnormal region (*D*, from *black box* in *A*) shows decrease in height of all peaks, particularly NAA, with a lipid/lactate peak at 1.3 ppm (*white arrow*).

MRS has performed similar or better than other advanced techniques for evaluating potential radiation necrosis.[52] MR perfusion has shown promise in evaluating necrosis, with hyperperfusion associated with tumor recurrence.[46] PET with both fludeoxyglucose F 18 and ^{11}C-methionine, an amino acid tracer, have had intermediate results. Quantitative diffusion imaging has also been relatively promising (sensitivity 75%, specificity 88.9%), with radiation necrosis having greater reduction in central apparent diffusion coefficient values.[53] Combined approaches using MRS in conjunction with other advanced imaging may have the best performance.

LIMITATIONS

Use of MRS in evaluation and follow-up of brain tumors has several significant limitations. The primary limitation is the considerable overlap between the spectroscopic appearance of different pathology. Each pathology has characteristic features that may occur most commonly, but typical diagnostic accuracy may range from 60% to 80%. However, because of overlapping appearance, many times short-term follow-up imaging (4–6 weeks) or surgical biopsy are required to confirm a diagnosis. The lack of definitive imaging findings has been the primary reason MRS is not used more frequently. Other technical limitations also confound implementation of MRS. Imaging sites and scanners vary widely in their implementation, and there is little widespread standardization of imaging techniques. Artifacts and noise are common and further limit interpretation. Susceptibility from adjacent bone or air limit signal from portions of the brain near the skull base and calvarium. Averaging of all signal within relatively large voxels limits evaluation of small lesions, and incomplete water and lipid suppression can completely obscure the diagnostic signal. Imaging can also be time-consuming and require technologist or radiologist intervention. All these limitations are the subject of ongoing research and development.

FUTURE DIRECTIONS

Research is currently under way to improve current technology and develop and new applications to increase the clinical usefulness of MRS in brain tumor diagnosis and treatment. Sequence development is geared toward improving resolution, brain coverage, and speed while decreasing artifacts. Conventional Cartesian 2D or 3D phase-encoding approaches can give excellent quality data, but they rapidly become too time-consuming with increasing spatial resolution and brain coverage. A number of methods to accelerate MRS have been described, include parallel imaging and compressed sensing.[54–56] Alternative strategies are required to increase acquisition speed by an order of magnitude or more; echo-planar spectroscopic imaging (EPSI) is one of the oldest but also one of the fastest acceleration methods for MRS.[57–60] In EPSI, k-space is traversed in a rectilinear manner by the oscillating read gradient that is, applied simultaneously with spectral data acquisition. For a 3D acquisition, the other 2 dimensions are encoded using conventional (or elliptical) phase-encoding. Scan times can be reduced even further through undersampling approaches such as SENSE or GRAPPA in these dimensions.[61–63] When combined with advanced water and lipid suppression techniques, EPSI can be used to obtain high-resolution wholebrain spectroscopic maps with scan times ranging from 10 to 18 minutes.[58,64,65] Smaller voxel sizes result in decreased artifact from surrounding structures and less partial volume artifact. Whole-brain coverage further allows novel applications such as biopsy[66] and treatment planning. These applications are not limited by overlap between different pathology, as the disease of often already known and MRS is being used to define the involved region.

Using MRS to choose optimal biopsy sites is made possible by whole-brain spectroscopic imaging. Brain tumors are highly infiltrative, and diagnosis of grade II and III gliomas can be particularly challenging because they are heterogeneous tumors that can lack well-defined enhancement.[67] Biopsy is taken from areas of hyperintensity on T2/FLAIR images, but this does not account for areas of tumor heterogeneity and can result in undersampling of high-grade or anaplastic areas.[68–70] Whole-brain EPSI can be a useful adjunct to conventional imaging to guide biopsy target selection, with Cho or Cho/NAA maps overlaid on anatomic images and uploaded to surgical guidance software to choose a biopsy site (**Fig. 7**) (Zhong et al., manuscript in preparation). Greater metabolite abnormalities are associated with more proliferative areas, and sampling these regions maximizes the chance of sampling highgrade areas.[44,71]

Advanced treatment planning is also a potential application of whole-brain MRS.[72–75] In grade IV tumors, high-dose radiation is targeted to the resection cavity and areas of residual contrast enhancement that may underrepresent areas of infiltrative tumor.[71] Recurrence can then occur in

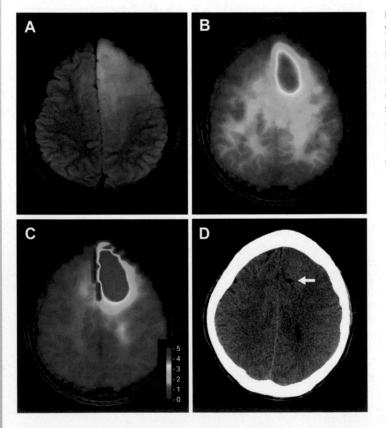

Fig. 7. Grade 3 astrocytoma. A 31-year-old man with a left frontal expansile, nonenhancing mass seen on FLAIR (*A*). T1-weighted images overlaid with 3D Cho map (*B*) and Cho/NAA ratio (*C*), showing areas of greatest metabolic abnormality. Scale in (*C*) shows the ratio between Cho/NAA and normal white matter. Stereotactic biopsy was targeted to a region with maximal metabolic abnormality, as seen on post-biopsy CT (*D*).

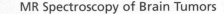

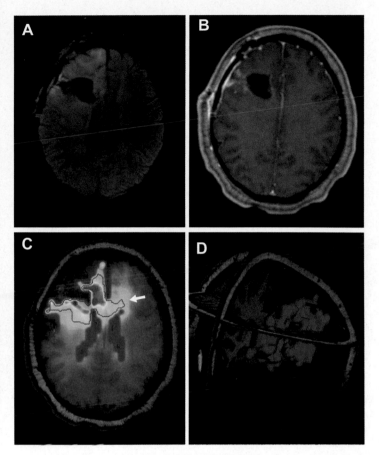

Fig. 8. Glioblastoma. Right frontal glioblastoma, status post resection. FLAIR abnormality surrounds the cavity in the right middle and superior frontal gyri (A). A small amount of nodular enhancement is present around the cavity on postcontrast T1-weighted imaging (B). T1-weighted images overlaid with 3D Cho/NAA ratio (C) show tumor extending beyond the area of abnormal enhancement and FLAIR (*white arrow*). The red line outlines the area with a Cho/NAA ratio 2 times normal white matter, a threshold associated with 30% tumor in previous biopsy studies. Three-dimensional rendering of area of MRS abnormality surrounding the resection cavity (D).

surrounding areas undertreated by existing radiation plans. An improved strategy might be to treat areas of greater spectroscopic abnormality, such as those with elevated Cho/NAA ratio, with high-dose radiation to the area meeting a threshold difference from normal white matter (**Fig. 8**). A multisite clinical trial recently completed patient enrollment to test this approach (NCT03137888) and is currently in the follow-up period.[76]

SUMMARY

MRS is an advanced technique that allows for molecular evaluation of tissue composition without contrast or radiation. It has a valuable role in the diagnosis, treatment, and subsequent evaluation of patients with brain tumor, particularly as a troubleshooting tool when conventional imaging findings of 2 diagnoses overlap. Unfortunately, overlap between spectroscopy findings and technical considerations limit its accuracy, MRS is most useful when interpreted in conjunction with MR imaging findings and other advanced techniques. Future developments promise faster and more accurate MRS, which can be applied to novel applications such as biopsy and treatment planning.

CLINICS CARE POINTS

- Magnetic resonance spectroscopy (MRS) is a useful troubleshooting tool which can be used in advanced imaging of brain tumors to differentiate tumor from other pathology and estimate tumor grade.

- Tumors are characterized by high cell turnover, resulting in elevated choline (Cho), and replacement of normal neurons, resulting in decreased N-acetyl aspartate (NAA).

- Greater elevation in choline (Cho) is associated with more aggressive tumors and other neoplastic pathologies such as lymphoma, while non neoplastic pathologies often manifest other peaks including lactate/lipids and myo-inositol.

- Because of considerable overlap between spectroscopic findings between a variety of pathology, spectroscopy results should be interpreted in the context of other imaging findings and clinical presentation.

DISCLOSURE

Funding for this project includes NIH/NCI R01 CA214557 and NIH/NIBIB U01 EB028145 (PI: Shim) and RSNA Scholar grant (PI: Weinberg).

REFERENCES

1. Proctor WG, Yu FC. The dependence of a nuclear magnetic resonance frequency. Phys Rev 1950;77:717.
2. Julia-Sape M, Candiota AP, Arus C. Cancer metabolism in a snapshot: MRS(I). NMR Biomed 2019; 32(10):e4054.
3. Ernst RR, Anderson WA. Application of Fourier transform spectroscopy to magnetic resonance. Rev Sci Instrum 1966;37:93–102.
4. Ernst RR, Bodenhausen G, Wokaun A. Principles of nuclear magnetic resonance in one and two dimensions, vol. 1. New York: Oxford University Press; 1990.
5. Behar KL, Ogino T. Characterization of macromolecule resonances in the 1H NMR spectrum of rat brain. Magn Reson Med 1993;30(1):38–44.
6. Barker PB, Gillard JH, van Zijl PC, et al. Acute stroke: evaluation with serial proton MR spectroscopic imaging. Radiology 1994;192(3):723–32.
7. Lin DD, Crawford TO, Barker PB. Proton MR spectroscopy in the diagnostic evaluation of suspected mitochondrial disease. AJNR Am J Neuroradiol 2003;24(1):33–41.
8. Remy C, Grand S, Lai ES, et al. 1H MRS of human brain abscesses in vivo and in vitro. Magn Reson Med 1995;34(4):508–14.
9. Luyten PR, den Hollander JA. Observation of metabolites in the human brain by MR spectroscopy. Radiology 1986;161(3):795–8.
10. Hanstock CC, Rothman DL, Prichard JW, et al. Spatially localized 1H NMR spectra of metabolites in the human brain. Proc Natl Acad Sci U S A 1988;85(6):1821–5.
11. Bottomley PA, Edelstein WA, Foster TH, et al. In vivo solvent-suppressed localized hydrogen nuclear magnetic resonance spectroscopy: a window to metabolism? Proc Natl Acad Sci U S A 1985;82(7): 2148–52.
12. Bax A, Freeman R. Enhanced NMR resolution by restricting the effective sample volume. J Magn Reson 1980;37:177–81.
13. Aue WP. Localization Methods for in vivo NMR spectroscopy. Rev Magn Reson Med 1986;1:21–72.
14. Frahm J. Localized Proton Spectroscopy using stimulated echoes. J Magn Reson 1987;72(3):502–8.
15. Frahm J, Bruhn H, Gyngell ML, et al. Localized high-resolution proton NMR spectroscopy using stimulated echoes: initial applications to human brain in vivo. Magn Reson Med 1989;9(1):79–93.
16. Granot J. Selected Volume Excitation Using Stimulated Echoes (VEST). Applications to spatially localized spectroscopy and imaging. J Magn Reson 1986;70(3):488–92.
17. Kimmich R, Hoepfel D. Volume-selective multipulse spin-echo spectroscopy. J Magn Reson 1987; 72(2):379–84.
18. Bottomley PA, Inventor; General Electric Company, assignee. Selective volume method for performing localized NMR spectroscopy. US patent 4480228. October 30th 1984, 1984.
19. Ordidge RJ, Gordon RE, Inventors; Oxford Research Systems Limited, assignee. Methods and apparatus of obtaining NMR spectra. US patent 45310941983.
20. van Zijl PC, Moonen CT, Alger JR, et al. High field localized proton spectroscopy in small volumes: greatly improved localization and shimming using shielded strong gradients. Magn Reson Med 1989; 10(2):256–65.
21. Nelson SJ. Analysis of volume MRI and MR spectroscopic imaging data for the evaluation of patients with brain tumors. Magn Reson Med 2001;46(2): 228–39.
22. Brandão LA, Castillo M. Adult brain tumors: clinical applications of magnetic resonance spectroscopy. Magn Reson Imaging Clin N Am 2016;24(4): 781–809.
23. Shimizu H, Kumabe T, Shirane R, et al. Correlation between choline level measured by proton MR spectroscopy and Ki-67 labeling index in gliomas. AJNR Am J Neuroradiol 2000;21(4):659–65.
24. Server A, Josefsen R, Kulle B, et al. Proton magnetic resonance spectroscopy in the distinction of high-grade cerebral gliomas from single metastatic brain tumors. Acta Radiol 2010;51(3):316–25.
25. Fan G. Comments and controversies: magnetic resonance spectroscopy and gliomas. Cancer Imaging 2006;6:113–5.
26. Lai PH, Ho JT, Chen WL, et al. Brain abscess and necrotic brain tumor: discrimination with proton MR spectroscopy and diffusion-weighted imaging. AJNR Am J Neuroradiol 2002;23(8):1369–77.
27. Yamasaki F, Takaba J, Ohtaki M, et al. Detection and differentiation of lactate and lipids by single-voxel proton MR spectroscopy. Neurosurg Rev 2005; 28(4):267–77.
28. Brandão LA, Castillo M. Adult brain tumors: clinical applications of magnetic resonance spectroscopy. Neuroimaging Clin N Am 2013;23(3):527–55.
29. Castillo M, Smith JK, Kwock L. Correlation of myo-inositol levels and grading of cerebral astrocytomas. AJNR Am J Neuroradiol 2000;21(9):1645–9.
30. Suh CH, Kim HS, Jung SC, et al. Imaging prediction of isocitrate dehydrogenase (IDH) mutation in patients with glioma: a systemic review and meta-analysis. Eur Radiol 2019;29(2):745–58.

31. Grist JT, Miller JJ, Zaccagna F, et al. Hyperpolar-ized (13)C MRI: A novel approach for probing ce-rebral metabolism in health and neurological disease. J Cereb Blood Flow Metab 2020;40(6): 1137–47.

32. Wenger KJ, Hattingen E, Franz K, et al. In vivo meta-bolic profiles as determined by (31)P and short TE (1)H MR-spectroscopy : no difference between pa-tients with IDH wildtype and IDH mutant gliomas. Clin Neuroradiol 2019;29(1):27–36.

33. Pope WB. Brain metastases: neuroimaging. Handb Clin Neurol 2018;149:89–112.

34. Durmo F, Rydelius A, Cuellar Baena S, et al. Multi-voxel (1)H-MR spectroscopy biometrics for preop-rerative differentiation between brain tumors. Tomography 2018;4(4):172–81.

35. Chiang IC, Kuo YT, Lu CY, et al. Distinction between high-grade gliomas and solitary metastases using peritumoral 3-T magnetic resonance spectroscopy, diffusion, and perfusion imagings. Neuroradiology 2004;46(8):619–27.

36. Nagashima H, Sasayama T, Tanaka K, et al. Myo-inositol concentration in MR spectroscopy for differ-entiating high grade glioma from primary central nervous system lymphoma. J Neurooncol 2018; 136(2):317–26.

37. Lu SS, Kim SJ, Kim HS, et al. Utility of proton MR spectroscopy for differentiating typical and atypical primary central nervous system lymphomas from tu-mefactive demyelinating lesions. AJNR Am J Neuro-radiol 2014;35(2):270–7.

38. Vallee A, Guillevin C, Wager M, et al. Added value of spectroscopy to perfusion MRI in the differential diagnostic performance of common malignant brain tumors. AJNR Am J Neuroradiol 2018;39(8): 1423–31.

39. Brandao LA, Castillo M. Lymphomas-Part 1. Neuro-imaging Clin N Am 2016;26(4):511–36.

40. Ikeguchi R, Shimizu Y, Abe K, et al. Proton magnetic resonance spectroscopy differentiates tumefactive demyelinating lesions from gliomas. Mult Scler Relat Disord 2018;26:77–84.

41. Saindane AM, Cha S, Law M, et al. Proton MR spec-troscopy of tumefactive demyelinating lesions. AJNR Am J Neuroradiol 2002;23(8):1378–86.

42. Kim SH, Chang KH, Song IC, et al. Brain abscess and brain tumor: discrimination with in vivo H-1 MR spectroscopy. Radiology 1997;204(1):239–45.

43. Pal D, Bhattacharyya A, Husain M, et al. In vivo pro-ton MR spectroscopy evaluation of pyogenic brain abscesses: a report of 194 cases. AJNR Am J Neu-roradiol 2010;31(2):360–6.

44. Bulik M, Jancalek R, Vanicek J, et al. Potential of MR spectroscopy for assessment of glioma grading. Clin Neurol Neurosurg 2013;115(2):146–53.

45. Wang Q, Zhang H, Zhang J, et al. The diagnostic performance of magnetic resonance spectroscopy in differentiating high-from low-grade gliomas: A systematic review and meta-analysis. Eur Radiol 2016;26(8):2670–84.

46. Siu A, Wind JJ, Iorgulescu JB, et al. Radiation necro-sis following treatment of high grade glioma–a re-view of the literature and current understanding. Acta Neurochir (Wien) 2012;154(2):191–201 [dis-cussion: 201].

47. Parvez K, Parvez A, Zadeh G. The diagnosis and treatment of pseudoprogression, radiation necrosis and brain tumor recurrence. Int J Mol Sci 2014; 15(7):11832–46.

48. Brandes AA, Franceschi E, Tosoni A, et al. MGMT promoter methylation status can predict the inci-dence and outcome of pseudoprogression after concomitant radiochemotherapy in newly diag-nosed glioblastoma patients. J Clin Oncol 2008; 26(13):2192–7.

49. Wen PY, Macdonald DR, Reardon DA, et al. Up-dated response assessment criteria for high-grade gliomas: response assessment in neuro-oncology working group. J Clin Oncol 2010;28(11):1963–72.

50. Zhang H, Ma L, Wang Q, et al. Role of magnetic resonance spectroscopy for the differentiation of recurrent glioma from radiation necrosis: a system-atic review and meta-analysis. Eur J Radiol 2014; 83(12):2181–9.

51. Nakajima T, Kumabe T, Kanamori M, et al. Differen-tial diagnosis between radiation necrosis and glioma progression using sequential proton magnetic reso-nance spectroscopy and methionine positron emis-sion tomography. Neurol Med Chir (Tokyo) 2009; 49(9):394–401.

52. van Dijken BRJ, van Laar PJ, Holtman GA, et al. Diagnostic accuracy of magnetic resonance imag-ing techniques for treatment response evaluation in patients with high-grade glioma, a systematic re-view and meta-analysis. Eur Radiol 2017;27(10): 4129–44.

53. Zakhari N, Taccone MS, Torres C, et al. Diagnostic accuracy of centrally restricted diffusion in the differ-entiation of treatment-related necrosis from tumor recurrence in high-grade gliomas. AJNR Am J Neu-roradiol 2018;39(2):260–4.

54. Nassirpour S, Chang P, Avdievitch N, et al. Com-pressed sensing for high-resolution nonlipid sup-pressed (1) H FID MRSI of the human brain at 9.4T. Magn Reson Med 2018;80(6):2311–25.

55. Strasser B, Povazan M, Hangel G, et al. (2 + 1)D-CAIPIRINHA accelerated MR spectroscopic imag-ing of the brain at 7T. Magn Reson Med 2017; 78(2):429–40.

56. Thomas MA, Nagarajan R, Huda A, et al. Multidi-mensional MR spectroscopic imaging of prostate cancer in vivo. NMR Biomed 2014;27(1):53–66.

57. Ebel A, Soher BJ, Maudsley AA. Assessment of 3D proton MR echo-planar spectroscopic imaging

using automated spectral analysis. Magn Reson Med 2001;46(6):1072–8.

58. Ebel A, Maudsley AA. Improved spectral quality for 3D MR spectroscopic imaging using a high spatial resolution acquisition strategy. Magn Reson Imaging 2003;21(2):113–20.

59. Mansfield P. Spatial mapping of chemical shift in NMR. Magn Reson Med 1984;1:370–86.

60. Posse S, Cuenod CA, Risinger R, et al. Anomalous transverse relaxation in 1H spectroscopy in human brain at 4 Tesla. Magn Reson Med 1995;33(2): 246–52.

61. Lin FH, Tsai SY, Otazo R, et al. Sensitivity-encoded (SENSE) proton echo-planar spectroscopic imaging (PEPSI) in the human brain. Magn Reson Med 2007; 57(2):249–57.

62. Tsai SY, Otazo R, Posse S, et al. Accelerated proton echo planar spectroscopic imaging (PEPSI) using GRAPPA with a 32-channel phased-array coil. Magn Reson Med 2008;59(5):989–98.

63. Zhu X, Ebel A, Ji JX, et al. Spectral phase-corrected GRAPPA reconstruction of three-dimensional echo-planar spectroscopic imaging (3D-EPSI). Magn Reson Med 2007;57(5):815–20.

64. Ebel A, Maudsley AA. Comparison of methods for reduction of lipid contamination for in vivo proton MR spectroscopic imaging of the brain. Magn Reson Med 2001;46(4):706–12.

65. Nelson SJ, Li Y, Lupo JM, et al. Serial analysis of 3D H-1 MRSI for patients with newly diagnosed GBM treated with combination therapy that includes bevacizumab. J Neurooncol 2016;130(1):171–9.

66. Jin T, Ren Y, Zhang H, et al. Application of MRS- and ASL-guided navigation for biopsy of intracranial tumors. Acta Radiol 2019;60(3):374–81.

67. Scott JN, Brasher PM, Sevick RJ, et al. How often are nonenhancing supratentorial gliomas malignant? A population study. Neurology 2002;59(6):947–9.

68. Henson JW, Gaviani P, Gonzalez RG. MRI in treatment of adult gliomas. Lancet Oncol 2005;6(3): 167–75.

69. Jacobs AH, Kracht LW, Gossmann A, et al. Imaging in neurooncology. NeuroRx 2005;2(2):333–47.

70. Weber MA, Giesel FL, Stieltjes B. MRI for identification of progression in brain tumors: from morphology to function. Expert Rev Neurother 2008;8(10): 1507–25.

71. Cordova JS, Shu HK, Liang Z, et al. Whole-brain spectroscopic MRI biomarkers identify infiltrating margins in glioblastoma patients. Neuro Oncol 2016;18(8):1180–9.

72. Nelson SJ, Graves E, Pirzkall A, et al. In vivo molecular imaging for planning radiation therapy of gliomas: an application of 1H MRSI. J Magn Reson Imaging 2002;16(4):464–76.

73. Pirzkall A, McKnight TR, Graves EE, et al. MR-spectroscopy guided target delineation for high-grade gliomas. Int J Radiat Oncol Biol Phys 2001;50(4): 915–28.

74. Ken S, Vieillevigne L, Franceries X, et al. Integration method of 3D MR spectroscopy into treatment planning system for glioblastoma IMRT dose painting with integrated simultaneous boost. Radiat Oncol 2013;8:1.

75. Cordova JS, Kandula S, Gurbani S, et al. Simulating the effect of spectroscopic MRI as a metric for radiation therapy planning in patients with glioblastoma. Tomography 2016;2(4):366–73.

76. Gurbani S, Weinberg B, Cooper L, et al. The brain imaging collaboration suite (BrICS): a cloud platform for integrating whole-brain spectroscopic MRI into the radiation therapy planning workflow. Tomography 2019;5(1):184–91.

Cellular and Molecular Imaging with SPECT and PET in Brain Tumors

Mohammad S. Sadaghiani, MD, MPH, Sara Sheikhbahaei, MD, MPH,
Steven P. Rowe, MD, PhD, Martin G. Pomper, MD, PhD,
Lilja B. Solnes, MD, MBA*

KEYWORDS

• Brain tumor • PET • SPECT • Molecular imaging

KEY POINTS

• Molecular imaging provides functional information based on target detection, which can be helpful in management of brain tumors.
• There are multiple different radiotracers developed based on different mechanisms that can be used in neuro-oncology.
• These radiotracers can detect brain tumors, differentiate low-grade and high-grade lesions, determine eligibility for theranostics, estimate prognosis, and evaluate post-radiation changes.

INTRODUCTION

Brain neoplasms include a diverse group of primary tumors as well as secondary tumors or metastases from neoplasms outside the central nervous system (CNS), which occur more frequently than the primary brain tumors. The incidence rate of primary CNS tumors in adults in the United States is approximately 30 per 100,000 population, with approximately one-third of these tumors being malignant.[1]

Single-photon emission computed tomography (SPECT) and positron emission tomogarphy (PET) are the 2 major tomographic modalities in nuclear medicine that provide functional information regarding different tissues and disorders.[2] Different nuclear medicine radiotracers are utilized for evaluation of brain neoplasms.[3] Although most novel emerging molecular imaging radiotracers are compatible with PET imaging, SPECT remains an alternative modality with lower costs and wider availability.

The emergence of novel radiotracers provides major opportunities in the diagnosis and management of brain tumors. This review delineates the complementary role of conventional and novel molecular imaging radiotracers in neuro-oncology. Most emerging radiotracers are PET agents and, therefore, this review largely focuses on PET imaging agents.

SINGLE-PHOTON EMISSION COMPUTED TOMOGRAPHY

SPECT imaging provide a reasonable imaging alternative to PET, with higher affordability and availability.[4] In SPECT, the gamma camera rotates about the patient and acquires projections at different angles (**Fig. 1**). The main limitation of SPECT imaging is lower resolution and lack of precise anatomic details compared to PET imaging. Recent development of integrated hybrid SPECT/ computed tomography (CT), however, has

The Russell H. Morgan Department of Radiology and Radiological Science, Johns Hopkins University School of Medicine, 601 North Caroline Street, JHOC 3150, Baltimore, MD 21287, USA
* Corresponding author. Johns Hopkins Outpatient Center, 601 North Caroline Street, JHOC 3150, Baltimore, MD 21287.
E-mail address: lsolnes1@jhmi.edu

Radiol Clin N Am 59 (2021) 363–375
https://doi.org/10.1016/j.rcl.2021.01.005
0033-8389/21/© 2021 Elsevier Inc. All rights reserved.

improved the localization of tumor and increased the diagnostic accuracy.

Technetium-99m or [99mTc] labeled compounds and thallium-201 or [201Tl] are 2 example of SPECT radiotracers that have been evaluated in brain tumors.[5] [99mTc] labeled compounds are preferred over [201Tl] based on better contrast resolution; less radiation to the patient; universal availability; and favorable gamma emission characteristics of [99mTc], including the 140-keV gamma ray energy and high photon flux compared to [201Tl].

[99mTc]methoxy-2-isobutylisonitrile ([99mTc]MIBI) and [99mTc]tetrofosmin ([99mTc]TF) are passively accumulated in mitochondria and are considered markers of cellular transmembrane electrical potentials.[6] These features result in higher uptake in neoplastic cells in comparison with surrounding tissues.[5] [99mTc]MIBI and [99mTc]TF can help in improving diagnostic and prognostic accuracy of brain tumors.[5] Alexiou and colleagues showed that [99mTc]TF can provide helpful information to differentiate recurrence from radiation necrosis[6], with the best results observed in gliomas,[7] particularly when anatomic imaging is equivocal[8] (Fig. 2). Semiquantitative analysis of [201Tl] uptake can differentiate tumor recurrence and postradiation necrosis in metastatic brain tumors.[9] Novel SPECT radiotracers are under development for detection of brain tumors. For example, diethylenetriamine pentaacetic acid–conjugated CooP with indium-111 can detect gliomas in 85% of mice.[10]

POSITRON EMISSION TOMOGRAPHY

PET agents play a crucial role in understanding the pathophysiology of neoplasms, developing targeted therapies, and monitoring response to therapy. These agents play a valuable role in diagnosis, classification, staging, image-guided therapy planning, and post-therapeutic evaluation of brain tumors.[11] **Table 1** summarized different PET radiotracers in neuro-oncology. Current and emerging novel radiotracers are discussed within the context of their mechanisms of action.

TRACING GLUCOSE METABOLISM
2-Deoxy-2-[18F]fluoro-ᴅ-glucose

2-Deoxy-2-[18F]fluoro-ᴅ-glucose ([18F]FDG) is the most commonly used PET radiotracer in oncology. Its half-life is relatively longer than most other positron emitters (approximately 2 hours) and it is widely and readily available. Increased glucose metabolism is associated not only with growth but also with malignant transformation.[40]

The Response Assessment in Neuro-Oncology working group recently provided recommendations in using glucose and amino acid radiotracers in glioma as a complementary modality to MR imaging.[41] To improve the accuracy of [18F]FDG PET in detecting brain tumors, two critical steps are recommended. The first step is to coregister the images with MR imaging if a PET/CT was performed, and the second is to acquire delayed images to improve differentiation of brain neoplasm from cortical uptake.[42] PET/MR imaging provides simultaneous data acquisition which results in gathering functional and anatomic data with significant improvement of spatial and temporal resolution.[42] Few institutions have dedicated PET/MR imaging scanners, however, and,

A

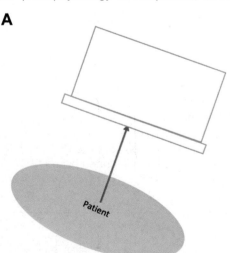

B

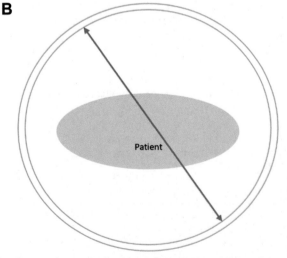

Fig. 1. Schematic acquisition of SPECT (*A*) and PET (*B*). For SPECT, the gamma camera rotates around the patient and acquires images at different angles. In PET, the patient is in the center of a ring of detectors, and positron annihilation results in 2 photons emitted at opposite directions.

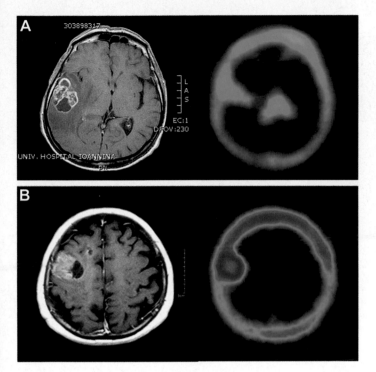

Fig. 2. Postcontrast T1-weighted MR images (*left*) and [99mTc]TF SPECT images (*right*) in glioblastoma showing low tracer uptake in 1 patient (*A*) and high uptake in another patient (*B*), This research originally was published in the *Journal of Nuclear Medicine.*[6] George A Alexiou, Spyridon Tsiouris, Athanasios P Kyritsis, George Fotakopoulos, Anna Goussia, Spyridon Voulgaris, Andreas D Fotopoulos. The value of 99mTc-tetrofosmin brain SPECT in predicting survival in patients with glioblastoma multiforme. *J Nucl Med.* 2010;51(12):1923-1926.

therefore, the importance of fusion software is critical.

2-Deoxy-2-[18F]Fluoro-D-Glucose PET in Neuro-Oncology

Delineating tumor boundaries
One of the challenges in neuro-oncology is delineation of the tumor margins at the edge of gray matter, which also intrinsically shows high activity. This can be addressed with coregistration with MR imaging or delayed PET imaging (**Fig. 3**).[43] Tumor demonstrates higher [18F]FDG avidity than gray matter on delayed acquisitions due to lower degradation of intracellular [18F]FDG-6-phosphate in tumor than in brain.[43]

Table 1
Selected PET radiotracers and their mechanism of action in neuro-oncology

Tracer	Mechanism	Tumor Type
[11C]acetate	Anabolism by acetyl-CoA synthesis, cell membrane	Glioma,[12] meningioma,[13] meningioma, schwannoma,[14] metastases[15]
[11C]CHO	Phospholipids synthesis	Glioma,[16] CNS metastases,[16] meningioma,[16] schwannoma[17]
[11C]MET	Amino acid uptake (methionine based)	Glioma,[12] germinoma,[18] CNS metastases,[19] meningioma,[20] CNS lymphoma[3]
[18F]FDOPA	Amino acid uptake	Glioma,[21] CNS metastases,[22] meningioma[23]
[18F]FAZA	Hypoxia	High-grade glioma[24]
[18F]FDG	Glucose metabolism	Glioma,[3] CNS metastases,[25] meningioma,[26] CNS lymphoma,[27] oligodendroglioma[28]
[18F]FET	Amino acid uptake (tyrosine based)	Glioma,[29] CNS metastases,[30] meningioma,[31] medulloblastoma,[32] ganglioglioma[32]
[18F]FMISO	Hypoxia	Glioma[33]
[68Ga]DOTA-TATE	somatostatin receptor up-regulation	Meningioma,[34] hemangioblastoma,[35] CNS neuroendocrine,[36] medulloblastoma[37]
[68Ga]PSMA	PSMA	Glioma,[38] metastasis,[38] meningioma[39]

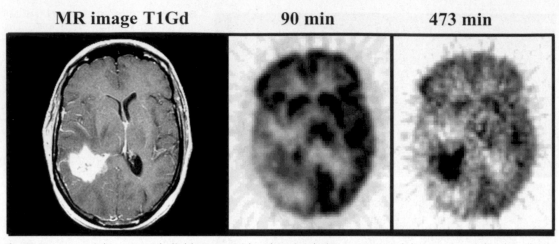

Fig. 3. Recurrent right temporal glioblastoma with enhancing lesion on post gadolinium T1-weighted MR imaging (T1Gd). There is an improvement of TBR in the [18F]FDG PET imaging at the delayed time point in comparison with earlier acquisition. This research originally was published in the *Journal of Nuclear Medicine*.[43] Alexander M Spence 1, Mark Muzi, David A Mankoff, S Finbarr O'Sullivan, Jeanne M Link, Thomas K Lewellen, Barbara Lewellen, Pam Pham, Satoshi Minoshima, Kristin Swanson, Kenneth A Krohn. 18F-FDG PET of gliomas at delayed intervals: improved distinction between tumor and normal gray matter. *J Nucl Med*. 2004;45(10):1653-1659.

Tumor grading

Some studies have shown that [18F]FDG PET can differentiate low-grade and high-grade gliomas based on glioma–to–white matter and glioma–to–gray matter ratios. Tumor–to–white matter ratio of greater than 1.5 and tumor–to–gray matter ratio of greater than 0.6 can differentiate high-grade from low-grade gliomas, with 94% sensitivity and 77% specificity,[44] although other studies have failed to differentiate high-grade and low-grade gliomas based on [18F]FDG uptake.[45]

Determining prognosis

Higher [18F]FDG uptake in a previously known low-grade glioma can indicate anaplastic transformation.[42] [18F]FDG PET can predict survival regardless of histologic classification.[42] Some studies show that [18F]FDG uptake is the most powerful predictor of progression-free survival and overall survival in comparison with other variables, such as histologic grade.[46]

Guiding post-therapy evaluation

One of the major advantages of [18F]FDG PET compared with structural imaging is differentiating radiation necrosis from recurrent disease.[47] This feature is more reliable in gliomas in contrast to metastatic disease. A meta-analysis regarding the diagnostic accuracy of [18F]FDG PET in detecting recurrences in gliomas showed heterogeneous diagnostic accuracies across the studies, with sensitivity of 0.77 (95% CI, 0.66–0.85) and specificity of 0.78 (95% CI, 0.54–0.91). [18F]FDG PET can be used in planning for stereotactic biopsy

by improving delineation of higher-grade foci within a heterogeneous tumor. This improves the diagnostic yield of brain biopsy.[48]

AMINO ACID METABOLISM

Amino acids are required in the synthesis of proteins and can indicate level of metabolism and proliferation. Amino acids generally demonstrate a low background uptake in gray matter and white matter, which improves tumor-to-background ratio (TBR). TBR is used to compare the uptake in tumor to the contralateral lobe. The uptake of amino acid–based radiotracers in tumoral cells is based on overexpression of amino acid transporters,[49] which correlates with malignant phenotype and angiogenesis.[50]

Methyl-[11C]-L-Methionine

The most commonly used radiolabeled amino acid in detecting brain tumors is methyl-[11C]-L-methionine ([11C]MET). The relatively short half-life of carbon-11 ([11C]MET), approximately 20 minutes, limits its usage to institutions with an on-site cyclotron. This radiotracer can be synthesized rapidly without requirement for purification.[19] The intracellular uptake happens through transmembrane transport by sodium independent L-transporter based on a concentration gradient. [11C]MET brain uptake generally is lower than brain tumors, resulting in high detection rate and sharp delineation of the tumor.

[11C]MET PET can detect primary gliomas with high sensitivity and specificity, with sensitivities ranging from 76% to 100%.[19] Besides neoplasms, however, inflammatory cells have increased uptake, making this radiotracer an unideal method in differentiating tumor from inflammation.[51]

The results of quantitative analysis among different [11C]MET PET studies have been controversial in grading primary gliomas. Low-grade gliomas generally show lower uptake in contrast to high-grade gliomas.[19] A meta-analysis in 2019 showed that [11C]MET PET can differentiate low-grade from high-grade gliomas with higher sensitivity than [18F]FDG PET.[52]

Some studies have shown that [11C]MET PET can be used as a prognostic tool with higher uptake values associated with worse outcome. For example, Nariai and colleagues[53] showed significant correlation between survival and pretreatment TBR. In contrast, Ceyssens and colleagues[54] showed that [11C]MET PET does not predict survival in patients with brain tumors.

[11C]MET PET has been shown to improve tumor delineation with higher accuracy in comparison to CT or MR imaging and can identify areas with highest risk of recurrence.[19] This radiotracer can improve biopsy planning by identifying the regions with higher grades and determining better target regions in contrast to structural imaging modalities.[19]

O-(2-[18F]fluoroethyl)-L-Tyrosine

O-(2-[18F]fluoroethyl)-L-tyrosine ([18F]FET) is a tyrosine analogue that can be used in detection of brain tumors. This molecule is not incorporated into proteins; hence, it has greater intracellular stability in contrast to other amino acid radiotracers.[55]

[18F]FET PET can diagnose[29] brain tumors and grade gliomas[52] with higher sensitivities than [18F]FDG. It can differentiate low-grade from high-grade gliomas[29] as well as low-grade and high-grade meningiomas based on TBR.[31] In untreated metastatic lesions, [18F]FET PET uptake is increased in only two-thirds of lesions less than 1.0 cm whereas all lesions greater than 1.0 cm show pathologic uptake independent of tumor size.[30] Fig. 4 shows [18F]FET uptake in metastatic melanoma lesions, which demonstrate high variability.[30]

This radiotracer can be helpful for target selection and biopsy guidance as well as tumor resection planning.[55] A cost-effectiveness analysis showed that [18F]FET PET and MR imaging may be superior to MR imaging alone in determining the biopsy site in glioma.[56]

[18F]FET also is useful in detection of residual brain tumor after surgery. Early evaluation of the resection status in high-grade glioma is feasible with [18F]FET PET, and PET findings have been shown to correlate with intraoperative assessment with 5-aminolevulinic acid as well as MR imaging results.[57] Multiple studies have shown the role of [18F]FET PET in differentiating recurrence from post therapeutic changes.[55] In a related study, Galldiks and colleagues[58] concluded that [18F]FET PET parameters can differentiate progressive or recurrent glioma from post treatment changes with higher accuracy than MR imaging.

[18F]FET PET also can predict prognosis and survival in gliomas. Early time to peak in dynamic [18F]FET PET is associated with worse outcome in newly diagnosed high-grade gliomas.[59] Maximum and mean TBRs are significant and independent predictors for progression-free survival and overall survival.[60]

l-3,4-Dihydroxy-6-[18F]fluoro-phenyl-alanine

l-3,4-Dihydroxy-6-[18F]fluoro-phenyl-alanine ([18F]FDOPA) is transported into cells through large amino acid transporter and then is decarboxylated by DOPA decarboxylase to [18F]dopamine that is trapped intracellularly in storage granules by vesicular monoamine transporters.[61] Chen and colleagues[62] compared [18F]FDOPA with [18F]FDG PET in 81 patients with brain tumor. [18F]FDOPA had higher sensitivity (96%) in identifying brain tumors compared with [18F]FDG (61%), with similar specificities (43%). [18F]FDOPA is more accurate than [18F]FDG PET for diagnosing low-grade tumors and evaluating recurrent tumors (Fig. 5). Moreover, it was able to distinguish tumor recurrence from radiation necrosis.[62]

A recent meta-analysis showed that this radiotracer has pooled sensitivity of 0.90 (95% CI, 0.86–0.93) and pooled specificity of 0.75 (95% CI, 0.65–0.83) for diagnosis of glioma.[21] Pooled sensitivity and specificity to differentiate high-grade from low-grade gliomas were 88% (95% CI, 0.81–0.93) and 73% (95% CI, 0.64–0.81) respectively.

TARGETING CELL MEMBRANE COMPONENTS
[11C]Choline

[11C]choline ([11C]CHO) can be integrated into lecithin, which is a component of cell membrane phospholipid. In neoplasms, there is increased cell membrane turnover, which results in higher choline uptake as a marker of metabolite activity.[42]

In a prospective trial [11C]CHO PET was compared with [18F]FDG PET for various types of malignancies, including 25 patients with brain tumor. [11C]CHO PET was able to differentiate benign and malignant tumors, with area under the curve (AUC) of 0.79, which was significantly higher than [18F]FDG PET (0.58). [11C]CHO PET provides high contrast images of brain tumors in comparison with [18F]FDG PET because of lower background

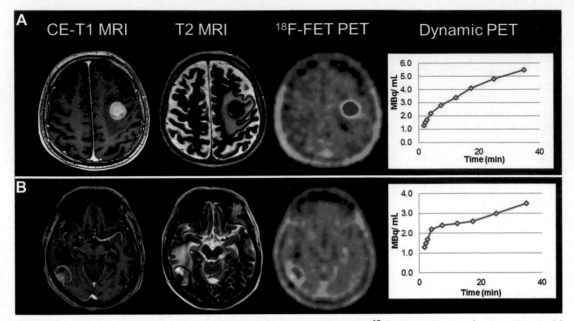

Fig. 4. Contrast enhanced T1-weighted (CE-T1), T2-weighted MR, and [^{18}F]FET PET images for 2 patients with metastatic melanoma (*A, B*). There is high variability in [^{18}F]FET PET avidity in metastatic melanoma. This research originally was published in the *Journal of Nuclear Medicine*.[30] Marcus Unterrainer, Norbert Galldiks, Bogdana Suchorska, Lara-Caroline Kowalew, Vera Wenter, Christine Schmid-Tannwald, Maximilian Niyazi, Peter Bartenstein, Karl-Josef Langen, Nathalie L Albert. 18F-FET PET Uptake Characteristics in Patients with Newly Diagnosed and Untreated Brain Metastasis. *J Nucl Med.* 2017;58(4):584-589.

uptake. [^{11}C]CHO PET is superior to [^{18}F]FDG PET in properly delineating the border of brain tumors, likely because of higher background uptake in [^{18}F]FDG PET.[63]

[^{11}C]acetate

The radiotracer [^{11}C]acetate is a precursor of fatty acids in cell membrane, being transformed to acetyl coenzyme A (CoA) and entering the tricarboxylic acid cycle. It can detect high-grade glioma with sensitivity of 90%.[12] In a prospective study, Kim and colleagues[64] showed that [^{11}C]acetate can differentiate low-grade and high-grade gliomas. [^{11}C]acetate may be helpful in detection of meningiomas, assessing tumor extent, and evaluating response to radiosurgery.[13]

TARGETING HYPOXIA

Detection of hypoxia in solid tumors is associated with more aggressive phenotype and worse prognosis. Hypoxia-specific PET can help in therapeutic decision making and provide tumor prognostication.[42] The initial uptake of the radiotracer is determined by blood flow; however, in the later phase (2–4 hours from injection), hypoxia regulates the uptake.[42]

[^{18}F]fuoromisonidazole

[^{18}F]fuoromisonidazole ([^{18}F]FMISO) is the most extensively used and studied hypoxia radiotracer in brain tumors.[33] A major drawback regarding [^{18}F]FMISO is the slow clearance of the unbound radiotracer from normal tissue, resulting in low TBR and slow plasma clearance.[33] There is a positive correlation between radiotracer uptake and expression of biomarkers of hypoxia (carbonic anhydrase IX, hypoxia-inducible factor carbonic anhydrase IX, and hypoxia-inducible factor 1α) and angiogenesis (vascular endothelial growth factor, angiopoietin-2, and relative cerebral blood volume).[65]

In a prospective clinical study in patient with gliomas [^{18}F]FMISO uptake was associated with different grades, with higher uptake in glioblastoma.[65] In another study, hypoxia determined based on [^{18}F]FMISO PET was found to be a negative prognostic marker.[66]

[^{18}F]flouroazomycin arabinoside

[^{18}F]flouroazomycin arabinoside ([^{18}F]FAZA) is one of the most promising hypoxia radiotracers introduced after [^{18}F]FMISO. [^{18}F]FAZA is less lipophilic in comparison with [^{18}F]FMISO, hence its improved biodistribution.[67] [^{18}F]FAZA retention is

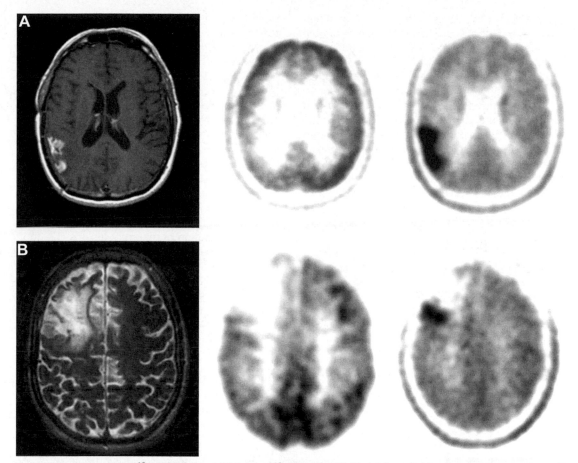

Fig. 5. MR image (*left*), [^{18}F]FDG PET (*middle*), and [^{18}F]FDOPA PET (*right*) for glioblastoma (*A*) and grade II oligodendroglioma (*B*). The lesions show high FDOPA uptake without [^{18}F]FDG avidity. This research originally was published in the *Journal of Nuclear Medicine*.[62] Wei Chen, Daniel H S Silverman, Sibylle Delaloye, Johannes Czernin, Nirav Kamdar, Whitney Pope, Nagichettiar Satyamurthy, Christiaan Schiepers, Timothy Cloughesy. 18F-FDOPA PET imaging of brain tumors: comparison study with 18F-FDG PET and evaluation of diagnostic accuracy. *J Nucl Med*. 2006;47(6):904-911.

dependent on reducing processes, which occur in hypoxic conditions. It has more rapid clearance from normal tissues that results in high TBR.[68] [^{18}F]FAZA is highly representative of hypoxia in glioblastoma.[24]

This radiotracer has been studied for treatment planning and guiding tailored radiotherapy as well as evaluation of tumor response to radiotherapy.[24] Identification of hypoxic regions in tumors can provide guidance by detecting areas with highest aggressive potential.[69]

TRACING SOMATOSTATIN RECEPTOR

Three different Gallium-68 or [^{68}Ga] labeled 1,4,7,10-tetraazacyclo-dodecane-N,N′,N″,N‴-tetraacetic-acid (DOTA) conjugated peptides are available for clinical imaging, namely [^{68}Ga]DOTA-Phe^1-Tyr^3-octreotide ([^{68}Ga]DOTA-TOC), [^{68}Ga]DOTA-Nal^3-

octreotide ([^{68}Ga]DOTA-NOC), and [^{68}Ga]DOTA-Tyr^3-octreotate ([^{68}Ga]DOTA-TATE).

The somatostatin receptor (SSTR) affinity of these radiotracers is different. [^{68}Ga]DOTA-TATE provides the highest affinity to SSTR2. [^{68}Ga]DOTA-NOC has the broadest SSTR affinity, including to SSTR2, SSTR3, SSTR4, and SSTR5, which makes it an agent of choice to detect intracranial tumors.[70]

Meningiomas express SSTR2, demonstrating excellent TBR uptake.[42] [^{68}Ga]DOTA-conjugated peptides can confirm with presence of meningioma if the MR imaging results are equivocal.[71] One study found that the combination of [^{68}Ga]DOTA-TOC PET/CT and MR imaging changes the target volume definition for radiotherapy in 73% of patients compared with planning with only MR imaging or CT.[72] Moreover, [^{68}Ga]DOTA-conjugated peptides PET can predict response to radiopeptide therapy in meningioma.[34] **Fig. 6** shows an incidental meningioma in a patient being imaged for neuroendocrince tumor.

Besides meningioma, several studies showed the utility of [^{68}Ga]DOTA-conjugated peptides in CNS neuroendocrine,[36] medulloblastoma, and hemangioblastoma[35] (see **Table 1**). In high-grade glioma, the uptake of this radiotracer is associated with blood-brain barrier disruption, which limits its value in detecting these tumors.[73] Moreover, radiotracer uptake cannot be predicted by SSTR2 expression on immunohistochemistry.

PROSTATE-SPECIFIC MEMBRANE ANTIGEN–EXPRESSING TUMORS

Prostate-specific membrane antigen (PSMA) is a transmembrane enzyme that is overexpressed in prostate adenocarcinoma.[74] The overexpression of PSMA is observed in tumor-associated neovasculature of many solid tumors.[75] PSMA is expressed in primary gliomas and breast cancer

brain metastases.[38] These radiotracers are likely to be Food and Drug Administration (FDA) approved in the near future for prostate cancer evaluation.

Glu-NH-CO–NH-Lys-(Ahx)-[^{68}Ga(HBED-CC)] ([^{68}Ga]PSMA-11) and 2-(3-{1-carboxy-5-[(6-[^{18}F] fluoro-pyridine-3-carbonyl)-amino]-pentyl}-ureido)-pentanedioic acid ([^{18}F]DCFPyL) are radiotracers that can be used for a variety of indications in patients with prostate cancer.[76] [^{68}Ga]PSMA-11 can detect brain metastasis in prostate carcinoma.[77] Sasikumar and colleagues[78] compared [^{18}F]FDG and [^{68}Ga]PSMA-11 brain PET in patients with glioblastoma. According to their study, [^{68}Ga]PSMA-11 showed better visualization of recurrent lesions due to its high TBR. There have been reports of incidental meningiomas detected by [^{68}Ga]PSMA-11.[39,79] Similarly, [^{18}F]DCFPyL can detect high-grade gliomas[80] and schwannomas[81] (**Fig. 7**), although there is some question as to the specificity of uptake of PSMA-targeted radiotracers in patients with previously treated brain tumors.[82]

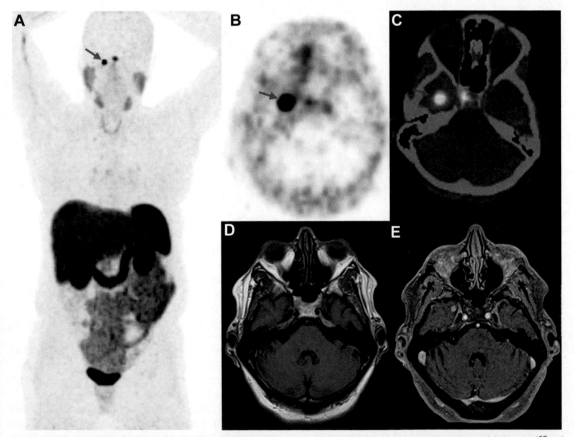

Fig. 6. A 57-year-old woman with incidental note of DOTA-TATE-avid lesion in the right temporal lobe on [^{68}Ga] DOTA-Tyr[3] -octreotide ([^{68}Ga]DOTA-TATE) PET, including coronal view (*A*), axial view (*B*), PET/CT fusion axial view (*C*) Subsequent precontrast MR (*D*) and postcontrast MR (*E*) images show 0.7-cm dural-based enhancing mass in the right middle cranial fossa, with MR characteristics favoring meningioma.

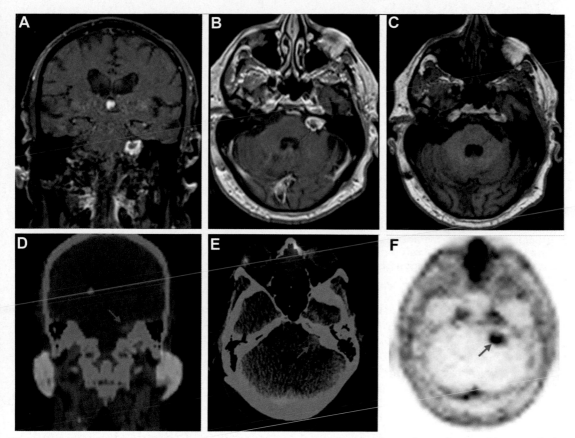

Fig. 7. An 80-year-old man with left cerebellopontine angle lesion (*red arrow*), consistent with a vestibular schwannoma. Coronal (*A*) and axial (*B*) views, postcontrast T1 MR imaging of the brain, show peripherally enhancing lesion in left cerebellopontine angle. Fluid-attenuated axial inversion recovery axial view (*C*) shows low signal intensity within the lesion. Coronal (*D*) and axial (*E*) views, [¹⁸F]DCFPyL PET/CT, and axial [¹⁸F]DCFPyL PET image (*F*) show radiotracer avidity in the lesion.

SUMMARY

Structural imaging, such as CT or MR imaging, is crucial in initial diagnosis of brain tumors; however, emerging molecular imaging techniques can provide additional information, including tumor grade, tumor composition, and tumor extent. Functional imaging can differentiate tumor recurrence from post-therapeutic changes based on metabolic activity at the surgical bed. Different SPECT and PET radiotracers have been developed that can be used in diagnosis, grading, surgical and radiation planning, post-therapeutic residual tumor detection, recurrence detection, and determining prognosis. Although [¹⁸F]FDG is the most commonly used PET radiotracer in neuro-oncology, it has multiple intrinsic limitations, including low TBR and broad differential diagnosis. Other radiotracers, such as amino acid–based agents, provide better TBRs. More novel radiotracers, such as [⁶⁸Ga]DOTA-conjugated peptide compounds, provide more specific

targeting and a narrower differential diagnosis for lesions with avid uptake.

Among the radiotracers discussed previously, only [¹⁸F]FDG is approved by the FDA and included in US Pharmacopeia (USP) whereas most are enlisted in European Pharmacopoeia (EP).[83] In Europe, radiotracers are recognized as a special group of medicines. EP is based on the drug quality and is independent of clinical utility or licensing status. In the United States, the clinical use of all radiotracers is regulated by FDA. USP monographs typically are developed based on FDA-approved medicines and are considered as one basis of reimbursements; 8 FDA-unapproved tracers were included in USP monologues until 2014 (including [¹¹C]MET, [¹¹C] sodium acetate, and [¹⁸F]FDOPA). These FDA-unapproved drugs were omitted from USP monologues in 2014 based on Society of Nuclear Medicine and Molecular Imaging (SNMMI) committee recommendations in 2013. According to SNMMI, the data regarding these tracers were unvalidated and the analytical methods were outdated.[84]

CLINICS CARE POINTS

- Different SPECT and PET radiotracers have been developed that can be used in neuro-oncology

- PET provides better imaging resolution; however, SPECT provides greater availability and affordability

- Molecular imaging tracers can be used in diagnosis, grading, therapeutic planning, residual tumor detection, recurrence detection, and determination of prognosis.

- [18F]FDG is the most commonly used PET radiotracer in neuro-oncology, with intrinsic limitations, including low TBR and broad differential diagnosis.

- Others PET radiotracers, such as amino acid–based agents, provide higher TBRs.

DISCLOSURE

L.B. Solnes is a consultant for Progenics and AAA/Novartis Pharmaceuticals.

REFERENCES

1. Ostrom QT, Gittleman H, Truitt G, et al. CBTRUS statistical report: primary brain and other central nervous system tumors diagnosed in the United States in 2011-2015. Neuro Oncol 2018;20(suppl_4):iv1–86.

2. Rahmim A, Zaidi H. PET versus SPECT: strengths, limitations and challenges. Nucl Med Commun 2008;29(3):193–207.

3. Pruis IJ, van Dongen GAMS, Veldhuijzen van Zanten SEM. The Added Value of Diagnostic and Theranostic PET Imaging for the Treatment of CNS Tumors. Int J Mol Sci 2020;21(3). https://doi.org/10.3390/ijms21031029.

4. Fotopoulos AD, Alexiou GA. Is there still a place for SPET in the era of PET brain imaging? Hell J Nucl Med 2012;15(2):89–91.

5. Tsitsia V, Svolou P, Kapsalaki E, et al. Multimodality-multiparametric brain tumors evaluation. Hell J Nucl Med 2017;20(1):57–61.

6. Alexiou GA, Tsiouris S, Kyritsis AP, et al. The value of 99mTc-tetrofosmin brain SPECT in predicting survival in patients with glioblastoma multiforme. J Nucl Med 2010;51(12):1923–6.

7. Schillaci O, Filippi L, Manni C, et al. Single-photon emission computed tomography/computed tomography in brain tumors. Semin Nucl Med 2007;37(1):34–47.

8. Alexiou GA, Fotopoulos AD, Papadopoulos A, et al. Evaluation of brain tumor recurrence by (99m)Tc-tetrofosmin SPECT: a prospective pilot study. Ann Nucl Med 2007;21(5):293–8.

9. Matsunaga S, Shuto T, Takase H, et al. Semiquantitative analysis using thallium-201 SPECT for differential diagnosis between tumor recurrence and radiation necrosis after gamma knife surgery for malignant brain tumors. Int J Radiat Oncol Biol Phys 2013;85(1):47–52.

10. Hyvönen M, Enbäck J, Huhtala T, et al. Novel target for peptide-based imaging and treatment of brain tumors. Mol Cancer Ther 2014;13(4):996–1007.

11. Horky LL, Hsiao EM, Weiss SE, et al. Dual phase FDG-PET imaging of brain metastases provides superior assessment of recurrence versus post-treatment necrosis. J Neurooncol 2011;103(1):137–46.

12. Yamamoto Y, Nishiyama Y, Kimura N, et al. 11C-acetate PET in the evaluation of brain glioma: comparison with 11C-methionine and 18F-FDG-PET. Mol Imaging Biol 2008;10(5):281–7.

13. Liu R-S, Chang C-P, Guo W-Y, et al. 1-11C-acetate versus 18F-FDG PET in detection of meningioma and monitoring the effect of gamma-knife radiosurgery. J Nucl Med 2010;51(6):883–91.

14. Lee SM, Kim T-S, Kim S-K. Cerebellopontine angle schwannoma on C-11 acetate PET/CT. Clin Nucl Med 2009;34(11):831–3.

15. Park J-W, Kim JH, Kim SK, et al. A prospective evaluation of 18F-FDG and 11C-acetate PET/CT for detection of primary and metastatic hepatocellular carcinoma. J Nucl Med 2008;49(12):1912–21.

16. Giovannini E, Lazzeri P, Milano A, et al. Clinical applications of choline PET/CT in brain tumors. Curr Pharm Des 2015;21(1):121–7.

17. Ohtani T, Kurihara H, Ishiuchi S, et al. Brain tumour imaging with carbon-11 choline: comparison with FDG PET and gadolinium-enhanced MR imaging. Eur J Nucl Med 2001;28(11):1664–70.

18. Okochi Y, Nihashi T, Fujii M, et al. Clinical use of (11)C-methionine and (18)F-FDG-PET for germinoma in central nervous system. Ann Nucl Med 2014;28(2):94–102.

19. Glaudemans AWJM, Enting RH, Heesters MAAM, et al. Value of 11C-methionine PET in imaging brain tumours and metastases. Eur J Nucl Med Mol Imaging 2013;40(4):615–35.

20. Arita H, Kinoshita M, Okita Y, et al. Clinical characteristics of meningiomas assessed by 11C-methionine and 18F-fluorodeoxyglucose positron-emission tomography. J Neurooncol 2012;107(2):379–86.

21. Xiao J, Jin Y, Nie J, et al. Diagnostic and grading accuracy of 18F-FDOPA PET and PET/CT in patients

with gliomas: a systematic review and meta-analysis. BMC Cancer 2019;19(1):767.

22. Lizarraga KJ, Allen-Auerbach M, Czernin J, et al. (18)F-FDOPA PET for differentiating recurrent or progressive brain metastatic tumors from late or delayed radiation injury after radiation treatment. J Nucl Med 2014;55(1):30–6.

23. Calabria FF, Chiaravalloti A, Calabria EN, et al. 18F-DOPA PET/CT and MRI Findings in a Patient With Multiple Meningiomas. Clin Nucl Med 2016;41(8):636–7.

24. Mapelli P, Zerbetto F, Incerti E, et al. 18F-FAZA PET/CT Hypoxia Imaging of High-Grade Glioma Before and After Radiotherapy. Clin Nucl Med 2017;42(12):e525–6.

25. Li H, Deng L, Bai HX, et al. Diagnostic accuracy of amino acid and FDG-PET in differentiating brain metastasis recurrence from radionecrosis after radiotherapy: a systematic review and meta-analysis. AJNR Am J Neuroradiol 2018;39(2):280–8.

26. Lee JW, Kang KW, Park S-H, et al. 18F-FDG PET in the assessment of tumor grade and prediction of tumor recurrence in intracranial meningioma. Eur J Nucl Med Mol Imaging 2009;36(10):1574–82.

27. Kawai N, Miyake K, Yamamoto Y, et al. 18F-FDG PET in the diagnosis and treatment of primary central nervous system lymphoma. Biomed Res Int 2013;2013:247152.

28. Ambinder EB, Rowe SP. A case of anaplastic oligodendroglioma with extensive extraneural metastases imaged with FDG PET. Clin Nucl Med 2017;42(12):968–70.

29. Dunet V, Pomoni A, Hottinger A, et al. Performance of 18F-FET versus 18F-FDG-PET for the diagnosis and grading of brain tumors: systematic review and meta-analysis. Neuro Oncol 2016;18(3):426–34.

30. Unterrainer M, Galldiks N, Suchorska B, et al. 18F-FET PET uptake characteristics in patients with newly diagnosed and untreated brain metastasis. J Nucl Med 2017;58(4):584–9.

31. Cornelius JF, Stoffels G, Filß C, et al. Uptake and tracer kinetics of O-(2-(18)F-fluoroethyl)-L-tyrosine in meningiomas: preliminary results. Eur J Nucl Med Mol Imaging 2015;42(3):459–67.

32. Misch M, Guggemos A, Driever PH, et al. 18)F-FET-PET guided surgical biopsy and resection in children and adolescence with brain tumors. Childs Nerv Syst 2015;31(2):261–7.

33. Quartuccio N, Laudicella R, Mapelli P, et al. Hypoxia PET imaging beyond 18 F-FMISO in patients with high-grade glioma: 18 F-FAZA and other hypoxia radiotracers. Clin Transl Imaging 2020;8(1):11–20.

34. Bartolomei M, Bodei L, De Cicco C, et al. Peptide receptor radionuclide therapy with (90)Y-DOTATOC in recurrent meningioma. Eur J Nucl Med Mol Imaging 2009;36(9):1407–16.

35. Sharma P, Dhull VS, Bal C, et al. Von Hippel-Lindau syndrome: demonstration of entire disease spectrum with (68)Ga-DOTANOC PET-CT. Korean J Radiol 2014;15(1):169–72.

36. Carreras C, Kulkarni HR, Baum RP. Rare metastases detected by (68)Ga-somatostatin receptor PET/CT in patients with neuroendocrine tumors. Recent Results Cancer Res 2013;194:379–84.

37. Arunraj ST, Parida GK, Damle NA, et al. 68Ga-DOTANOC PET/CT in Medulloblastoma. Clin Nucl Med 2018;43(5):e145–6.

38. Nomura N, Pastorino S, Jiang P, et al. Prostate specific membrane antigen (PSMA) expression in primary gliomas and breast cancer brain metastases. Cancer Cell Int 2014;14(1):26.

39. Bilgin R, Ergül N, Çermik TF. Incidental meningioma mimicking metastasis of prostate adenocarcinoma in 68Ga-Labeled PSMA Ligand PET/CT. Clin Nucl Med 2016;41(12):956–8.

40. Hatanaka M, Augl C, Gilden RV. Evidence for a functional change in the plasma membrane of murine sarcoma virus-infected mouse embryo cells. Transport and transport-associated phosphorylation of 14C-2-deoxy-D-glucose. J Biol Chem 1970;245(4):714–7.

41. Albert NL, Weller M, Suchorska B, et al. Response Assessment in Neuro-Oncology working group and European Association for Neuro-Oncology recommendations for the clinical use of PET imaging in gliomas. Neuro Oncol 2016;18(9):1199–208.

42. Basu S, Alavi A. Molecular imaging (PET) of brain tumors. Neuroimaging Clin N Am 2009;19(4):625–46.

43. Spence AM, Muzi M, Mankoff DA, et al. 18F-FDG PET of gliomas at delayed intervals: improved distinction between tumor and normal gray matter. J Nucl Med 2004;45(10):1653–9.

44. Delbeke D, Meyerowitz C, Lapidus RL, et al. Optimal cutoff levels of F-18 fluorodeoxyglucose uptake in the differentiation of low-grade from high-grade brain tumors with PET. Radiology 1995;195(1):47–52.

45. Tsuchida T, Takeuchi H, Okazawa H, et al. Grading of brain glioma with 1-11C-acetate PET: comparison with 18F-FDG PET. Nucl Med Biol 2008;35(2):171–6.

46. Colavolpe C, Chinot O, Metellus P, et al. FDG-PET predicts survival in recurrent high-grade gliomas treated with bevacizumab and irinotecan. Neuro Oncol 2012;14(5):649–57.

47. Kim EE, Chung SK, Haynie TP, et al. Differentiation of residual or recurrent tumors from post-treatment changes with F-18 FDG PET. Radiographics 1992;12(2):269–79.

48. Pirotte B, Goldman S, Brucher JM, et al. PET in stereotactic conditions increases the diagnostic yield of brain biopsy. Stereotact Funct Neurosurg 1994;63(1–4):144–9.

49. Galldiks N, Langen K-J, Albert NL, et al. PET imaging in patients with brain metastasis-report of the RANO/PET group. Neuro Oncol 2019;21(5):585–95.

50. Haining Z, Kawai N, Miyake K, et al. Relation of LAT1/4F2hc expression with pathological grade, proliferation and angiogenesis in human gliomas. BMC Clin Pathol 2012;12:4.

51. Stöber B, Tanase U, Herz M, et al. Differentiation of tumour and inflammation: characterisation of [methyl-3H]methionine (MET) and O-(2-[18F]fluoroethyl)-L-tyrosine (FET) uptake in human tumour and inflammatory cells. Eur J Nucl Med Mol Imaging 2006;33(8):932–9.

52. Katsanos AH, Alexiou GA, Fotopoulos AD, et al. Performance of 18F-FDG, 11C-Methionine, and 18F-FET PET for Glioma Grading: A Meta-analysis. Clin Nucl Med 2019;44(11):864–9.

53. Nariai T, Tanaka Y, Wakimoto H, et al. Usefulness of L-[methyl-11C] methionine-positron emission tomography as a biological monitoring tool in the treatment of glioma. J Neurosurg 2005;103(3):498–507.

54. Ceyssens S, Van Laere K, de Groot T, et al. [11C] methionine PET, histopathology, and survival in primary brain tumors and recurrence. AJNR Am J Neuroradiol 2006;27(7):1432–7.

55. Muoio B, Giovanella L, Treglia G. Recent Developments of 18F-FET PET in Neuro-oncology. Curr Med Chem 2018;25(26):3061–73.

56. Heinzel A, Stock S, Langen K-J, et al. Cost-effectiveness analysis of FET PET-guided target selection for the diagnosis of gliomas. Eur J Nucl Med Mol Imaging 2012;39(7):1089–96.

57. Kläsner B, Buchmann N, Gempt J, et al. Early [18F] FET-PET in Gliomas after Surgical Resection: Comparison with MRI and Histopathology. PLoS One 2015;10(10):e0141153.

58. Galldiks N, Stoffels G, Filss C, et al. The use of dynamic O-(2-18F-fluoroethyl)-l-tyrosine PET in the diagnosis of patients with progressive and recurrent glioma. Neuro Oncol 2015;17(9):1293–300.

59. Jansen NL, Suchorska B, Wenter V, et al. Prognostic significance of dynamic 18F-FET PET in newly diagnosed astrocytic high-grade glioma. J Nucl Med 2015;56(1):9–15.

60. Galldiks N, Langen K-J, Holy R, et al. Assessment of treatment response in patients with glioblastoma using O-(2-18F-fluoroethyl)-L-tyrosine PET in comparison to MRI. J Nucl Med 2012;53(7):1048–57.

61. Treglia G, Muoio B, Trevisi G, et al. Diagnostic Performance and Prognostic Value of PET/CT with Different Tracers for Brain Tumors: A Systematic Review of Published Meta-Analyses. Int J Mol Sci 2019; 20(19). https://doi.org/10.3390/ijms20194669.

62. Chen W, Silverman DHS, Delaloye S, et al. 18F-FDOPA PET imaging of brain tumors: comparison study with 18F-FDG PET and evaluation of diagnostic accuracy. J Nucl Med 2006;47(6):904–11.

63. Tian M, Zhang H, Oriuchi N, et al. Comparison of 11C-choline PET and FDG PET for the differential diagnosis of malignant tumors. Eur J Nucl Med Mol Imaging 2004;31(8):1064–72.

64. Kim S, Kim D, Kim SH, et al. The roles of 11C-acetate PET/CT in predicting tumor differentiation and survival in patients with cerebral glioma. Eur J Nucl Med Mol Imaging 2018;45(6):1012–20.

65. Bekaert L, Valable S, Lechapt-Zalcman E, et al. [18F]-FMISO PET study of hypoxia in gliomas before surgery: correlation with molecular markers of hypoxia and angiogenesis. Eur J Nucl Med Mol Imaging 2017;44(8):1383–92.

66. Gerstner ER, Zhang Z, Fink JR, et al. ACRIN 6684: Assessment of Tumor Hypoxia in Newly Diagnosed Glioblastoma Using 18F-FMISO PET and MRI. Clin Cancer Res 2016;22(20):5079–86.

67. Busk M, Mortensen LS, Nordsmark M, et al. PET hypoxia imaging with FAZA: reproducibility at baseline and during fractionated radiotherapy in tumour-bearing mice. Eur J Nucl Med Mol Imaging 2013; 40(2):186–97.

68. Lopci E, Grassi I, Chiti A, et al. PET radiopharmaceuticals for imaging of tumor hypoxia: a review of the evidence. Am J Nucl Med Mol Imaging 2014;4(4): 365–84.

69. Mapelli P, Incerti E, Bettinardi V, et al. Hypoxia 18 F-FAZA PET/CT imaging in lung cancer and high-grade glioma: open issues in clinical application. Clin Transl Imaging 2017;5(4):389–97.

70. Sharma P, Mukherjee A, Bal C, et al. Somatostatin receptor-based PET/CT of intracranial tumors: a potential area of application for 68 Ga-DOTA peptides? AJR Am J Roentgenol 2013;201(6):1340–7.

71. Afshar-Oromieh A, Giesel FL, Linhart HG, et al. Detection of cranial meningiomas: comparison of 68Ga-DOTATOC PET/CT and contrast-enhanced MRI. Eur J Nucl Med Mol Imaging 2012;39(9): 1409–15.

72. Milker-Zabel S, Zabel-du Bois A, Henze M, et al. Improved target volume definition for fractionated stereotactic radiotherapy in patients with intracranial meningiomas by correlation of CT, MRI, and [68Ga]-DOTATOC-PET. Int J Radiat Oncol Biol Phys 2006; 65(1):222–7.

73. Kiviniemi A, Gardberg M, Frantzén J, et al. Somatostatin receptor subtype 2 in high-grade gliomas: PET/CT with (68)Ga-DOTA-peptides, correlation to prognostic markers, and implications for targeted radiotherapy. EJNMMI Res 2015;5:25.

74. Ghosh A, Heston WDW. Tumor target prostate specific membrane antigen (PSMA) and its regulation in prostate cancer. J Cell Biochem 2004;91(3): 528–39.

75. Chang SS, Reuter VE, Heston WD, et al. Five different anti-prostate-specific membrane antigen (PSMA) antibodies confirm PSMA expression in

tumor-associated neovasculature. Cancer Res 1999; 59(13):3192–8.

76. Sterzing F, Kratochwil C, Fiedler H, et al. 68)Ga-PSMA-11 PET/CT: a new technique with high potential for the radiotherapeutic management of prostate cancer patients. Eur J Nucl Med Mol Imaging 2016; 43(1):34–41.

77. Dureja S, Thakral P, Pant V, et al. Rare sites of metastases in prostate cancer detected on Ga-68 PSMA PET/CT scan—a case series. Indian J Nucl Med 2017;32(1):13.

78. Sasikumar A, Joy A, Pillai MRA, et al. Diagnostic Value of 68Ga PSMA-11 PET/CT Imaging of Brain Tumors-Preliminary Analysis. Clin Nucl Med 2017; 42(1):e41–8.

79. Salas Fragomeni RA, Amir T, Sheikhbahaei S, et al. Imaging of nonprostate cancers using PSMA-targeted radiotracers: rationale, current state of the field, and a call to arms. J Nucl Med 2018;59(6):871–7.

80. Salas Fragomeni RA, Menke JR, Holdhoff M, et al. Prostate-specific membrane antigen-targeted imaging With [18F]DCFPyL in High-Grade Gliomas. Clin Nucl Med 2017;42(10):e433–5.

81. Sheikhbahaei S, Werner RA, Solnes LB, et al. Prostate-specific membrane antigen (PSMA)-Targeted PET imaging of prostate cancer: an update on important pitfalls. Semin Nucl Med 2019;49(4): 255–70.

82. Salas Fragomeni RA, Pienta KJ, Pomper MG, et al. Uptake of Prostate-Specific Membrane Antigen-Targeted 18F-DCFPyL in Cerebral Radionecrosis: Implications for Diagnostic Imaging of High-Grade Gliomas. Clin Nucl Med 2018;43(11): e419–21.

83. Huang, Ya-Yao. An overview of PET radiopharmaceuticals in clinical use: regulatory, quality and pharmacopeia monographs of the United States and Europe. In: Shahzad A, Bashir S, editors. Nuclear medicine Physics. United Kingdom: IntechOpen; 2019. p. 35–58.

84. Schwarz S, Norenberg J, Berridge M, et al. The future of USP monographs for PET drugs. J Nucl Med 2013;54(3):472–5.

Role of Functional Magnetic Resonance Imaging in the Presurgical Mapping of Brain Tumors

Rozita Jalilianhasanpour, MD[a], Elham Beheshtian, MD[a], Daniel Ryan, MD[a], Licia P. Luna, MD, PhD[a], Shruti Agarwal, PhD[a], Jay J. Pillai, MD[a,b], Haris I. Sair, MD[a,c], Sachin K. Gujar, MBBS[a,*]

KEYWORDS

- Brain mapping • Functional MR imaging • Task fMR imaging • Resting state fMR imaging
- Presurgical mapping

KEY POINTS

- Functional neuroimaging has been shown to be a valuable tool in preoperative mapping of brain functions in patients with tumors and provides reliable in vivo assessment of the eloquent cortex to minimize the risk of postsurgical morbidity.
- Task-based functional magnetic resonance (tb-fMR) imaging is the most commonly used method for noninvasive assessment of eloquent cortex and can reliably display cortical activity, including sensorimotor, language, and visual functions.
- Emerging evidence suggests that resting state functional MR imaging is a promising tool in addition to tb-fMR imaging in clinical settings, and it has the potential to become the noninvasive standard tool for surgical planning and a biomarker of prognosis in patients with brain tumor.
- Although functional MR imaging is a powerful tool that can significantly influence the planning for brain tumor surgery, there are some limitations to this technique that should be addressed in order to optimally perform and interpret the results in clinical practice.

INTRODUCTION

When approached with the task of brain tumor resection, finding a balance between maximizing resection and minimizing injury to eloquent brain parenchyma is paramount. Technological advances have enabled the functional mapping of regions of the brain, which can be used for many clinical applications and investigative opportunities. Specifically, the advent of blood oxygenation level–dependent (BOLD) functional magnetic resonance (fMR) imaging has allowed researchers and clinicians to measure physiologic fluctuations in brain oxygenation related to neuronal activity with good spatial resolution. When coupled with intraoperative awake functional mapping, an avoidance of unanticipated resection-related deficits can substantially reduce the risk of morbidity of neurosurgical procedures.[1] This article highlights the benefits that task-based fMR (tb-fMR) imaging has provided to surgical therapeutic practice.

[a] Division of Neuroradiology, The Russell H. Morgan Department of Radiology and Radiological Science, Johns Hopkins University School of Medicine, 600 North Wolfe Street, Baltimore, MD 21287, USA; [b] Department of Neurosurgery, Johns Hopkins University School of Medicine, 1800 Orleans Street, Baltimore, MD 21287, USA; [c] The Malone Center for Engineering in Healthcare, The Whiting School of Engineering, Johns Hopkins University, 3400 North Charles Street, Baltimore, MD 21218, USA
* Corresponding author. Department of Radiology and Radiological Science, Division of Neuroradiology, Johns Hopkins University School of Medicine, 600 North Wolfe Street, Phipps B-100, Baltimore, MD 21287.
E-mail address: sgujar1@jhmi.edu

Radiol Clin N Am 59 (2021) 377–393
https://doi.org/10.1016/j.rcl.2021.02.001
0033-8389/21/© 2021 Elsevier Inc. All rights reserved.

BACKGROUND OF FUNCTIONAL MAGNETIC RESONANCE IMAGING (BLOOD OXYGENATION LEVEL–DEPENDENT SIGNAL, FUNCTIONAL MAGNETIC RESONANCE IMAGING STUDY DESIGN)

fMR imaging is typically performed using the BOLD contrast technique, described by Ogawa and colleagues[2] in 1990. Deoxygenated hemoglobin, being paramagnetic, results in increased local susceptibility changes. In contrast, oxygenated hemoglobin is diamagnetic. Gradient echo techniques sensitive to these susceptibility changes can be used to determine relative oxyhemoglobin versus deoxyhemoglobin concentrations in blood. The variation of BOLD signal changes as a function of time in response to neural activity is called the hemodynamic response function.[3] The principle of neurovascular coupling states that, for a given set of neurons that are active, there are changes in local field potential that induce regional neurovascular changes, which result in an overall influx of local oxygenated blood, thus increasing relative signal on BOLD magnetic resonance (MR) imaging. Therefore, during acquisition of BOLD MR imaging, a patient that is actively engaging in a particular task shows increased relative signal in brain areas subserving the task.

Using this principle, investigators designed specific functional tasks presented at regular or random intervals to study patients under alternating blocks of exposure or under the condition of sporadic measured events. Simple task-based experimental design allows the control of behavior in a manner that may be easily reproduced and from which clinicians can assign cortical functional regions. Through task structure previously measured in healthy persons, the same experimental design can be applied to patients that may have a lesion in the region responsible for a particular task.

FUNCTIONAL MAGNETIC RESONANCE IMAGING: CURRENT CLINICAL APPLICATIONS

Clinical use of fMR imaging is a recent phenomenon with about 20 years of collective experience. The main clinical application is in the presurgical evaluation and mapping of patients with structural lesions such as brain tumors, and in patients with epilepsy.[4] Preoperative fMR imaging studies have been shown to be helpful to surgeons for mapping of eloquent cortex and proximity to the target lesion, allowing informed decisions to be made regarding potential risks or safety of surgical resection and the surgical trajectory, and may influence the need for intraoperative cortical

mapping.[5] When fMR imaging is used for presurgical planning, the choice of task paradigms to be used depends mainly on the location of the lesion.[6] For example, if the tumor is located in the posterior frontal lobe, motor paradigms can be used to map the motor strip.

Presurgical mapping has also been extensively used in patients with epilepsy, primarily for hemispheric language lateralization. In patients with epilepsy, a higher percentage of patients show atypical language lateralization than in normal individuals. Sometimes there is discordance between expressive and receptive language lateralization. It has also been used for motor and visual cortical mapping in cases where malformations of cortical development or other resectable epileptogenic lesions are thought to be in close spatial proximity to such eloquent cortical regions.[7]

This evolution of fMR imaging in clinical practice has been facilitated by the development of a CPT (Current Procedural Terminology) code for this technique by the American Society of Functional Neuroradiology (ASFNR) as well as several other studies on this topic. Notwithstanding, it is not the scope of this article to discuss the clinical applications of presurgical fMR imaging mapping in patients with epilepsy, cortical developmental lesions, as well as cortical plasticity in patients with vascular malformations (such as arteriovenous malformations and cavernomas), which are amply reviewed by the authors and others elsewhere.[8–10]

FUNCTIONAL MAGNETIC RESONANCE IMAGING APPLICATIONS IN BRAIN TUMOR SURGERY

The clinical application of fMR imaging has been well established in preoperative brain tumor surgery planning and it is currently part of routine preoperative work-up in patients with brain tumors that are close to areas of presumed selected eloquent brain function.[5,11] In this context, it is essential to maximize the lesion resection while preserving the adjacent eloquent cortex to minimize the postoperative neurologic and functional deficits.[12,13] Beyond significant anatomic variations of the individual human brains, lesions may result in mass effect, with anatomic distortion limiting assessment of normal anatomic landmarks; furthermore, slow-growing lesions may result in brain plasticity and recruitment of brain regions that are not typically associated with a specific task or function. As a result, the eloquent cortex areas adjacent to the tumor may not be localized accurately merely by structural brain imaging.[14–16] Clinical fMR imaging can identify the critical brain regions that are associated with patients' daily functions, such as motor, language, and visual functions. Preoperative identification of eloquent cortices could help neurosurgeons to select the best surgical approach, to plan the extent of the resection, and to optimize intraoperative direct cortical stimulation (DCS).[17–19] Notably, an important question for surgeons is to determine whether the lesion is ipsilateral or contralateral to the dominant language areas. Intraoperative DCS remains the gold standard in localizing the dominant language areas; however, this procedure is time consuming and has considerable procedural challenges and limitations. Taking these into consideration, using preoperative fMR imaging to determine the lesion and language laterality is a useful noninvasive alternative tool that is complementary to intraoperative DCS.[17–19]

Preoperative fMR imaging has several other advantages in addition to determining language laterality. The anatomic relationship of the lesion to adjacent eloquent areas can be examined using fMR imaging; the data can be processed to optimize visualization of essential cortical structures, including three-dimensional displays to guide resection; and fMR imaging maps can be incorporated into the neurosurgical navigation systems to guide the operation.[20]

THE GENERAL WORKFLOW FOR CLINICAL FUNCTIONAL MAGNETIC RESONANCE IMAGING

To obtain fMR imaging brain maps effectively, several key measures should be considered in the process.[21] The selection of the fMR imaging paradigms to be used is largely determined by the location of the lesion or intended surgical target, and the relevant local brain function at risk.[22] Assessment of any existing neurologic deficits may inform the possibility of infiltrative neoplasm causing functional deficits that may not be recoverable. Alternatively, intact neurologic function could aid in cautious interpretation of signal voids in peritumoral regions that may be affected by neurovascular uncoupling (NVU), whereby underlying neuronal activity remains intact but the vascular response is attenuated or absent. This topic is discussed later in this article.

Prescan Interview and Training

Reviewing recent and prior imaging studies is crucial for accurate lesion location and spread assessment, planning of the fMR imaging study, and selection of paradigms tailored to the individual patient. Patients' cooperation and performance are essential to achieve an optimal fMR imaging dataset.[23] Therefore, preprocedure patient training involves necessary steps, including interviewing and assessing the clinical status of the patient, giving detailed instructions, and modifying the paradigm practice to fit the patient's abilities and limitations, before the scan. MR imaging–compatible corrective glasses may be considered at this time if it is evident that the patient has a refractive error. A detailed explanation of the fMR imaging task commensurate with patient understanding is beneficial, serving to alleviate patient anxiety and increase patient compliance for the study. The incorporation of patient instruction before the fMR imaging scan has been shown to increase the reliability of the data.[24]

Data Acquisition

Because current fMR imaging techniques are limited in spatial resolution, a high-resolution anatomic scan, typically T1 weighted, is necessary to subsequently map the functional activations to structural images.[25] The inclusion of white matter imaging, most commonly diffusion tensor imaging, can be complementary to BOLD fMR imaging.

The stimulus paradigm is typically administered visually by displaying text or instructions via projector-mirror system or via specialized goggles, or by using specialized headphones for tasks with auditory presentation. During fMR imaging studies, patients may be monitored using a video camera to determine compliance for movement tasks, specifically the various motor tasks. Performance on selected language tasks may also be determined by using response systems such as button boxes.[23,26] However, the performance of covert language tasks cannot be monitored directly and should be assumed based on the patient performance during the prescan training.[27] Real-time activation maps can be used for a general quality control check (**Fig. 1**); motion or other artifacts can be readily discerned on real-time maps, and any suboptimal task paradigms may be repeated at this time.

Clinical fMR imaging uses a block design, whereby a specific task is performed for a sustained period of time (routinely 20–30 seconds), called the active period (or task phase), followed by the same period of rest (control phase), where the subject is instructed to stay still (as in a motor task) or performed a control task; the active and rest blocks are then repeated for a specified number of times to generate ample signal. Block designs are generally easier to perform, more efficient, and produce more statistically robust results compared with event-related designs.[28]

Because BOLD fMR imaging is inherently noisy and the signal changes caused by activation are

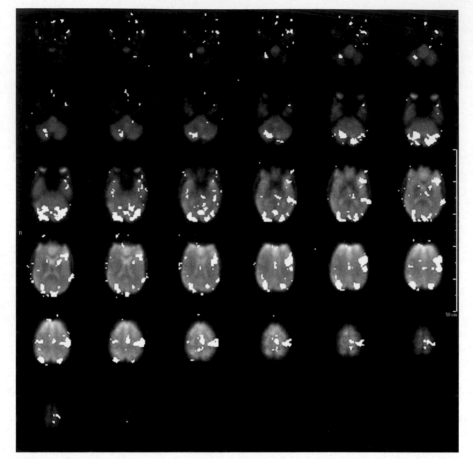

Fig. 1. Real-time BOLD fMR imaging maps obtained during scanning can alert the supervising radiologist if motion or other artifact necessitates repeating the study. However, the real-time maps only show absolute signal change over a certain threshold; therefore, both positive and negative signal changes would be highlighted. To determine positive changes, calculated t scores immediately following the task may be used. Images showing areas of positive signal change correlated with the task, t>4 in this case (images showing the combined signal changes and negative signal changes t<4 are not displayed).

on the order of 3% to 5% from baseline, the repetition of the tasks is necessary to ensure adequate signal to noise.[6,21,22,29] The use of a high field strength is essential; although a 1.5-T MR system is acceptable, the current standard is the use of a 3-T MR imaging scanner. Most functional MR imaging performed clinically uses acquisition of ultrafast images; for example, single shot T2* gradient recalled echo echo-planar technique, with a temporal resolution of approximately 2000 milliseconds and spatial resolution of 3 to 5 mm. A typical fMR imaging study paradigm generally acquires between 90 and 120 whole brain volumes in 3 to 4 minutes.

Postprocessing and Quality Control

After data acquisition, several preprocessing steps are needed before the statistical analysis

and creation of activation maps. Quality control (QC) analysis is also an essential step, which includes assessment of patient head motion, functional-anatomic alignment, susceptibility artifacts, and data outlier volumes.[30,31]

The minimum processing steps for fMR imaging analysis are motion correction and spatial smoothing. Motion correction is performed on each fMR imaging volume, with the first acquired volume typically as the target. Spatial smoothing is performed using a spatial gaussian filter, typically of the order of 1.5 to 3 times full width at half maximum the native voxel size. fMR imaging data are often detrended to account for linear drifts during scanning. If field maps are obtained, they can be used to correct for susceptibility-related distortion. As an alternative to gradient echo–based imaging, spin echo methods can also be used to minimize these susceptibility artifacts; however, they provide lower BOLD effect and lower contrast and have not been widely used.[26] Slice timing correction can be useful to correct for temporal shifts of image acquisition within a repetition time; however, in clinical practice with block paradigm design, this is not necessary.[32–34]

Functional Magnetic Resonance Imaging Data Analysis

A regression analysis using a general linear model (GLM) is most commonly used for fMR imaging analysis. From the fMR imaging data, a signal intensity curve is generated over time for each voxel within the brain.[35] As noted, any area of the brain that is active during the task period results in slightly increased BOLD signal because of relative increase in oxyhemoglobin compared with deoxyhemoglobin. An idealized hemodynamic response curve is convolved with the task design to generate a task-specific reference waveform across the acquisition period. Simply put, any voxel that shows similar modulation of signal with the reference curve is determined to be correlated with the task. For each voxel, this reference curve is fitted and those voxels exceeding a preset statistical threshold are considered active. During this regression analysis, additional regressors may be added as confounds. In clinical practice, motion confounds are often not included, because motion time courses may be highly correlated with a task. A design matrix is then constructed that designates beta coefficients of the variables of interest, followed by calculation of contrasts, or weighted combinations of the beta coefficients, to determine the signal of interest.[6,21,22] For example, in a typical motor task, the contrast of interest is the time period during which the patient moved a specific part of the body. If 2 different active states are present in the task (for example, a widely used 3-phase hand motor task paradigm described later in this article), the contrast may specify activation during movement of 1 of the hands, or activation during movement of either hand.

A typical fMR imaging study comprises approximately 100,000 voxels. A separate GLM analysis is performed for each voxel, which is also referred to as a massive univariate analysis. Given the large number of calculations performed, various methods are used to minimize the activation errors because the surgical resection of areas labeled as no activation may result in significant morbidity. These methods include (but are not limited to) multiple correction methods, such as family-wise error, Bonferroni correction, and false discovery rate, or cluster-based thresholding methods.[36]

Following statistical analysis, activation maps can then be created, and the fMR imaging data coregistered to the patient's high-resolution anatomic images for localization. At this point, the final activation maps are thresholded, to strike a balance between sensitivity of localization and specificity. No single method of thresholding is widely used, and typically the activation maps are thresholded in a qualitative fashion, to visualize robust activation in an area of interest while minimizing depiction of noisy spurious foci. There have been methods to attempt to standardize the thresholding of activation maps, such as using a percentage of the maximum activation in a region.[37]

Role of Streamlined Postprocessing Tools

Research-level BOLD fMR imaging postprocessing software is very accurate but requires significant experience in image processing as well as computer programming for generation of custom-made scripts for postprocessing; the main disadvantage of using this software is the lack of built in functions to export postprocessed images to PACS (Picture Archiving and Communication System) servers and neuronavigation systems efficiently. There are several commercial US Food and Drug Administration–approved software packages available that are more user friendly, allow better image overlays on high-resolution anatomic images, and are compatible with both PACS servers and neuronavigation software. The coregistered images can be downloaded to the neurosurgical computer. The neurosurgeon can then visualize three-dimensional reconstructions that define the relationship between the lesion and the eloquent cortices to guide the brain tumor resection. Many of these packages, being built on top of research software engines, also provide multiple options for customization such as statistical thresholding, image registration, as well as for QC analysis. At the same time, research software allows for additional processing in situations where the processing with the commercially available packages is inadequate.[30,31]

COMMONLY USED TASKS
Motor Tasks

tb-fMR imaging for motor function is frequently used to identify the primary motor cortex, by localizing the 3 main motor areas: foot, hand or fingers, and face/tongue. These areas are arranged in the precentral gyrus medially to laterally following the motor homunculus. Because the hand motor tasks are relatively easy to perform and show robust activation of the motor cortex, these tasks should be performed if the primary motor cortex is to be localized. There are also secondary motor areas that may be important for preoperative planning (ie, the supplementary motor area [SMA] along the medial surface of the frontal lobe) that are also shown on these motor tasks.[38]

Most of the motor tasks that we use at our institution have a block design paradigm with 30 seconds of rest alternating with 30 seconds of activity within each cycle, with visual instructions to stop or go. For foot motor activation, we instruct patients to continuously and gently plantar flex and dorsiflex the foot at the ankle bilaterally during the task period. Occasionally, this causes motion transfer to the head. As an alternative, patients may be instructed to curl their toes (or perform flexion and extension of the toes bilaterally) to minimize bulk body motion. Orofacial tasks can also be challenging because of induction of head motion during the task. We usually perform a vertical tongue movement task where the patient is asked to perform continuous gentle up and down movement of the tongue (alternately touching the roof and floor of the mouth with the tongue), taking care not to move the jaw. If the patient has difficulty with this task, lip puckering may be used as an alternative for eliciting activation in the lower face sensorimotor cortex. For hand sensorimotor activation, a finger movement task including bilateral simultaneous sequential finger tapping is performed with a similar block design, eliciting activation of the somatosensory cortex. The movement tasks often show good activation of the supplemental motor areas in addition to the primary motor cortex in the precentral gyrus. We often use a more complex 3-phase hand-grasp task as an alternative or complementary task for hand motor activation while minimizing sensory activation. In this task, we use a dynamic visual display and the patient is instructed to gently open and close each hand sequentially corresponding with the block length (typically 20 seconds), with an identical rest period following these, repeated multiple times. **Fig. 2** shows activation in the primary hand motor area and SMA in addition to the premotor SMA (language).

Language Tasks

fMR imaging has been shown to be reliable for the prediction of hemispheric language dominance.[39–41] Numerous paradigms are typically used to elicit the activation in the eloquent cortex related to language function. Certain paradigms have been specially designed to elicit activation primarily in the speech production areas (expressive paradigms), and in the receptive language regions (receptive paradigms), whereas others may activate both regions. Language activation paradigms may be further divided into semantic, phonological, or verbal fluency paradigms.

Data published on language presurgical fMR imaging studies are varied because of the complexity of language function and different paradigms applied for this purpose in different institutions. Recent studies emphasize the need to evaluate all components of linguistic functions in preoperative mapping, because language evaluations do not account for particular aspects of grammar, even if patients may have postoperative language deficits. Therefore, it is necessary to identify a specific battery of linguistic tests to characterize cortical language representation at the individual level.[42,43] It may be necessary to perform additional tasks in multilingual patients.

Based on recent clinical experience using lexical semantic tasks, at least 6 core clinically relevant language areas can be identified using fMR imaging: (1) the Broca's area, in the posterior third of the inferior frontal gyrus; (2) the Exner's area, in the posterior middle frontal gyrus; (3) Supplementary speech area (pre-SMA); (4) angular gyrus; (5) the Wernicke's area, inferior (mid to anterior superior temporal gyrus [STG]) and superior (posterior STG and supramarginal gyrus) components; and (6) basal temporal language area.

In 2017, Benjamin and colleagues[44] studied 22 patients with epilepsy and tumor who underwent Wada test and fMR imaging to determine a clinician-driven individualized thresholding, to reliably identify these 6 language regions. Their results suggest that experienced clinicians can form conjunctions from 2 sets of 3 language tasks to generate equivalent maps by individualized thresholding which these maps differ from and are rated as of better quality than those generated with a fixed threshold. They concluded that a fixed threshold, without expert clinician input, may lead to inaccurate mapping in presurgical planning for language localization.[44]

Language tasks may differ in their sensitivity and specificity, which is another important factor to consider during paradigm selection. Some studies suggest that the use of expressive language paradigms could be associated with greater specificity than receptive and semantic tasks based on this study.[45]

Choice of task paradigm may need to be adjusted for patients with neurologic deficits such as speaking and reading difficulties. Specifically, in patients with reading or visual difficulties,

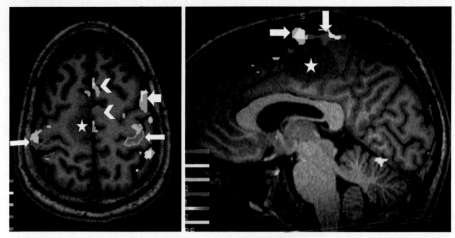

Fig. 2. Patient with tumor centered (*star*) in the posterior aspect of the right superior frontal gyrus. Primary functional area of concern is supplemental motor area and pre-supplemetary motor area. An area of activation is seen in the posterior aspect of the left superior frontal gyrus contralateral to the lesion, representing SMA activation (shown by chevrons on axial and arrows on sagittal images) during hand motor (*orange and blue*), finger motor (*light blue*), and foot motor (*pink*) tasks. Anterior to this, an area of convergent activation is seen with sentence completion (*yellow*) and silent word generation (*green*) tasks. The primary hand motor cortex (*arrows*) and dorsolateral prefrontal cortex (*short arrow*) are seen.

a language task paradigm could be tested via auditory input rather than visual, still activating language, visual, and auditory pathways. Although language dominance is usually left sided, many variations may occur. Surgery involving the mesial temporal lobe ipsilateral to the side of language dominance can result in postoperative memory-related word-finding difficulty, highlighting the value of preoperative fMR imaging assessment.[46]

The ASFNR recommended task algorithms with the aim of balancing varying levels of sensitivity and specificity as well as strengths in lateralization and localization and balancing paradigms that primarily activate frontal/expressive regions (silent word generation [SWG], antonym generation, object naming) and those that primarily activate temporal/receptive areas (sentence completion [SC], passive story listening).[47] In a study using the ASFNR paradigm, SC and SWG tasks were used for language localization and hemispheric lateralization to identify the primary language cortex. The standardized language tasks used were shown to have a high level of intrasubject intrascan repeatability for language mapping in a large cohort of patients undergoing presurgical fMR imaging across several years using both threshold-dependent and threshold-independent approaches. On the ASFNR Web site, parameters for language tasks paradigms are listed, as well as direct download of relevant task PowerPoint files for ASFNR members that can be directly incorporated into the stimulus presentation software.

As per the ASFNR recommendations, the most robust task for language activation is the sentence completion task, which shows good expressive and receptive language activation. The SWG task is a good choice for productive language activation as well as for language lateralization. Additional tasks include the rhyming task, noun-verb association task for productive language activation, and several tasks that preferentially activate receptive areas such as the reading comprehension, listening comprehension, or the passive story listening tasks. The object naming task is also an expressive task that can be used to elicit activation in visual recognition areas centered in the fusiform gyrus; however, this activation can be inconsistent.

There have been recent review articles discussing the current standards of presurgical language mapping using task-based fMR imaging in greater detail.[48] **Figs. 3** and **4** show convergent activation on these maps performed with a battery of expressive (productive) and receptive tasks in patients with inferior frontal gyrus (see **Fig. 3**) and STG (see **Fig. 4**) lesions.

Visual Paradigms

The primary visual cortex is organized to regionally correspond with the receptor field of the retina. As such, the visual cortex can be mapped through systematic visual stimulation. Typically, this is done via a visual stimulus that produces a spreading wave of activity such as an expanding

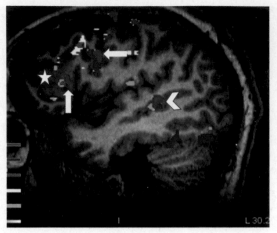

Fig. 3. Patient with infiltrative tumor in the left inferior frontal gyrus pars triangularis and orbitalis (*star*). Primary area of concern is primary productive language. An area of convergent productive language activation (*up arrow*) is seen in the pars triangularis related to the rhyming task (*red*), verb-noun association task (*pink*), and SWG task (*green*). Receptive language activation is also seen as a convergent area of activation along the posterior aspect of the superior temporal sulcus (*chevron*) related to the rhyming task, the SWG task, and the reading comprehension task (*blue*). Additional secondary language-related activation noted in the middle frontal gyrus and prefrontal cortex (*left arrow*).

ring or rotating wedge pattern, elucidating primary visual cortices and distinguishing between areas involved in central or peripheral vision. Often, visual fMR imaging is used to delineate eloquent visual cortex from the planned margin of surgical resection, and preoperative maps correspond well with intraoperative cortical stimulation.[49]

In addition, essential to vision are the networks that facilitate synchronized eye movements, image comprehension, and the understanding of spatial relationships. Areas involved in these networks include the frontal eye fields (precentral sulcus), supplementary eye fields (medial frontal cortex), visuospatial attention region (intraparietal sulcus), visuospatial processing region (temporoparietal junction), visual motion detection (middle temporal cortex/V5), visual cortex (occipital lobes: V1 to V4), and executive working memory (dorsolateral

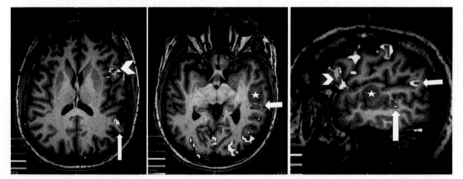

Fig. 4. Patient with mass lesion (*star*) in the left superior temporal gyrus, with primary area of concern being the primary receptive language areas. Axial image on left shows left lateralized productive language areas in the inferior frontal gyrus (*chevron*). The sentence completion task (*yellow*) shows activation in the left inferior frontal gyrus, as well as in the left supramarginal gyrus (*up arrow*) consisting of receptive language region often referred to as the Geschwind region, in this case also lateralized to the left. SWG (*green*) shows productive language activation, whereas listening comprehension (*pink*) shows primarily receptive activation. The axial image on the right shows additional convergent receptive language activation in the left temporal lobe (*block arrow*) immediately posterior to the lesion. The sagittal image shows the relationship of the lesion to the left posterior temporal receptive language activation (*up arrow*), as well as convergent inferior frontal gyrus productive language activation (*chevron*), and finally convergent receptive language activation in the left supramarginal gyrus (*left arrow*).

prefrontal cortex). Although clinical task fMR imaging has not attempted to routinely characterize these regions, the advent of resting state fMR imaging described later in this article has allowed delineation of these regions for potential operative planning.

Visual pathways are so clearly shown by fMR imaging that they can even be evaluated in patients under light sedation, as has been done during presurgical planning in young or uncooperative children to minimize risk of vision loss during resection. In 1 case series, preoperative fMR imaging data were synchronized with frameless stereotactic guidance to determine visual structure–sparing approaches in 6 children who ultimately underwent surgery. No cases of unexpected visual field deficits resulting from false-negative visual cortex delineation occurred.[50]

Memory Paradigm

Memory paradigms have not gained general acceptance for clinical fMR imaging, although much work has been performed at a research level using such paradigms.[7,39] These paradigms can be difficult to perform and interpret, and susceptibility artifacts near the skull base can be a major limitation.

Breath-Hold Cerebrovascular Reactivity Mapping

A major limitation of blood oxygen level fMR imaging in the clinical setting is NVU. As described earlier, BOLD fMR imaging is an indirect measure of neuronal activity based on related hemodynamic changes.[7] This measure requires the presence of a physiologic vascular response to performance of a task.

Hypercapnic challenges have been used to effectively evaluate brain cerebrovascular reactivity with exogenous carbon dioxide gas administration during MR imaging. However breath-hold tasks have been proved equivalent in evaluating the hemodynamic reserve capacity with BOLD fMR imaging.[51]

At our institution, we routinely perform a breath-hold task with all fMR imaging studies for mapping cerebrovascular reactivity. This breath-hold technique includes short-duration breath holds with a longer duration of normal relaxed breathing (16 seconds of a breath hold following inspiration alternating with a 40-second block of normal breathing), repeated multiple times. Monitoring of this task performance is performed by the use of a standard respiratory belt. Postprocessing is performed with specific modeling to account for the differing durations of the task and the control blocks.[23] The derived information is used to validate the ability of a perfusion bed to respond to the physiologic stimulus and reliability of the fMR imaging mapping.[23] This task is another important quality metric that is used in clinical fMR imaging.

Limitations of Task-Base Functional Magnetic Resonance Imaging

Foremost among limitations of task fMR imaging for network localization and lateralization is the need to use tasks appropriate to the relevant anatomic structures of concern. Language and memory networks in particular are complex, involving multiple discrete sites and the connections between them, necessitating the use of multiple tasks in presurgical fMR imaging protocols to increase the sensitivity of fMR imaging language mapping.[52] Tasks used in their localization must have sufficient discriminating power, and the potential for the introduction of bias or artifact must be recognized. Many potential causes of task paradigm failure exist. For example, a large cohort study of patients with tumor and epilepsy with more than 2300 attempted paradigms found that failures were mostly related to problems in patient compliance, or tumor-induced neurologic disorder, especially from deficits affecting speech paradigms (likely caused by longer examination times, and increased cooperation, cognitive demand, and patience required from the patient). Other failures resulted from technical issues such as motion or foreign body artifacts, or scanner problems (system crash, head-coil defect). Physiologic limitations in BOLD imaging occur in the diagnostic power of the BOLD signal, which largely depends on changes of hemoglobin oxygenation state.[53] Intratumoral hemorrhage, tumor mass effect, hyperperfusion, steal phenomena, or drug effects may modify local hemodynamics and thereby produce failures and false-negative results.[45,54]

Another problem associated with fMR imaging in the clinical setting is NVU. As mentioned earlier, BOLD fMR imaging is an indirect measure of neuronal activity based on the related hemodynamic changes. The absence of activation on BOLD fMR imaging does not always imply the lack of neuronal activity. There are conditions under which the BOLD response may be disturbed, such as with large vascular malformations; brain tumors with associated neovascularity, including some low-grade tumors; and in situations with severe proximal arterial stenosis or strokes. This NVU may give rise to false-negative activation.[23,28,55] NVU can result in underrepresentation or nondetection of eloquent cortex (**Fig. 5**). In such settings, the detection of NVU may necessitate the use of complementary electrophysiologic intraoperative mapping.[23]

In contrast, false-positive results on fMR imaging mapping depict an incorrectly large area compared with actual eloquent structures established via direct electrical stimulation testing. Use

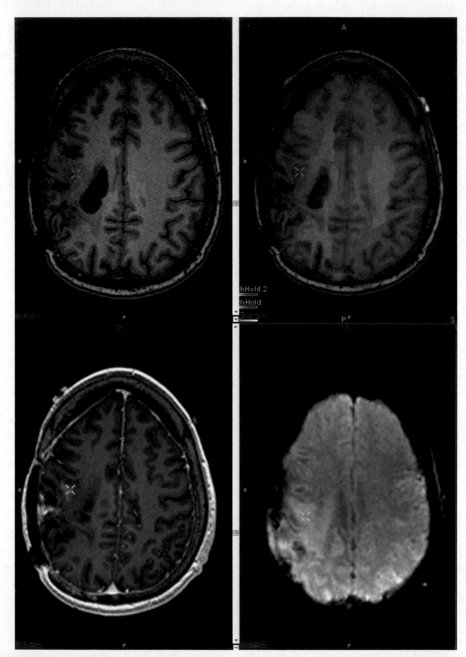

Fig. 5. Demonstration of NVU in a patient with a right parietal lesion, previously resected, with recurrent enhancement and consideration of reresection. The crosshairs localize to the enhancing lesion of interest. The bottom right raw echo-planar images show no significant susceptibility in this region, despite overlying craniotomy. The top right breath-hold cerebrovascular reactivity maps overlaid onto T1-weighted images show absence of cerebrovascular reactivity in the location of the lesion and posterior to it. (*Top left*) Precontrast T1; (*bottom left*) postcontrast T1.

of such an fMR imaging map could lead to a lesser extent of resection, reducing the benefits of cytoreduction.[53]

RESTING STATE FUNCTIONAL MAGNETIC RESONANCE IMAGING

In recent years, resting-state fMR (rs-fMR) imaging has emerged as a powerful adjunct tool to tb-fMR imaging in neuroscience research.[56–58] Significant progress has also been made in attempting to use rs-fMR imaging as a clinical tool.[59–61] The greatest potential of rs-fMR imaging in clinical practice is in presurgical mapping. There are several advantages of rs-fMR imaging compared with tb-fMR imaging in this setting, because there is no need to perform a specific task. This technique is most helpful in situations where patients cannot fully comply with performing the tb-fMR imaging because of cognitive deficits, language barriers, and/or physical disability.[29,62,63]

rs-fMR imaging assesses low-frequency fluctuations (0.1–0.01 Hz) in the BOLD signal while the patient is at rest. Functionally connected regions of the brain show synchronous spontaneous neural activity even if they are anatomically distant.[64] rs-fMR imaging analysis methods can be categorized as model-dependent and model-free methods. Seed-based correlation analysis is a model-dependent method that examines correlations between the time series of a predefined region of interest (ROI), called seed region, and its relationship to other brain regions. Model-free or data-driven computational methods include independent component analysis (ICA). ICA decomposes rs-fMR imaging data into a sum of independent components, each component corresponding with a spatial representation and a time course, without the need of an a priori ROI.[65,66]

APPLICATION OF RESTING-STATE FUNCTIONAL MAGNETIC RESONANCE IMAGING IN PRESURGICAL MAPPING

An initial experimental study by Zhang and colleagues[57] assessed the use of rs-fMR imaging in presurgical planning of 4 patients with tumors located near motor and somatosensory cortices. Their result showed spatial reliability and specificity of the rs-fMR imaging technique for mapping the sensorimotor cortex. To date, several rs-fMR imaging studies have investigated the feasibility of this technique for preoperative mapping in the clinical setting, as well comparing rs-fMR imaging with tb-fMR imaging or intraoperative DCS.[53] Overall, rs-fMR imaging has shown

comparable results with other techniques in the assessment of functional connectivity (FC), and several studies showed the efficacy of rs-fMR imaging in mapping the motor, sensorimotor, and language network, using both seed-based analysis and ICA. However, some investigators focused their interest on the evaluation of FC changes in motor networks during the postoperative period, as well as the FC alterations in default mode network and its relationship with the intellectual decline in patients with glioma.[67–69]

A study by Ding and colleagues[70] used an improved component automatic identification method to localize the common resting state networks (RSNs) in patients with brain metastases. They showed that ICA can effectively and reliably identify RSNs from rs-fMR imaging data in both individual patients and controls. In addition, the RSNs in the patients showed a distinct spatial shift compared with those in the control group, and the spatial shift of specific brain regions was correlated to the tumor location, suggesting functional disruptions and reorganizations caused by the lesions. Furthermore, higher cognitive networks, including default mode, executive control, dorsal attention, and language networks, showed significantly larger spatial shifts than perceptual networks (somatomotor, auditory, and visual networks), supporting a functional dichotomy between the 2 networks even in abnormal alterations associated with the lesions. Overall, their findings suggested that ICA is a promising method for presurgical localization of multiple RSNs from rs-fMR imaging data in patients.

A study by Tie and colleagues[71] in healthy individuals showed that language networks obtained from rs-fMR imaging showed significant similarities with language networks obtained from tb-fMR imaging, especially in the left frontal and temporal/parietal regions. These results were also reproduced in patients with brain tumors and epilepsy.[72] Rosazza and colleagues[73] reported a similar significant correlation of the results of ROI rs-fMR imaging and ICA in 40 healthy individuals. Kumar and colleagues[74] retrospectively reviewed a cohort of patients with brain tumor who underwent preoperative fMR imaging language mapping. Their results showed that rs-fMR imaging can be a valuable tool for clinical preoperative language mapping when a patient cannot perform tasks or if the tb-fMR imaging results are inadequate for accurate brain mapping.

Although rs-fMR imaging has shown potential to localize primary motor and sensory regions equally to tb-fMR imaging in patients with brain tumors,[63,75–77] the data-driven resting-derived sensorimotor networks typically cannot specify and differentiate functional subregions along the central sulcus. Recent developments in accelerated image acquisition techniques may improve the specificity of clinical rs-fMR imaging scans. In healthy volunteers scanned for the Human Connectome Project, high-temporal-resolution rs-fMR imaging has provided separation between the hand, foot, and mouth motor regions; however, the extent to which these advantages might support presurgical planning is yet to be determined.[76,78] In a study by Voets and colleagues,[76] presurgical localization of the primary sensorimotor cortex using fMR imaging was assessed in patients with gliomas. Sensorimotor network was successfully identified in 60.9% of rs-fMR imaging and in 97.9% of patients when using accelerated rs-fMR imaging. The investigators concluded that rs-fMR imaging offers benefits when tb-fMR imaging is not feasible but the data require rapid (or prohibitively long) sampling to attain similar statistical sensitivity.

A recent study by Leuthardt and colleagues[79] using a supervised machine learning approach for rs-fMR imaging reported a significantly higher failure rate of tb-fMR imaging compared with rs-fMR imaging. Studies in patients with neurologic diseases reported high consistency between rs-fMR imaging and tb-fMR imaging in identification of the motor network.[57,80,81] Similarly, high concordance of cortical stimulation mapping, and reproducibility of rs-fMR imaging–derived motor maps comparable with that of tb-fMR imaging in healthy subjects, have been reported in some studies.[57,75,80,82] However, rs-fMR imaging results in language mapping have been variable among studies on this topic. An investigation by Sair and colleagues[83] in patients with brain tumors showed moderate group-level consistency in rs-fMR imaging versus tb-fMR imaging language network identification, and a significant subject-level variability. Also, several studies have reported infiltration and abnormal NVU, which are associated with higher tumor grade but also can be present in the low-grade gliomas, and can alter the BOLD contrast and FC both in rs-fMR imaging and tb-fMR imaging.[84–88] A recent study by Lemée and colleagues compared the preoperative language mapping using rs-fMR and tb-fMR imaging for cortical mapping during awake craniotomies. They suggested that rs-fMR imaging is an easy technique to implement, allowing the identification of functional brain language areas with a greater sensitivity than the tb-fMR imaging, although it might have lower specificity.[89] Furthermore, Park and colleagues[90] conducted a study to compare a supervised classifier-based analysis of rs-fMR imaging data with the tb-fMR imaging in presurgical language mapping. Their results showed that presurgical language mapping with rs-fMR imaging is comparable with, and to some extent superior to, tb-fMR imaging. They reported that language tb-fMR imaging also activated the task-general brain networks (ie, not language specific) in addition to the Broca and Wernicke areas, whereas classifier-based analysis of rs-fMR imaging generated maps confined to language-specific brain regions.[90]

A recent study by Vakamudi and colleagues[81] has shown the feasibility of the real-time rs-fMR imaging of the sensorimotor and language networks in patients with brain tumors. The investigators suggested that this novel approach not only allows real-time monitoring of data quality but also has the potential for real-time presurgical mapping of eloquent cortex in patients with brain tumors with high concordance relative to task activation and DCS localization, within the constraints of impaired neurovascular coupling and/or cortical reorganization.

A major limitation of rs-fMR imaging in clinical practice has been the lack of standardization among studies. Despite advances, there is a lack of standardization of physiologic parameters, pharmacologic interventions, and characterization of disease-related vascular changes, with limited existing data on how these changes might affect the BOLD signal.[91] There are also some limitations within analysis methods. Seed-based analysis is based on predetermined ROIs, which can be arbitrary or driven by tb-fMR imaging.[92] Given that some patients have brain-distorting lesions, the collective database of ROIs may not be useable.[20] Although task versus rs-fMR imaging techniques differ in terms of reliability in functional mapping, certain approaches show similar reliability with respect to mapping the sensorimotor network, and rs-fMR imaging has shown promising results as a noninvasive diagnostic and prognostic tool. However, it is important to address other drawbacks of this technique, such as NVU and artifact susceptibility, to provide the most accurate functional assessment in clinical practice.[91,93]

Overall, rs-fMR imaging has shown concordant results with other techniques such as tb-fMR imaging or DCS in brain network identification.[59,61,94–96] Current evidence shows great promise for the future application of rs-fMR imaging in presurgical planning. rs-fMR imaging may also represent an opportunity for preoperative planning in pediatric patients.[53] So far, only a limited number of studies have been conducted in pediatric populations using passive motor, language, and visual stimuli in candidates for tumor or epilepsy surgery. Other areas of future rs-fMR imaging in patients with brain tumors may also include postsurgery longitudinal follow-up,[97,98] as well as the relationship between presurgery and postsurgery rs-fMR imaging data and patients' neuropsychological battery for evaluation of brain plasticity.[53,99,100]

SUMMARY

Significant advances have been made in the assessment of brain FC since the discovery of synchronous BOLD signals. Functional neuroimaging has been shown to be a valuable tool in preoperative mapping of the eloquent cortex in neurosurgical patients, minimizing the risk of postsurgical morbidity. tb-fMR imaging is the most commonly used method for noninvasive assessment of brain function in clinical settings and can reliably show cortical activity, including sensorimotor, language, and visual functions. rs-fMR imaging has also shown great promise in preoperative brain mapping, as well as postoperative neuroplasticity and functional recovery. Nonetheless, it is important to be aware of the limitations of these techniques, such as patient compliance, artifact susceptibility, and NVU, in order to provide the most accurate functional assessment of the brain.

CLINICS CARE POINTS

- Functional MR (fMR) Imaging is an integral part of presurgical planning in patients with brain tumors and it provides reliable in vivo assessment of the eloquent cortex to help minimize the risk of postsurgical morbidity.

- Task-based fMRI (tb-fMRI) is the most commonly used technique for noninvasive assessment of eloquent cortex and can reliably demonstrate brain regions involved in sensorimotor, language, and visual functions.

- Resting state fMRI (rs-fMRI) is increasingly being used in addition to tb-fMRI and has the potential to become the noninvasive standard tool for surgical planning in patients with brain tumor.

- Although fMRI has been shown to be a reliable tool, there are some limitations to this technique, such as neurovascular uncoupling and susceptibility artifact, that should be addressed in order to provide the most accurate functional assessment in clinical practice.

DISCLOSURE

The authors have no disclosures.

REFERENCES

1. Saito T, Muragaki Y, Maruyama T, et al. Intraoperative functional mapping and monitoring during glioma surgery. Neurol Med Chir (Tokyo) 2015;55(1):1–13.
2. Ogawa S, Lee TM, Kay AR, et al. Brain magnetic resonance imaging with contrast dependent on blood oxygenation. Proc Natl Acad Sci U S A 1990;87(24):9868–72.
3. Heeger DJ, Ress D. What does fMRI tell us about neuronal activity? Nat Rev Neurosci 2002;3(2):142–51.
4. Pillai JJ. The evolution of clinical functional imaging during the past 2 decades and its current impact on neurosurgical planning. AJNR Am J Neuroradiol 2010;31(2):219–25.
5. Petrella JR, Shah LM, Harris KM, et al. Preoperative functional MR imaging localization of language and motor areas: effect on therapeutic decision making in patients with potentially resectable brain tumors. Radiology 2006;240(3):793–802.
6. Bogomolny DL, Petrovich NM, Hou BL, et al. Functional MRI in the brain tumor patient. Top Magn Reson Imaging 2004;15(5):325–35.
7. Gujar SK, Sair HI, Pillai JJ. Functional magnetic resonance imaging. CT and MRI of the whole body. 6th edition. Elsevier; 2017. p. 489–98. Chapter 16.
8. Chaudhary UJ, Duncan JS. Applications of blood-oxygen-level-dependent functional magnetic resonance imaging and diffusion tensor imaging in epilepsy. Neuroimaging Clin N Am 2014;24(4):671–94.
9. Pillai JJ, Williams HT, Faro S. Functional imaging in temporal lobe epilepsy. Semin Ultrasound CT MR 2007;28(6):437–50.
10. Soldozy S, Akyeampong DK, Barquin DL, et al. Systematic review of functional mapping and cortical reorganization in the setting of arteriovenous malformations, redefining anatomical eloquence. Front Surg 2020;7:514247.
11. Gabriel M, Brennan NP, Peck KK, et al. Blood oxygen level dependent functional magnetic resonance imaging for presurgical planning. Neuroimaging Clin N Am 2014;24(4):557–71.
12. Gupta A, Shah A, Young RJ, et al. Imaging of brain tumors: functional magnetic resonance imaging and diffusion tensor imaging. Neuroimaging Clin N Am 2010;20(3):379–400.
13. Brennan NP, Peck KK, Holodny A. Language mapping using fMRI and direct cortical stimulation for brain tumor surgery: the good, the bad, and the questionable. Top Magn Reson Imaging 2016;25(1):1–10.

14. Fisicaro RA, Jost E, Shaw K, et al. Cortical plasticity in the setting of brain tumors. Top Magn Reson Imaging 2016;25(1):25–30.

15. Holodny AI, Schulder M, Ybasco A, et al. Translocation of Broca's area to the contralateral hemisphere as the result of the growth of a left inferior frontal glioma. J Comput Assist Tomogr 2002;26(6):941–3.

16. Li Q, Dong JW, Del Ferraro G, et al. Functional translocation of broca's area in a low-grade left frontal glioma: graph theory reveals the novel, adaptive network connectivity. Front Neurol 2019;10:702.

17. Ille S, Sollmann N, Hauck T, et al. Combined noninvasive language mapping by navigated transcranial magnetic stimulation and functional MRI and its comparison with direct cortical stimulation. J Neurosurg 2015;123(1):212–25.

18. Picht T, Krieg SM, Sollmann N, et al. A comparison of language mapping by preoperative navigated transcranial magnetic stimulation and direct cortical stimulation during awake surgery. Neurosurgery 2013;72(5):808–19.

19. Babajani-Feremi A, Narayana S, Rezaie R, et al. Language mapping using high gamma electrocorticography, fMRI, and TMS versus electrocortical stimulation. Clin Neurophysiol 2016;127(3):1822–36.

20. Lang S, Duncan N, Northoff G. Resting-state functional magnetic resonance imaging: review of neurosurgical applications. Neurosurgery 2014;74(5):453–64 [discussion 464–5].

21. Belyaev AS, Peck KK, Brennan NM, et al. Clinical applications of functional MR imaging. Magn Reson Imaging Clin N Am 2013;21(2):269–78.

22. Brennan NP. Preparing the patient for the fMRI study and optimization of paradigm selection and delivery. Informa Healthcare Inc; 2008. p. 13–22.

23. Pillai JJ, Mikulis DJ. Cerebrovascular reactivity mapping: an evolving standard for clinical functional imaging. AJNR Am J Neuroradiol 2015;36(1):7–13.

24. Silva MA, See AP, Essayed WI, et al. Challenges and techniques for presurgical brain mapping with functional MRI. Neuroimage Clin 2018;17:794–803.

25. Zacá D, Pillai JJ. BOLD fMRI for presurgical planning: Part I. In: Pillai JJ, editor. Functional brain tumor imaging. New York (N Y): Springer; 2014. p. 59–78.

26. Jones RA, Brooks JA, Moonen CTW. Ultra-fast fMRI. Functional MRI: An introduction to methods. 2001. p. 93.

27. Peck KK, Cho NS, Holodny AI. Methods of analysis: functional MRI for presurgical planning. Neuroimaging Clin N Am 2021;31(1):23–32.

28. Zaca D, Pillai JJ. BOLD fMRI for presurgical planning: part 1. Functional Brain Tumor Imaging. 2014. p. 59–78.

29. Fox MD, Snyder AZ, Vincent JL, et al. The human brain is intrinsically organized into dynamic, anti-correlated functional networks. Proc Natl Acad Sci U S A 2005;102(27):9673–8.

30. González-Ortiz S, Oleaga L, Pujol T, et al. Simple fMRI postprocessing suffices for normal clinical practice. AJNR Am J Neuroradiol 2013;34(6):1188–93.

31. Pillai JJ. The significance of streamlined postprocessing approaches for clinical FMRI. AJNR Am J Neuroradiol 2013;34(6):1194–6.

32. Friston KJ, Ashburner J, Frith CD, et al. Spatial registration and normalization of images. Hum Brain Mapp 1995;3(3):165–89.

33. Murphy K, Birn RM, Bandettini PA. Resting-state fMRI confounds and cleanup. Neuroimage 2013;80:349–59.

34. Muschelli J, Nebel MB, Caffo BS, et al. Reduction of motion-related artifacts in resting state fMRI using aCompCor. Neuroimage 2014;96:22–35.

35. Friston KJ, Holmes AP, Worsley KJ, et al. Statistical parametric maps in functional imaging: a general linear approach. Hum Brain Mapp 1994;2(4):189–210.

36. Loring DW, Meador KJ, Allison JD, et al. Now you see it, now you don't: statistical and methodological considerations in fMRI. Epilepsy Behav 2002;3(6):539–47.

37. Voyvodic JT. Reproducibility of single-subject fMRI language mapping with AMPLE normalization. J Magn Reson Imaging 2012;36(3):569–80.

38. Boecker H, Kleinschmidt A, Requardt M, et al. Functional cooperativity of human cortical motor areas during self-paced simple finger movements. A high-resolution MRI study. Brain 1994;117(Pt 6):1231–9.

39. Gaillard WD. Functional MR imaging of language, memory, and sensorimotor cortex. Neuroimaging Clin N Am 2004;14(3):471–85.

40. Rutten GJ, Ramsey NF, van Rijen PC, et al. FMRI-determined language lateralization in patients with unilateral or mixed language dominance according to the Wada test. Neuroimage 2002;17(1):447–60.

41. Sabbah P, Chassoux F, Leveque C, et al. Functional MR imaging in assessment of language dominance in epileptic patients. Neuroimage 2003;18(2):460–7.

42. Połczyńska MM, Japardi K, Bookheimer SY. Lateralizing language function with pre-operative functional magnetic resonance imaging in early proficient bilingual patients. Brain Lang 2017;170:1–11.

43. Rofes A, Miceli G. Language mapping with verbs and sentences in awake surgery: a review. Neuropsychol Rev 2014;24(2):185–99.

44. Benjamin CF, Walshaw PD, Hale K, et al. Presurgical language fMRI: mapping of six critical regions. Hum Brain Mapp 2017;38(8):4239–55.

45. Weng HH, Noll KR, Johnson JM, et al. Accuracy of presurgical functional MR imaging for language mapping of brain tumors: a systematic review and meta-analysis. Radiology 2018;286(2):512–23.

46. van Heerden J, Desmond PM, Phal PM. Functional MRI in clinical practice: a pictorial essay. J Med Imaging Radiat Oncol 2014;58(3):320–6.

47. Black DF, Vachha B, Mian A, et al. American society of functional neuroradiology-recommended fMRI Paradigm Algorithms for presurgical language assessment. AJNR Am J Neuroradiol 2017;38(10):E65–73.

48. Agarwal S, Sair HI, Gujar S, et al. Language mapping with fMRI: current standards and reproducibility. Top Magn Reson Imaging 2019;28(4):225–33.

49. Black DF, Little JT, Johnson DR. Neuroanatomical considerations in preoperative functional brain mapping. Top Magn Reson Imaging 2019;28(4):213–24.

50. Li W, Wait SD, Ogg RJ, et al. Functional magnetic resonance imaging of the visual cortex performed in children under sedation to assist in presurgical planning. J Neurosurg Pediatr 2013;11(5):543–6.

51. Kastrup A, Krüger G, Neumann-Haefelin T, et al. Assessment of cerebrovascular reactivity with functional magnetic resonance imaging: comparison of CO_2 and breath holding. Magn Reson Imaging 2001;19(1):13–20.

52. Unadkat P, Fumagalli L, Rigolo L, et al. Functional MRI task comparison for language mapping in neurosurgical patients. J Neuroimaging 2019;29(3):348–56.

53. Castellano A, Cirillo S, Bello L, et al. Functional MRI for surgery of gliomas. Curr Treat Options Neurol 2017;19(10):34.

54. Tyndall AJ, Reinhardt J, Tronnier V, et al. Presurgical motor, somatosensory and language fMRI: technical feasibility and limitations in 491 patients over 13 years. Eur Radiol 2017;27(1):267–78.

55. Zaca D, Hua J, Pillai JJ. Cerebrovascular reactivity mapping for brain tumor presurgical planning. World J Clin Oncol 2011;2(7):289–98.

56. Stufflebeam SM, Liu H, Sepulcre J, et al. Localization of focal epileptic discharges using functional connectivity magnetic resonance imaging. J Neurosurg 2011;114(6):1693–7.

57. Zhang D, Johnston JM, Fox MD, et al. Preoperative sensorimotor mapping in brain tumor patients using spontaneous fluctuations in neuronal activity imaged with functional magnetic resonance imaging: initial experience. Neurosurgery 2009;65(6 Suppl):226–36.

58. Mitchell TJ, Hacker CD, Breshears JD, et al. A novel data-driven approach to preoperative mapping of functional cortex using resting-state functional magnetic resonance imaging. Neurosurgery 2013;73(6):969–82 [discussion 982–3].

59. Tanaka N, Stufflebeam SM. Presurgical mapping of the language network using resting-state functional connectivity. Top Magn Reson Imaging 2016;25(1):19–24.

60. Kokkonen SM, Nikkinen J, Remes J, et al. Preoperative localization of the sensorimotor area using independent component analysis of resting-state fMRI. Magn Reson Imaging 2009;27(6):733–40.

61. Lee MH, Miller-Thomas MM, Benzinger TL, et al. Clinical resting-state fMRI in the preoperative setting: are we ready for prime time? Top Magn Reson Imaging 2016;25(1):11–8.

62. Gusnard DA, Raichle ME, Raichle ME. Searching for a baseline: functional imaging and the resting human brain. Nat Rev Neurosci 2001;2(10):685–94.

63. Liu H, Buckner RL, Talukdar T, et al. Task-free presurgical mapping using functional magnetic resonance imaging intrinsic activity. J Neurosurg 2009;111(4):746–54.

64. van den Heuvel MP, Hulshoff Pol HE. Exploring the brain network: a review on resting-state fMRI functional connectivity. Eur Neuropsychopharmacol 2010;20(8):519–34.

65. Yeh CJ, Tseng YS, Lin YR, et al. Resting-state functional magnetic resonance imaging: the impact of regression analysis. J Neuroimaging 2015;25(1):117–23.

66. Wu L, Caprihan A, Bustillo J, et al. An approach to directly link ICA and seed-based functional connectivity: application to schizophrenia. Neuroimage 2018;179:448–70.

67. Esposito R, Mattei PA, Briganti C, et al. Modifications of default-mode network connectivity in patients with cerebral glioma. PLoS One 2012;7(7):e40231.

68. Zhang H, Shi Y, Yao C, et al. Alteration of the intra- and cross- hemisphere posterior default mode network in frontal lobe glioma patients. Sci Rep 2016;6:26972.

69. Xu H, Ding S, Hu X, et al. Reduced efficiency of functional brain network underlying intellectual decline in patients with low-grade glioma. Neurosci Lett 2013;543:27–31.

70. Ding JR, Zhu F, Hua B, et al. Presurgical localization and spatial shift of resting state networks in patients with brain metastases. Brain Imaging Behav 2019;13(2):408–20.

71. Tie Y, Rigolo L, Norton IH, et al. Defining language networks from resting-state fMRI for surgical

planning–a feasibility study. Hum Brain Mapp 2014;35(3):1018–30.

72. Branco P, Seixas D, Deprez S, et al. Resting-state functional magnetic resonance imaging for language preoperative planning. Front Hum Neurosci 2016;10:11.

73. Rosazza C, Minati L, Ghielmetti F, et al. Functional connectivity during resting-state functional MR imaging: study of the correspondence between independent component analysis and region-of-interest-based methods. AJNR Am J Neuroradiol 2012;33(1):180–7.

74. Kumar VA, Heiba IM, Prabhu SS, et al. The role of resting-state functional MRI for clinical preoperative language mapping. Cancer Imaging 2020;20(1):47.

75. Smith SM, Fox PT, Miller KL, et al. Correspondence of the brain's functional architecture during activation and rest. Proc Natl Acad Sci U S A 2009; 106(31):13040–5.

76. Voets NL, Plaha P, Parker Jones O, et al. Presurgical localization of the primary sensorimotor cortex in gliomas. Clin Neuroradiol 2021;31:245–56. https://doi. org/10.1007/s00062-020-00879-1.

77. Rosazza C, Aquino D, D'Incerti L, et al. Preoperative mapping of the sensorimotor cortex: comparative assessment of task-based and resting-state FMRI. PLoS One 2014;9(6):e98860.

78. Smith SM, Beckmann CF, Andersson J, et al. Resting-state fMRI in the human connectome project. Neuroimage 2013;80:144–68.

79. Leuthardt EC, Guzman G, Bandt SK, et al. Integration of resting state functional MRI into clinical practice - a large single institution experience. PLoS One 2018;13(6):e0198349.

80. Shimony JS, Zhang D, Johnston JM, et al. Resting-state spontaneous fluctuations in brain activity: a new paradigm for presurgical planning using fMRI. Acad Radiol 2009;16(5):578–83.

81. Vakamudi K, Posse S, Jung R, et al. Real-time pre-surgical resting-state fMRI in patients with brain tumors: Quality control and comparison with task-fMRI and intraoperative mapping. Hum Brain Mapp 2020;41(3):797–814.

82. Mannfolk P, Nilsson M, Hansson H, et al. Can resting-state functional MRI serve as a complement to task-based mapping of sensorimotor function? A test-retest reliability study in healthy volunteers. J Magn Reson Imaging 2011;34(3):511–7.

83. Sair HI, Yahyavi-Firouz-Abadi N, Calhoun VD, et al. Presurgical brain mapping of the language network in patients with brain tumors using resting-state fMRI: Comparison with task fMRI. Hum Brain Mapp 2016;37(3):913–23.

84. Hou BL, Bradbury M, Peck KK, et al. Effect of brain tumor neovasculature defined by rCBV on BOLD fMRI activation volume in the primary motor cortex. Neuroimage 2006;32(2):489–97.

85. Jiang Z, Krainik A, David O, et al. Impaired fMRI activation in patients with primary brain tumors. Neuroimage 2010;52(2):538–48.

86. Holodny AI, Schulder M, Liu WC, et al. The effect of brain tumors on BOLD functional MR imaging activation in the adjacent motor cortex: implications for image-guided neurosurgery. AJNR Am J Neuroradiol 2000;21(8):1415–22.

87. Agarwal S, Sair HI, Airan R, et al. Demonstration of brain tumor-induced neurovascular uncoupling in resting-state fMRI at ultrahigh field. Brain Connect 2016;6(4):267–72.

88. Pak RW, Hadjiabadi DH, Senarathna J, et al. Implications of neurovascular uncoupling in functional magnetic resonance imaging (fMRI) of brain tumors. J Cereb Blood Flow Metab 2017;37(11): 3475–87.

89. Lemée JM, Berro DH, Bernard F, et al. Resting-state functional magnetic resonance imaging versus task-based activity for language mapping and correlation with perioperative cortical mapping. Brain Behav 2019;9(10):e01362.

90. Park KY, Lee JJ, Dierker D, et al. Mapping language function with task-based vs. resting-state functional MRI. PLoS One 2020;15(7):e0236423.

91. Chen JE, Glover GH. Functional magnetic resonance imaging methods. Neuropsychol Rev 2015; 25(3):289–313.

92. Caballero-Gaudes C, Reynolds RC. Methods for cleaning the BOLD fMRI signal. Neuroimage 2017;154:128–49.

93. Agarwal S, Lu H, Pillai JJ. Value of frequency domain resting-state functional magnetic resonance imaging metrics amplitude of low-frequency fluctuation and fractional amplitude of low-frequency fluctuation in the assessment of brain tumor-induced neurovascular uncoupling. Brain Connect 2017;7(6):382–9.

94. Hou BL, Bhatia S, Carpenter JS. Quantitative comparisons on hand motor functional areas determined by resting state and task BOLD fMRI and anatomical MRI for pre-surgical planning of patients with brain tumors. Neuroimage Clin 2016; 11:378–87.

95. Cochereau J, Deverdun J, Herbet G, et al. Comparison between resting state fMRI networks and responsive cortical stimulations in glioma patients. Hum Brain Mapp 2016;37(11):3721–32.

96. Qiu TM, Yan CG, Tang WJ, et al. Localizing hand motor area using resting-state fMRI: validated with direct cortical stimulation. Acta Neurochir (Wien) 2014;156(12):2295–302.

97. Boyer A, Deverdun J, Duffau H, et al. Longitudinal changes in cerebellar and thalamic spontaneous neuronal activity after wide-awake surgery of brain tumors: a resting-state fMRI study. Cerebellum 2016;15(4):451–65.

98. Ives-Deliperi VL, Butler JT. Functional mapping in pediatric epilepsy surgical candidates: functional magnetic resonance imaging under sedation with chloral hydrate. Pediatr Neurol 2015;53(6): 478–84.

99. Vassal M, Charroud C, Deverdun J, et al. Recovery of functional connectivity of the sensorimotor network after surgery for diffuse low-grade gliomas involving the supplementary motor area. J Neurosurg 2017;126(4):1181–90.

100. Kristo G, Raemaekers M, Rutten GJ, et al. Inter-hemispheric language functional reorganization in low-grade glioma patients after tumour surgery. Cortex 2015;64:235–48.

Imaging Surveillance of Gliomas
Role of Basic and Advanced Imaging Techniques

Jayapalli Rajiv Bapuraj, MD[a], Krishna Perni, MD[a],
Diana Gomez-Hassan, MD[b], Ashok Srinivasan, MD[a],*

KEYWORDS

- Glioma surveillance • Advanced imaging • RANO • Perfusion imaging • Diffusion imaging
- MR spectroscopy • 11C-Met-PET • FDG-PET

KEY POINTS

- The 2016 revised World Health Organization classification and grading system of gliomas includes additional information obtained from molecular biomarkers.
- Modified Response Assessment in Neuro-oncology (RANO) criteria divide treatment response in gliomas into complete response, partial response, progressive disease, and stable disease based on assessment of measurable and nonmeasurable lesions.
- Pseudoprogression is identified radiographically when tumors undergo growth similar to true disease progression defined by RANO criteria but occurring between 3 and 6 months' after treatment, typically with concurrent radiation treatment and temozolomide.
- Pseudoprogression has been shown to involve reduced relative cerebral blood volume (rCBV) on gadolinium-based dynamic susceptibility contrast perfusion magnetic resonance imaging scans in contrast with increase in the rCBV index in true progression.

INTRODUCTION

Gliomas are the most ubiquitous neoplasms of the central nervous system. According to the Central Brain Tumor Registry of the United States (CBTRUS), the reported average age-adjusted incidence rate for all benign and malignant central nervous system (CNS) tumors is 23.41, with glioblastomas being the most common malignant tumor. Glioblastomas account for 14.6% of all tumors of the CNS.[1] Before 2016, prognosis was based on the interpretation of hematoxylin-eosin–stained sections observed on light microscopy. The revised World Health Organization (WHO) classification and grading system of 2016 was based on the added information obtained from molecular biomarkers.[2,3] The major molecular markers that differentiate the histologic types of gliomas and their prognostic significance are summarized in **Table 1**.

Grading of gliomas combines the observed prognosis from histologic data and expected course of the tumors. Grade I tumors can be excised with low potential for recurrence. Grade II tumors show low levels of proliferative activity but are infiltrative with a potential to dedifferentiate to higher grades of the tumor. Grade III lesions show cellular atypia with higher proliferative indices and are frequently associated with recurrence. Grade IV tumors are associated with active

[a] Division of Neuroradiology, Department of Radiology, University of Michigan Medical School, Michigan Medicine, 1500 East Medical Center Drive, UMHS, B2-A209, Ann Arbor, MI 48109, USA; [b] Division of Neuroradiology, Department of Radiology, University of Michigan Medical School, Michigan Medicine, 4260 Plymouth Road, Ann Arbor, MI 48105, USA
* Corresponding author.
E-mail address: ashoks@med.umich.edu

Radiol Clin N Am 59 (2021) 395–407
https://doi.org/10.1016/j.rcl.2021.01.006

Table 1
Molecular markers of gliomas and their prognostic significance

Molecular Marker	Implication for Follow-up Imaging and Treatment Strategies
IDH1 and IDH2 mutations	Marker for astrocytic tumors. IDH wild-type (without mutations) is associated with an aggressive course. IDH mutant tumors include diffuse and anaplastic astrocytic gliomas and oligodendroglial tumors
1p-19q codeletion	Confirming marker for oligodendroglial tumors if associated with IDH mutations
Alpha-thalassemia/mental retardation X-linked syndrome expression	Associated with IDH wild-type astrocytic tumors. Intermediate prognosis
TERT promotor mutations	IDH wild-type with TERT mutations is associated with poor prognosis
EGFR amplification	EGFR amplification and overexpression is seen in 40% of GBMs. EGFR-targeted therapies have led to a specific imaging techniques using PET-CT radiopharmaceuticals and experimental MR imaging contrast agents
MGMT promotor methylation	In the diagnostic schema for GBM, MGMT promoter methylation and IDH mutant GBMs denote better prognosis
Chromosome 7 gain and chromosome 10q loss	As in the TERTp mutations, the presence of this mutation is associated with poor prognosis in tumors that behave like GBMs
H3 K27M histone mutation	Identifier of diffuse midline gliomas, which are aggressive grade 4 tumors with no targeted therapies and universally poor outcomes

Abbreviations: CT, computed tomography; EGFR, epidermal growth factor receptor; GBM, glioblastoma; IDH, isocitrate dehydrogenase; MGMT, O^6-methylguanine-DNAmethlytransferase; MR, magnetic resonance; TERT, telomerase reverse transcriptase; TERTp, TERT promoter.

mitoses and a propensity for necrosis. Grade IV tumors are rapidly evolving tumors with a relentless progressive course and invariably have a fatal outcome.

TREATMENT AND RESPONSE ASSESSMENT OF HIGH-GRADE GLIOMAS

The International Society of Neuropathology established the Haarlem guidelines to consider how the molecular profile of a tumor can be incorporated into the current grading of tumors.[4] An understanding of this schematic diagnosis is essential because it reflects on the anticipated treatment protocols and hence the prognosis of the tumors.[5]

Preoperative functional imaging including tractography, precision surgical navigation techniques aided by magnetic resonance (MR) imaging studies, intraoperative MR imaging, ultrasonography, and 5-aminolevulinic acid are the

investigative tools available to neurosurgeons to aid in maximizing tumor excision.[6] MR imaging remains the mainstay in the assessment of residual tumor in the immediate postsurgical period and early in the follow-up following surgery. Studies with and without contrast are recommended together with diffusion scans.[7]

Treatment Strategies

Surgical management is considered after radiographic assessment and determining the functional risks to the patient. The Karnofsky Performance Scale is often used to help make this determination. Although surgical intervention is needed to establish a diagnosis with biopsy, gross total resection reduces the bulk of tumor and is the goal before initiating pharmacotherapy. The age of the patient and the performance scores dictate the clinical outcomes.

Radiotherapy and chemotherapy are the next line of defense to mitigate the progression of malignant gliomas. The age of the patient, extent of tumor resection, and the performance score play key roles in choosing the treatment paradigm before commencement of radiotherapy. MR imaging examinations performed after surgical resection are used to determine the extent of residual tumor (ie, gross tumor volume, based on the enhancing portions that remain in the surgical bed). T2-weighted and fluid-attenuated inversion recovery (FLAIR) sequences play key roles in the demarcation of the irradiated margin. Inclusion of this zone surrounding the tumor bed is defined as the clinical target volume.[6,8] Functional correlation using F[18]-fluorodeoxyglucose (FDG)-PET is increasingly being advocated to accurately delineate metabolic activity beyond the enhancing margin of the tumor or included in the radiation field.[9,10]

Alkylating agents and nitrosourea compounds are the mainstay of cytotoxic chemotherapy for malignant gliomas. The oral alkylating agent temozolomide is the frontline chemotherapeutic agent for the treatment of astrocytic tumors such as diffuse astrocytomas, glioblastomas, and diffuse midline gliomas because of its favorable penetration through the blood-brain barrier, good safety profile, and documented favorable effect on the median progression-free survival (PFS) and median overall survival.[11]

Nitroureas are the second line of chemotherapeutic agents and include lomustine, carmustine, nimustine, and fotemustine. Of these agents, lomustine (together with procarbazine and vincristine) and carmustine (used as a wafer placed locally on the margins of the surgical cavity) have been used successfully with WHO grade III and IV gliomas and recurrent gliomas.[12,13]

Antiangiogenic agents inhibit vascular endothelial growth factors (VEGFs) and play an important role in the treatment of recurrent glioblastoma. The titular representative of this class of drugs, bevacizumab (Avastin, a synthetic monoclonal antibody that inhibits tumor neoangiogenesis by targeting VEGF), often results in misleading decrease in enhancement of the treated tumors, termed tumor pseudoresponse.[14]

Immunotherapy is an emerging frontier in the management of gliomas.[15] Several agents have been included in clinical trials and research is still ongoing. Immune checkpoint inhibitors primarily target immunosuppressive factors such as programmed cell death 1 ligand (PD-L1), cytotoxic T-lymphatic antigen-4 (CTLA-4), and indolamine 2,3-dioxygenase (IDO). Nivolumab and pembrolizumab are PD-L1 pathway inhibitors. Ipilimumab is an anti-CTLA-4 antibody currently approved by the US Food and Drug Administration (FDA). IDO

in combination with temozolomide has shown promise in experimental studies. Dendritic cell vaccines are composed of dendritic cells generated in vitro and then loaded with tumor antigen developed from tumor lysate or cells cultured from surgical specimens. At present, only 1 vaccine (sipuleucel-T) has been approved by the FDA. Other immunotherapeutic options include cytokine therapy, adaptive cell therapy, and oncolytic viruses derived from strains of the herpes simplex virus, polio, and adenoviruses are under investigation. Large-scale population studies for assessing the efficacy of immunotherapy are ongoing.[16]

Response Assessment

MR imaging is essential for assessing treatment response and guiding management. The timing of serial imaging after the baseline pretreatment examination is important to assess structural changes in the brain. However, the temporal evolution of the changes is important and is taken into context relative to the patient's clinical status. The methodology used to measure response has evolved, but all of the following criteria are modifications from the WHO response criteria reported in 1981,[17] which measured tumors in 2 dimensions.

The Macdonald criteria

These criteria for glioblastoma treatment assessment in 1990[18] were established in clinical trials to standardize definitions of the imaging features combined with clinical assessments and the use of corticosteroids. Four criteria are summarized as follows:

- Complete response (CR): resolution of all enhancing lesions over 4 weeks without the concomitant appearance of new lesions. Patients needed to show clinical improvement with administration of corticosteroids.
- Partial response (PR): 50% or more decrease in the enhancement of all measurable lesions over 4 weeks without concomitant appearance of new lesions in patients and continued stability or improvement on reduced dosage of steroids.
- Stable disease (SD): clinical stability without features suggestive of progression of disease (PD), PR, or CR.
- PD: 25% or more increase in the enhancing lesions with or without appearance of new lesions, together with clinical deterioration.

The Macdonald criteria were limited for the following reasons. There was significant interobserver variability in their application. This methodology also did not take into account the difficulty in measuring residual tumors with irregular contours and the presence of new areas of enhancement after resection. Assessment of multifocal disease was also not included in these criteria. In addition, antiangiogenic therapy masks any potential residual enhancing disease.[7,19]

AVAglio criteria

The Avastin In Glioblastoma (AVAglio) study (BO21990) criteria were developed primarily to address the limitations of the Macdonald criteria.[19] In addition to assessing PD, these criteria consider pseudoprogression based on the MR imaging features on T2 and FLAIR sequences. According to this scheme, the index lesions are defined as all measurable contrast-enhancing lesions with clear borders greater than 10 mm in diameter. These criteria also include assessment of small or irregularly shaped enhancing lesions and lesions that do not enhance. Nonindex lesions were recorded in present, absent, or unable-to-assess categories. These categories were then used to fortify the criteria for CR where the nonindex lesions disappeared for more than 4 weeks, for SD when these lesions showed no significant change, and for PD when there was unequivocal increase in the size of the nonindex lesion or presence of a new nonindex lesion.

Response assessment in Neuro-oncology criteria

Given that the Macdonald criteria were developed for assessment of only glioblastomas and relied on two-dimensional (2D) measurements and the administration of corticosteroids, it was increasing evident that the criteria were deficient in the assessment of transient increase in tumor enhancement (pseudoprogression), development of nonenhancing tumor during antiangiogenic treatment, and the changes in the enhancing characteristics during such therapy (pseudoresponse). This realization led to the development of the Response Assessment in Neuro-oncology (RANO) criteria[20] in 2010 and their modification in 2017.[21] The modified RANO criteria rely on specific MR imaging sequences to assess for treatment response. These sequences include three-dimensional (3D) T1-weighted precontrast, axial 2D FLAIR, axial 2D diffusion-weighted imaging (DWI), axial 2D T2-weighted imaging, and 3D T1-weighted postcontrast sequences. Lesions were classified as measurable and nonmeasurable. Measurable lesions are those with contrast enhancement, with clear margins, that are visible, and that are measurable in 2 or more axial sections.

Measurements are performed in 2 perpendicular planes, each more than or equal to 10 mm in sections taken with interslice gaps of less than 5 mm. In those sequences where an interslice gap is greater than 5 mm, the minimum size of the lesions for both perpendicular measurements should be twice the sum of the slice thickness and interslice gap. Up to 5 target measurable lesions should be defined and ranked from largest to the smallest. Nonmeasurable lesions are those that do not meet the criteria of the measurable lesions, do not enhance, or lesions with poorly defined margins that cannot be measured with any degree of certainty.

Similar to the Macdonald criteria, the RANO criteria divide response into CR, PR, PD, and SD while incorporating additional features, as follows:

- CR: disappearance of all measurable and nonmeasurable lesions for at least 4 weeks. The patients are required to be off corticosteroids and should be clinically stable or improved since their baseline. The first MR study that shows these feature is termed the preliminary CR. Measurable lesions on any succeeding MR studies indicating unsustained response are termed preliminary PD (progression) or pseudoresponse. Durable CR is identified when the second scan shows continued absence of measurable lesions. Patients showing nonmeasurable lesions at baseline are best categorized as having SD.
- PR: defined as 50% or more decrease in measurable lesion, sustained for 4 weeks or more, with no progression of nonmeasurable lesions, and stable or improved nonenhancing FLAIR and T2 signals. Patients should be clinically stable, on reduced or unchanged dosage since baseline. No new lesions should be shown on follow-up studies.
- PD: defined as 25% or more increase in the product of perpendicular measurements or 40% increase in volume of the enhancing lesions in 2 successive scans. Measurements are compared with the baseline scan showing the smallest tumor measurement. This baseline study is termed the preliminary PD, and the first study that categorically shows the increase described earlier is termed the confirmed PD study. These criteria are applied 12 weeks or more after completion of radiotherapy. PD is also called when there are new lesions with clinical deterioration that cannot be attributed to radiation, ischemic injury, postoperative sequelae, demyelination, or infections. The findings also should not be attributable to changes in corticosteroid

dosage, adverse effects of medications, or seizures. Progression of nonmeasurable lesions is another criterion for PD.

- SD requires the patient to be clinically stable on a reduced or unchanged dose of steroids and without imaging criteria on the MR studies that qualify for other categories, such as CR, PR, or PD.

Immunotherapy response assessment for neuro-oncology criteria

With the advent of immunotherapy, the observed changes seen on imaging studies required reassessment of the criteria.[21] Therapy-induced changes showing increased dimensions of the lesions were deemed equivalent to PD. However, these patients remained clinically stable. Because this observed pseudoprogression was not similar to responses seen on standardized chemotherapies (Stupp protocol), patients were taken off these immunotherapy protocols. Modifications to the RANO criteria, Immunotherapy RANO (iRANO), take into account the adverse effects of immunotherapy and the occurrence of new enhancing lesions outside the radiation field. Clinical improvement on immunotherapy can be delayed, and repeat studies are needed to confirm stability or PD. Ideally, studies should be repeated 3 months or later after initiation of therapy as a baseline investigation. The principal diagnostic features of PD after immunotherapy include clinical deterioration caused by the primary tumor alone, or significant changes in measurable lesions after 6 months or more. If measurable changes are observed in a period less than 6 months after initiation of therapy, imaging at 3-month intervals is required to rule out pseudoprogression.

Pseudoprogression presumably occurs as a result of an immune-mediated inflammatory response or PD before treatment can take effect. In these cases, immunotherapy is not interrupted because of changes in lesion size provided that the patient does not show toxicity related to the ongoing therapeutic agent.[22]

Pseudoprogression and Assessment of Response to Combined Radiation and Alkylating Therapy

Pseudoprogression is identified radiographically when tumors undergo growth similar to true PD defined by RANO criteria but occurring between 3 and 6 months' after treatment, typically with concurrent radiation treatment and temozolomide. Unlike PD, pseudoprogression resolves spontaneously or improves without additional treatment. The incidence of pseudoprogression is reportedly around 36%,[23] making it a frequent occurrence in the treatment arc of gliomas. Pseudoprogression is thought to result from endothelial cell injury resulting from inflammation and upregulation of VEGF, leading on to increasing edema and vascular permeability.[24] Pseudoprogression is seen across the spectrum of low-grade and high-grade gliomas and has clinical implications in that manifestation of pseudoprogression is associated with better outcomes,[25] as is the presence of the O^6-methylguanine-DNAmethlytransferase (MGMT) promotor methylation.[26] The challenge of differentiating true tumor progression from pseudoprogression remains unresolved.[27]

Advanced imaging techniques

Advanced imaging techniques can play an important role in the differentiation of true tumor progression from pseudoprogression (Figs. 1 and 2). The temporal profile of treatment must be known to more accurately predict whether imaging changes represent PD versus pseudoprogression. The latter typically occurs within the first 3 months after completion of radiation treatment but has a range from a week to up to 6 months after treatment.[14]

Dynamic susceptibility contrast perfusion

Apart from showing changes in the nonspecific enhancement pattern (often described as Swiss cheese or soap bubble) and increase in the size of the lesions,[28] pseudoprogression is thought to show reduced relative cerebral blood volume (rCBV) on gadolinium-based dynamic susceptibility contrast (DSC) perfusion MR imaging scans,[29] in contrast with increase in the rCBV index in true progression.[30] The increase in this index is attributed to increased neovascularity, impeded flow through the collateral vasculature of the tumor bed, and increased microvascular density. DSC is based on the variations in the T2 and T2* parameters following the passage of gadolinium through a given volume of cerebral tissue. The passage of gadolinium decreases the susceptibility signals from the baseline with comparative ratios of change in this parameter between a portion of the tumor and the contralateral normal-appearing brain forming the basis of this perfusion study. The range of threshold values for rCBV has been studied by several investigators for pseudoprogression and true progression. For pseudoprogression, the range of thresholds for mean rCBV is reported to be 0.9 to 2.15 and the range of values for the maximum cerebral blood volume (CBV) is 1.49 mL /100 grams to 3.10 mL /100 grams.[31] Figs. 3 and 4 show how perfusion can play a role in the distinction between radiation-induced treatment changes from recurrent tumor. Fig. 5 shows

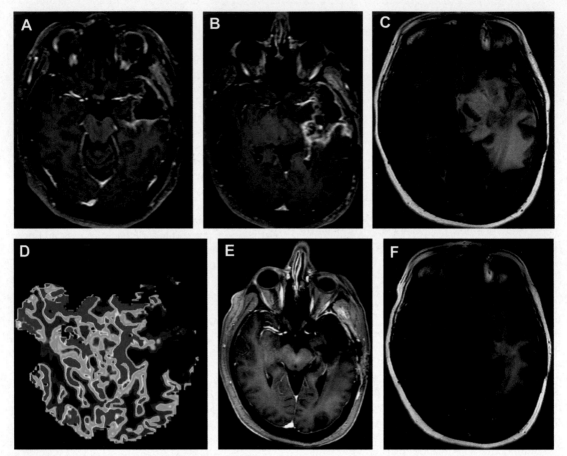

Fig. 1. A 41-year-old woman with new-onset spells was found to have a left frontal oligoastrocytoma and second-ary left subinsular/temporal lobe glioblastoma (isocitrate dehydrogenase [IDH] mutant, MGMT methylated). MR imaging acquired after gross total resection and chemoradiation therapy with Temodar shows progressive changes from postresection study (*A*) to 3 months posttreatment examination (*B–D*) and at 6 months posttreat-ment (*E, F*). Postresection MR imaging shows a rim-enhancing cavity in the left temporal lobe (*A*). Three months after treatment with Temodar, progressive enhancement lining the surgical bed (*B*) and surrounding hyperin-tense FLAIR signal (*C*) is seen but without increased relative cerebral blood volume (rCBV) (*D*), suggesting a higher likelihood of pseudoprogression than true progression. At 6 months posttreatment, the enhancement (*E*) and the FLAIR signal (*F*) have diminished, confirming the initial suspicion of pseudoprogression.

how perfusion imaging can be helpful in interval assessment of tumors during the course of treatment.

Dynamic contrast-enhanced perfusion

This technique relies on the microvascular perme-ability in the extracellular extravascular space. It is essentially a T1-weighted sequence using spoiled gradient techniques in which concentration-time curves are generated to calculate several parame-ters. Of these, K^{trans} (the rate of transfer of contrast between the plasma and extracellular space) and Vp (plasma volume) are higher in true progression compared with radiation necrosis and pseudo-progression. A cutoff value of a mean Vp measure-ment of 3.7 min^{-1} yielded a sensitivity of 85% and specificity of 85% for pseudoprogression, and a

K^{trans} greater than 3.6 min^{-1} had a specificity of 79% and a sensitivity of 69%.[32] Both gadolinium-based techniques do not at the pre-sent have well-defined, validated, and acceptable thresholds.[33]

Arterial spin labeling perfusion

These techniques can be applied to perfusion measurements without the use of gadolinium contrast. Arterial spin labeling (ASL) involves using a series of short radiofrequency pulses to tag a slab of flowing arterial blood in a pulsed or pseu-docontinuous fashion. Subtraction of the labeled and tagged images removes the static tissue and thus the flowing blood is imaged. Given the known volume of the tagged tissue, perfusion parameters can be calculated. The inherent low signal/noise

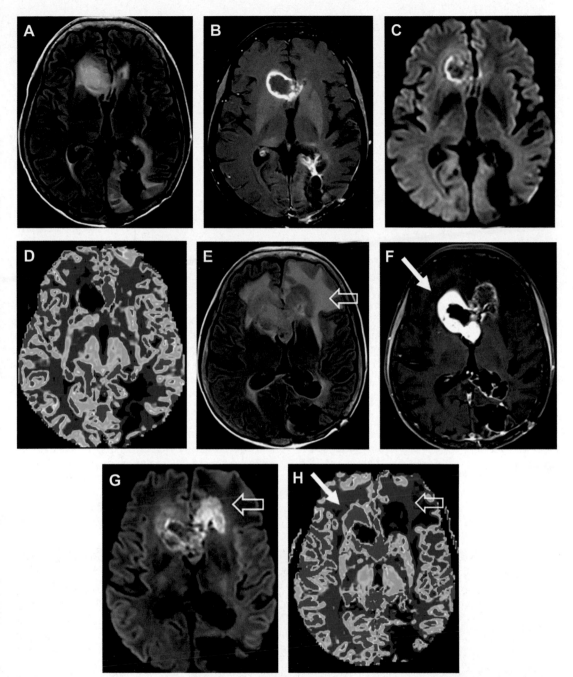

Fig. 2. A 52-year-old woman presented with blurred and double vision with headaches. A mass was identified in the left parieto-occipital region, which proved to be glioblastoma, IDH1 wild-type, MGMT positive. Despite surgical resection, radiation, and chemotherapy, radiographic stability was limited. MR imaging at completion of treatment showed hyperintense T2 FLAIR signal in the right frontal lobe (*A*) corresponding with a rim enhancing and central necrotic lesion in the right frontal horn (*B*). Limited rim of diffusion signal was seen along the periphery (*C*) with no increased rCBV (*D*). After 4 months, true progression is shown in 2 different ways. On the right, the frontal mass has grown, shows greater hyperintense signal and thicker rim enhancement (*solid arrow, F*), without significant change in diffusion in the right frontal region (*G*), but with significantly greater rCBV corresponding with the area of enhancement (*solid arrow, H*), suggesting progressive disease. Similar progressive disease is also shown in the left frontal lobe by significantly increased edema and restricted diffusion (*open arrow, G*) with increase in enhancement (*F*); however, perfusion MR imaging does not show increased rCBV (*open arrow, H*).

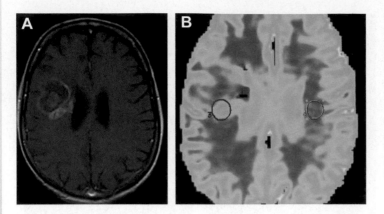

Fig. 3. A 65-year-old male patient with previously treated right frontal glioblastoma presented with new cognitive symptoms. T1 postcontrast MR imaging showed a new ring-enhancing lesion in the right frontal deep white matter (*A*) that could represent either radiation necrosis or recurrent tumor. (*B*) Corresponding perfusion map shows increased rCBV within the posterior enhancing wall, suspicious for tumor. Biopsy revealed tumor recurrence.

ratio of these perfusion techniques requires longer acquisition times and hypothetically is prone to motion artifacts. Echo planar sequences are required to acquire the ASL data and this adds to the distortion of images caused by high gradients. This technique is used primarily as an adjunct to DSC studies.[34] Note that the ASL sequences should be acquired before administration of contrast because the T1 shortening results in concomitant decrease in the ASL signal in the labeled and static images.

Diffusion-weighted imaging

DWI is uniformly included in the suite of conventional MR imaging sequences in almost all scanning protocols of the brain. Analysis of the apparent diffusion coefficient (ADC) was one of the first parameters used to differentiate tumor progression and pseudoprogression. Quantitative assessment of ADC maps has been shown to

reflect treatment response,[35] with further studies involving generation of functional diffusion maps, which can serially assess changes in ADC values in designated voxels in a volume of treated tumor over a period of time.[36] Increasing ADC measurements on these maps indicated higher survival at 1 year, whereas decreasing ADC values indicated worsening course and poorer prognosis.[37] DWI is not sensitive in differentiating pseudoprogression and true progression, with contradictory findings of increased and decreased ADC values reported in both entities.[38,39]

Magnetic resonance spectroscopy

MR spectroscopy is another technique available for assessment of treatment response. N-acetylaspartate (NAA), total choline (tCho), and total creatine (tCr), lactate, and lipids are well-known metabolites relevant to clinical imaging. NAA is an indicator for neuronal viability, cellular

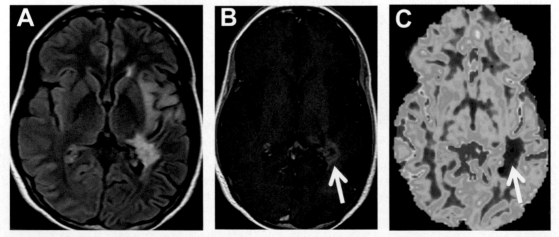

Fig. 4. MR imaging performed for surveillance in a 56-year-old man with previously resected and radiated oligoastrocytoma in the left temporal lobe (*arrows*) reveals new asymmetric FLAIR hyperintensity (*A*) and ring enhancement (*B*) within the left periatrial white matter. Although this could represent either radiation necrosis or recurrent tumor, the lack of increased rCBV on perfusion CBV map (*C*) favors the former as the likely diagnosis. This lesion was biopsied and was consistent with radiation-induced changes with no neoplastic cells.

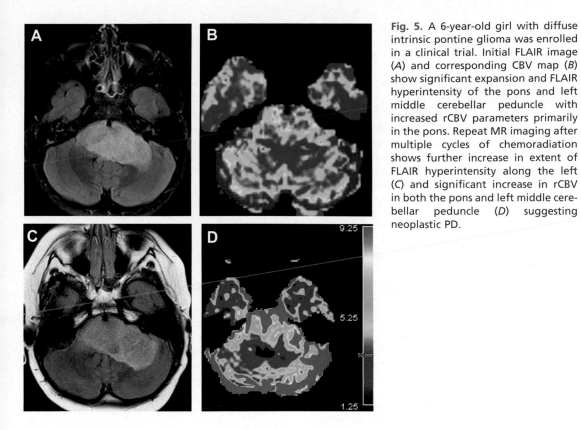

Fig. 5. A 6-year-old girl with diffuse intrinsic pontine glioma was enrolled in a clinical trial. Initial FLAIR image (*A*) and corresponding CBV map (*B*) show significant expansion and FLAIR hyperintensity of the pons and left middle cerebellar peduncle with increased rCBV parameters primarily in the pons. Repeat MR imaging after multiple cycles of chemoradiation shows further increase in extent of FLAIR hyperintensity along the left (*C*) and significant increase in rCBV in both the pons and left middle cerebellar peduncle (*D*) suggesting neoplastic PD.

proliferation is measured relative to the peak of tCho, tCr is related to the cellular energy turnover, lactates are a measure of anaerobic metabolism, and lipids are representative of necrosis and cell death. Given these basic presumptions, high-grade gliomas are associated with increased tCho and tCr peaks. Pseudoprogression has been shown with low choline peaks and increased lactate and lipid peaks together with a measured Cho/NAA ratio of less than or equal to 1.4.[40,41] Radiation necrosis is associated with expected broad peaks representing lipid, lactates, and amino acids. Radiation necrosis is seen to be represented by reduced NAA peaks. Increase in the ratio of Cho/Cr and Cho/NAA, and decrease in the NAA/Cr ratio, is considered to indicate PD or tumor recurrence.[22]

F[18]-fluorodeoxyglucose PET scan

Monitoring response by FDG-PET is limited by its availability and the related logistics of preparation and administration of the radiotracer. In the past, it was thought that increased standardized uptake values (SUVs) in FDG-PET studies were correlated with decrease in the overall survival and vice versa; however, the advent of newer agents, such as 18F-flourothymidine PET (FLT-PET), has changed the perception that PET has limited use

in the assessment of treatment response. FLT-PET has shown promise in that a persistent early decrease in SUV values is a predictor of long-term survival, and conversely an SUV increase to baseline pretreatment levels heralds a poor prognosis. Variations in the FLT-PET technique include dynamic imaging, and this technique has been used to measure the efficacy of treatment regimens.[42,43] Radiolabeled amino acids have been used as PET radiotracers. 11C-methionine (Met) PET in combination with FGD-PET is considered to be the gold standard.[44] 11C-Met-PET has been used to differentiate between tumor recurrence and radiation necrosis, with the former showing uptake of the tracer.[45]

Pseudoprogression and Immunotherapy

Patients having immunotherapy may undergo increase in size and enhancement, which may be related to a phase in time when the tumor is unresponsive to the treatment or may be a manifestation of localized inflammation termed a flare phenomenon. MR perfusion studies have been used to distinguish inflammation from true progression,[46,47] as has MR spectroscopy, because a lipid peak is thought to be associated with increase in lipids, which act as substrates to natural killer cells.[31,48] In the study by Stenberg and colleagues,[46] the investigators concluded that increased rCBV that corresponded to the contrast-enhancing lesion supported the diagnosis of recurrent malignant tumor and that a mismatch showing a volume of rCBV increase smaller than that of contrast enhancement could be identified in particularly aggressive tumor growth. In another study, by Vrabec and colleagues,[47] the investigators were able to show that the maximum lesional rCBV ratios and minimum ADC values in the contrast-enhancing area could serve as potential radiologic markers in differentiating between recurrent tumor growth and immune therapy–induced inflammatory response.

Pseudoresponse and Assessment of Response to Antiangiogenic Therapy

Pseudoresponse is a term for apparent decrease in the size and enhancement of a tumor, being treated by antiangiogenic therapy, on conventional MR imaging sequences in the absence of true treatment effect. Pseudoresponse is thought to occur secondary to stabilization of the blood-brain barrier early in the treatment with agents that target the VEGF signaling pathway. Bevacizumab, a monoclonal antibody that binds to the endothelial growth factor-A, which in turn inhibits neoangiogenesis, and cediranib, which inhibits a VEGF receptor tyrosine kinase, are the 2 principal agents used in clinical practice. Treatment by VEGF inhibitors is marked by significant early response to therapy but without corresponding overall survival. Rebound enhancement is seen in tumors when the patient is on a drug holiday, which again proves that the response is a manifestation of the stabilization of the blood-brain barrier. It is pertinent to note that there is often a concomitant increase in the nonmeasurable perifocal FLAIR hyperintense signals, which may indicate a shadowed progression.[49]

DSC perfusion has been studied as a potential tool for improving the identification of nonenhancing tumor compared with FLAIR signal images, which show both tumor and treatment response as bright signal. Although initial studies showed that decreased rCBV in bevacizumab-treated glioblastoma can distinguish vasogenic edema from infiltrative tumor and correlates with PFS, later studies showed that 8-week changes in rCBV were nonpredictive of overall survival.[14,19,22] Hence, the ability of posttherapy rCBV changes to predict overall survival probably depends on when the imaging is performed after treatment, and the overall role of DSC perfusion in this setting is still being investigated.

ADC maps were thought to be sensitive to the assessment of the presence of viable tumor in the background of pseudoresponse; however, studies have revealed that this does not occur.[50] A pretreatment ADC threshold of 1.24 μm^2/ms reportedly predicts an improved overall survival in patients with recurrent glioblastoma undergoing antiangiogenic treatment,[51] but this remains to be validated on larger trials.

Amino acid PET studies have exploited the fact that tumor viability is linked to increased demand for carbon. Therefore, the potential use of FET-PET and 3,4-dihydroxy-6-[18F]-fluoro-L-phenylalanine (18F-FDOPA) PET to show recurrent tumors previously treated with bevacizumab has been explored.[51,52]

TREATMENT RESPONSE ASSESSMENT AND SURVEILLANCE OF LOW-GRADE GLIOMAS

Diffuse low-grade gliomas (LGGs) are slow-growing indolent lesions, but approximately 70% have the potential for anaplastic transformation within 5 to 10 years of diagnosis.[53] In accordance with the revised 2016 WHO classification, the term low-grade glioma commonly includes grade II gliomas. These tumors often show little to no enhancement and are hyperintense with well-defined margins. However, these tumors require continued surveillance because they have infiltrative margins and can progress to grade II to IV tumors. With higher grades, these tumors are known to have poorer outcomes.[54]

Assessment of LGGs is challenging because they singularly lack the features of aggressive enhancement, which forms the bedrock of stratification by the Macdonald classification.[53] Furthermore, the imaging findings of these tumors are poorly correlated with clinical presentations with respect to quality of life and cognition. PFS is the parameter often used in clinical trials to assess the efficacy of therapeutic agents. Given these limitations, the RANO working group formulated separate and detailed criteria for treatment response in these patients. The criteria are[55]:

- CR: complete disappearance of the original lesion on T2 or FLAIR MR imaging sequences and the absence of any new lesions or imaging abnormalities other than those attributable to treatment. Patients should be clinically improved or stable and off steroids or on physiologic replacement doses only. CR status should be sustained for at least 4 weeks.
- PR: a greater than 50% decrease in the product of the perpendicular diameters on T2 or FLAIR MR imaging sequences without new

lesions, sustained for at least 4 weeks. Clinically, the patient should be stable or improved and there should be no increase in baseline steroid requirements.

- Minor response: a response of greater than 25% but less than 50% in the product of the perpendicular diameters on T2/FLAIR MR imaging sequences without new lesions. Clinically, the patient should be stable or improved and there should be no increase in baseline steroid requirements.
- SD: no change in imaging that meets the requirements for response (complete, partial, or minor) or progression. Clinically, the patient should be stable and there should be no increase in baseline steroid requirements.
- PD: progression based on imaging requires the development of new lesions, radiologic evidence of transformation to a high-grade glioma (increase in contrast enhancement), or a 25% increase in size on T2 or FLAIR MR imaging sequences of a nonenhancing lesion on stable or increasing doses of corticosteroids that is not attributable to treatment effect. Alternatively, progression is defined based on clinical criteria that include definite clinical deterioration that does not have other causes or to decreasing doses of corticosteroids.

The key point in the advanced imaging assessment of LGG includes accurate assessment of tumor growth rate by using velocity of diametric expansion (VDE). VDE is obtained by calculating a mean tumor diameter (MTD) and volume by segmentation of the tumor on axial images and then using linear regression of the MTD over time.[55] Before anaplastic conversion, LGG shows linear growth of VDE of 4 mm/y.

Advanced Imaging in Low-Grade Gliomas

Apart from assessment of growth, LGG also shows the following, which are important for appropriate surveillance strategies[56]:

- LGG has lower cellularity (ADC_{min}), angiogenesis ($rCBV_{max}$), capillary permeability (K^{trans}), and mitotic activity (Cho/Cr) than high-grade glioma.
- Initial low ADC_{min} with high CBV_{max} and K^{trans} values is consistent with poor prognosis.
- A gradual increase in Cho/Cr ratio and $rCBV_{max}$ values is well correlated with tumor progression.
- Critical distortions in quantifying parameters can be minimized by proper region of interest selection and voxel-based assessment.

- Quantitative multiparametric MR imaging can either improve the diagnostic accuracy of conventional MR imaging or provide a better assessment.

SUMMARY

It is important to keep updated with the latest recommendations for serial assessment of both high-grade gliomas and LGGs. Although conventional imaging-based metrics continue to be heavily used for surveillance of gliomas, there is an increasing role of advanced imaging modalities such as perfusion imaging in helping detect early recurrences and in prognostication.

CLINICS CARE POINTS

- The diagnosis of recurrence or progression of high grade gliomas is an essential aspect of management of these tumors.
- Treatment strategies are dependent on the accurate diagnosis of progressive disease and pseudoprogression.
- Advanced imaging techniques may be helpful in differentiating true progression and pseudoprogression.
- Advances in treatment have resulted in distinct changes in imaging morphologies of the tumors especially on MR studies which are the mainstay in the diagnosis and follow up of these lesion.

DISCLOSURE

The authors have nothing to disclose.

REFERENCES

1. Ostrom QT, Cioffi G, Gittleman H, et al. CBTRUS statistical report: primary brain and other central nervous system tumors diagnosed in the United States in 2012-2016. Neuro Oncol 2019;21(Suppl 5):v1–100.
2. Louis DN, Perry A, Reifenberger G, et al. The 2016 World Health Organization Classification of tumors of the central nervous system: a summary. Acta Neuropathol 2016;131(6):803–20.
3. Back M, Jayamanne DT, Brazier D, et al. Influence of molecular classification in anaplastic glioma for determining outcome and future approach to management. J Med Imaging Radiat Oncol 2019;63(2):272–80.
4. Back M, Rodriguez M, Jayamanne D, et al. Understanding the revised fourth edition of the World Health Organization Classification of Tumours of

the Central Nervous System (2016) for clinical decision-making: a guide for oncologists managing patients with glioma. Clin Oncol (R Coll Radiol) 2018;30(9):556–62.

5. Bates A, Gonzalez-Viana E, Cruickshank G, et al, Guideline Committee. Primary and metastatic brain tumours in adults: summary of NICE guidance. BMJ 2018;362:k2924.

6. Weller M, van den Bent M, Tonn JC, et al. European Association for Neuro-Oncology (EANO) guideline on the diagnosis and treatment of adult astrocytic and oligodendroglial gliomas. Lancet Oncol 2017;18(6):e315–29.

7. Vogelbaum MA, Jost S, Aghi MK, et al. Application of novel response/progression measures for surgically delivered therapies for gliomas: Response Assessment in Neuro-Oncology (RANO) working group. Neurosurgery 2012;70(1):234–43 [discussion: 43–4].

8. Niyazi M, Brada M, Chalmers AJ, et al. ESTRO-ACROP guideline "target delineation of glioblastomas. Radiother Oncol 2016;118(1):35–42.

9. Tralins KS, Douglas JG, Stelzer KJ, et al. Volumetric analysis of 18F-FDG PET in glioblastoma multiforme: prognostic information and possible role in definition of target volumes in radiation dose escalation. J Nucl Med 2002;43(12):1667–73.

10. Albert NL, Weller M, Suchorska B, et al. Response assessment in neuro-oncology working group and European Association for neuro-oncology recommendations for the clinical use of PET imaging in gliomas. Neuro Oncol 2016;18(9):1199–208.

11. Stupp R, Mason WP, van den Bent MJ, et al. Radiotherapy plus concomitant and adjuvant temozolomide for glioblastoma. N Engl J Med 2005;352(10):987–96.

12. Wick W, Roth P, Hartmann C, et al. Long-term analysis of the NOA-04 randomized phase III trial of sequential radiochemotherapy of anaplastic glioma with PCV or temozolomide. Neuro Oncol 2016; 18(11):1529–37.

13. Westphal M, Hilt DC, Bortey E, et al. A phase 3 trial of local chemotherapy with biodegradable carmustine (BCNU) wafers (Gliadel wafers) in patients with primary malignant glioma. Neuro Oncol 2003; 5(2):79–88.

14. Hygino da Cruz LC Jr, Rodriguez I, Domingues RC, et al. Pseudoprogression and pseudoresponse: imaging challenges in the assessment of posttreatment glioma. AJNR Am J Neuroradiol 2011;32(11):1978–85.

15. Xu S, Tang L, Li X, et al. Immunotherapy for glioma: current management and future application. Cancer Lett 2020;476:1–12.

16. Young JS, Dayani F, Morshed RA, et al. Immunotherapy for high grade gliomas: a clinical update and practical considerations for neurosurgeons. World Neurosurg 2019;S1878-8750(19)30106–8. https://doi.org/10.1016/j.wneu.2018.12.222.

17. Chukwueke UN, Wen PY. Use of the Response Assessment in Neuro-Oncology (RANO) criteria in clinical trials and clinical practice. CNS Oncol 2019;8(1):CNS28.

18. Macdonald DR, Cascino TL, Schold SC Jr, et al. Response criteria for phase II studies of supratentorial malignant glioma. J Clin Oncol 1990;8(7):1277–80.

19. Chinot OL, Macdonald DR, Abrey LE, et al. Response assessment criteria for glioblastoma: practical adaptation and implementation in clinical trials of antiangiogenic therapy. Curr Neurol Neurosci Rep 2013;13(5):347.

20. Wen PY, Macdonald DR, Reardon DA, et al. Updated response assessment criteria for high-grade gliomas: response assessment in neuro-oncology working group. J Clin Oncol 2010;28(11):1963–72.

21. Ellingson BM, Wen PY, Cloughesy TF. Modified criteria for radiographic response assessment in glioblastoma clinical trials. Neurotherapeutics 2017;14(2):307–20.

22. Margiewicz S, Cordova C, Chi AS, et al. State of the art treatment and surveillance imaging of glioblastomas. Semin Roentgenol 2018;53(1):23–36.

23. Abbasi AW, Westerlaan HE, Holtman GA, et al. Incidence of tumour progression and pseudoprogression in high-grade gliomas: a systematic review and meta-analysis. Clin Neuroradiol 2018;28(3):401–11.

24. Brandsma D, Stalpers L, Taal W, et al. Clinical features, mechanisms, and management of pseudoprogression in malignant gliomas. Lancet Oncol 2008;9(5):453–61.

25. Dworkin M, Mehan W, Niemierko A, et al. Increase of pseudoprogression and other treatment related effects in low-grade glioma patients treated with proton radiation and temozolomide. J Neurooncol 2019;142(1):69–77.

26. Brandes AA, Franceschi E, Tosoni A, et al. MGMT promoter methylation status can predict the incidence and outcome of pseudoprogression after concomitant radiochemotherapy in newly diagnosed glioblastoma patients. J Clin Oncol 2008;26(13):2192–7.

27. Radbruch A, Fladt J, Kickingereder P, et al. Pseudoprogression in patients with glioblastoma: clinical relevance despite low incidence. Neuro Oncol 2015;17(1):151–9.

28. Leao DJ, Craig PG, Godoy LF, et al. Response assessment in neuro-oncology criteria for gliomas: practical approach using conventional and advanced techniques. AJNR Am J Neuroradiol 2020;41(1):10–20.

29. Nasseri M, Gahramanov S, Netto JP, et al. Evaluation of pseudoprogression in patients with glioblastoma multiforme using dynamic magnetic resonance imaging with ferumoxytol calls RANO criteria into question. Neuro Oncol 2014;16(8):1146–54.

30. Sood S, Gupta A, Tsiouris AJ. Advanced magnetic resonance techniques in neuroimaging: diffusion, spectroscopy, and perfusion. Semin Roentgenol 2010;45(2):137–46.

31. Strauss SB, Meng A, Ebani EJ, et al. Imaging glioblastoma posttreatment: progression,

pseudoprogression, pseudoresponse, radiation necrosis. Radiol Clin North Am 2019;57(6):1199–216.

32. Thomas AA, Arevalo-Perez J, Kaley T, et al. Dynamic contrast enhanced T1 MRI perfusion differentiates pseudoprogression from recurrent glioblastoma. J Neurooncol 2015;125(1):183–90.

33. Heo YJ, Kim HS, Park JE, et al. Uninterpretable dynamic susceptibility contrast-enhanced perfusion MR images in patients with post-treatment glioblastomas: cross-validation of alternative imaging options. PLoS One 2015;10(8):e0136380.

34. Choi YJ, Kim HS, Jahng GH, et al. Pseudoprogression in patients with glioblastoma: added value of arterial spin labeling to dynamic susceptibility contrast perfusion MR imaging. Acta Radiol 2013;54(4):448–54.

35. Chenevert TL, Stegman LD, Taylor JM, et al. Diffusion magnetic resonance imaging: an early surrogate marker of therapeutic efficacy in brain tumors. J Natl Cancer Inst 2000;92(24):2029–36.

36. Moffat BA, Chenevert TL, Lawrence TS, et al. Functional diffusion map: a noninvasive MRI biomarker for early stratification of clinical brain tumor response. Proc Natl Acad Sci U S A 2005;102(15):5524–9.

37. Ellingson BM, Cloughesy TF, Zaw T, et al. Functional diffusion maps (fDMs) evaluated before and after radiochemotherapy predict progression-free and overall survival in newly diagnosed glioblastoma. Neuro Oncol 2012;14(3):333–43.

38. Sundgren PC, Fan X, Weybright P, et al. Differentiation of recurrent brain tumor versus radiation injury using diffusion tensor imaging in patients with new contrast-enhancing lesions. Magn Reson Imaging 2006;24(9):1131–42.

39. Asao C, Korogi Y, Kitajima M, et al. Diffusion-weighted imaging of radiation-induced brain injury for differentiation from tumor recurrence. AJNR Am J Neuroradiol 2005;26(6):1455–60.

40. Sawlani V, Taylor R, Rowley K, et al. Magnetic resonance spectroscopy for differentiating pseudo-progression from true progression in GBM on concurrent chemoradiotherapy. Neuroradiol J 2012;25(5):575–86.

41. Bulik M, Kazda T, Slampa P, et al. The diagnostic ability of follow-up imaging biomarkers after treatment of glioblastoma in the temozolomide era: implications from proton MR spectroscopy and apparent diffusion coefficient mapping. Biomed Res Int 2015;2015:641023.

42. Chen W, Delaloye S, Silverman DH, et al. Predicting treatment response of malignant gliomas to bevacizumab and irinotecan by imaging proliferation with [18F] fluorothymidine positron emission tomography: a pilot study. J Clin Oncol 2007;25(30):4714–21.

43. Wardak M, Schiepers C, Dahlbom M, et al. Discriminant analysis of (1)(8)F-fluorothymidine kinetic parameters to predict survival in patients with recurrent high-grade glioma. Clin Cancer Res 2011;17(20):6553–62.

44. Gulyas B, Halldin C. New PET radiopharmaceuticals beyond FDG for brain tumor imaging. Q J Nucl Med Mol Imaging 2012;56(2):173–90.

45. Ogawa T, Kanno I, Shishido F, et al. Clinical value of PET with 18F-fluorodeoxyglucose and L-methyl-11C-methionine for diagnosis of recurrent brain tumor and radiation injury. Acta Radiol 1991;32(3):197–202.

46. Stenberg L, Englund E, Wirestam R, et al. Dynamic susceptibility contrast-enhanced perfusion magnetic resonance (MR) imaging combined with contrast-enhanced MR imaging in the follow-up of immunogene-treated glioblastoma multiforme. Acta Radiol 2006;47(8):852–61.

47. Vrabec M, Van Cauter S, Himmelreich U, et al. MR perfusion and diffusion imaging in the follow-up of recurrent glioblastoma treated with dendritic cell immunotherapy: a pilot study. Neuroradiology 2011;53(10):721–31.

48. Pellegatta S, Eoli M, Frigerio S, et al. The natural killer cell response and tumor debulking are associated with prolonged survival in recurrent glioblastoma patients receiving dendritic cells loaded with autologous tumor lysates. Oncoimmunology 2013;2(3):e23401.

49. Norden AD, Young GS, Setayesh K, et al. Bevacizumab for recurrent malignant gliomas: efficacy, toxicity, and patterns of recurrence. Neurology 2008;70(10):779–87.

50. Auer TA, Breit HC, Marini F, et al. Evaluation of the apparent diffusion coefficient in patients with recurrent glioblastoma under treatment with bevacizumab with radiographic pseudoresponse. J Neuroradiol 2019;46(1):36–43.

51. Ellingson BM, Gerstner ER, Smits M, et al. Diffusion MRI phenotypes predict overall survival benefit from anti-VEGF monotherapy in recurrent glioblastoma: converging evidence from phase II trials. Clin Cancer Res 2017;23(19):5745–56.

52. Galldiks N, Rapp M, Stoffels G, et al. Earlier diagnosis of progressive disease during bevacizumab treatment using O-(2-18F-fluoroethyl)-L-tyrosine positron emission tomography in comparison with magnetic resonance imaging. Mol Imaging 2013;12(5):273–6.

53. van den Bent MJ, Wefel JS, Schiff D, et al. Response assessment in neuro-oncology (a report of the RANO group): assessment of outcome in trials of diffuse low-grade gliomas. Lancet Oncol 2011; 12(6):583–93.

54. Larsen J, Wharton SB, McKevitt F, et al. 'Low grade glioma': an update for radiologists. Br J Radiol 2017; 90(1070):20160600.

55. Pallud J, Taillandier L, Capelle L, et al. Quantitative morphological magnetic resonance imaging follow-up of low-grade glioma: a plea for systematic measurement of growth rates. Neurosurgery 2012; 71(3):729–39 [discussion: 39–40].

56. Bulakbasi N, Paksoy Y. Advanced imaging in adult diffusely infiltrating low-grade gliomas. Insights Imaging 2019;10(1):122.

Neoplastic Meningitis and Paraneoplastic Syndromes

Sangam Kanekar, MD[a,b,*], Thomas Zacharia, MD[a], Amit Agarwal, MD[c]

KEYWORDS

- Neoplastic meningitis • Paraneoplastic syndromes • Leptomeningeal metastasis
- Limbic encephalitis • Anti-NMDAR encephalitis

KEY POINTS

- Neoplastic meningitis (NM) is an uncommon metastatic manifestation of cancer, characterized by multifocal neurologic signs and symptoms.
- In a suspected case of NM, work-up includes detailed clinical examination, MR imaging of the brain and entire spine with and without contrast, cerebrospinal fluid analysis and pressure measurement, and systemic imaging, staging, and restaging of the primary tumor with PET–computed tomography or MR imaging.
- Paraneoplastic syndromes (PNSs) are a group of disorders present in patients with cancer, which may involve any part of the nervous system (central and peripheral nervous disorders) and simultaneously may affect multiple areas.
- PNSs encompass a variety of symptoms or syndromes, including limbic encephalitis, cerebellar degeneration, brainstem encephalitis, striatal encephalitis, and opsoclonus-myoclonus syndrome.

INTRODUCTION

Neoplastic meningitls (NM) is an uncommon metastatic manifestation of cancer, characterized by multifocal neurologic signs and symptoms and usually occurring late in the course of the disease. Diagnosis is challenging but essential to prevent progressive neurologic injury that substantially impairs cancer patients' quality of life. Clinical examination has a minimal role in the diagnosis of NM. The most common tests employed are the brain and spinal axis MR imaging and cerebrospinal fluid (CSF) cytology.

The incidence of NM varies, depending on the primary site of the tumor. NM is diagnosed in 4% to 15% of patients with solid tumors (carcinomatous meningitis), 5% to 15% of patients with hematological malignancies (leukemic or lymphomatous meningitis), and 1% to 2% of patients with primary brain tumors.[1–4] NM is associated with significant morbidity and short survival rates, ranging from several weeks to 8 months. Adenocarcinoma is the most frequent histology, whereas among the solid tumors, breast, lung, and skin are the most common primary sites of leptomeningeal metastasis. Although small cell lung carcinoma (SCLC) and melanoma have the highest rates of spread to the leptomeninges, with 11% and 20%, respectively, breast cancer, because of its higher incidence, accounts for most disorder cases despite a 5% metastatic rate.[5–7] Lymphomatous meningitis is reported most commonly with diffuse high-grade non-Hodgkin lymphoma. Prophylactic treatment commonly is considered in patients with aggressive non-Hodgkin lymphoma, such as Burkitt lymphoma and lymphoblastic lymphoma, because these diseases have a greater than 25% risk of meningeal relapse without central nervous system (CNS)-directed therapy. NM is the initial manifestation of systemic cancer in only 5% to 10% of patients.[2] Synchronous

[a] Department of Radiology, Penn State Health, Mail Code H066, 500 University drive, Hershey, PA 17033, USA;
[b] Department of Neurology, Penn State Health, Mail Code H066, 500 University drive, Hershey, PA 17033, USA;
[c] Department of Radiology, UT Southwestern Medical School and Parkland Hospital, 5323 Harry Hines Boulevard, Dallas, TX 75390, USA
* Corresponding author. Division of Neuroradiology, Penn State Milton Hershey Medical Center, Penn State College of Medicine, Mail Code H066, 500 University drive, Hershey, PA 17033.
E-mail address: skanekar@pennstatehealth.psu.edu

Radiol Clin N Am 59 (2021) 409–423
https://doi.org/10.1016/j.rcl.2021.01.007

intraparenchymal brain metastases are evident in 11% to 31% of patients with NM.[8]

PATHOPHYSIOLOGY

For NM to occur, tumor cells must reach the meninges and CSF. The invasion of the meninges occurs through different pathways, depending on the histology of the primary tumor. These include hematogenous (venous or arterial) spread, neural spread (endoneuronal and perineural), perivascular lymphatic spread, and iatrogenic spread.[9,10] In addition, spread may occur directly from brain parenchyma or bony tumor lesions in the skull, spine, or choroid plexus or from de novo tumors. All routes give tumor cells access to the subarachnoid space of the CNS. With regard to hematogenous spread, tumor cells in the bloodstream become lodged in small-caliber CNS vessels, resulting in ischemia distal to the affected vessel. This disrupts vessel endothelium and surrounding basement membranes, allowing tumor cells to access the CSF around the damaged vessel (the Virchow-Robin space) and the subarachnoid space.[9,10] Tumor cells can gain access to the ventricular system by invading the subependymal lining of the ventricular wall.

The threshold number of tumor cells necessary to reach the CSF and result in clinical NM is unknown. The location of the tumor, however, plays a vital role in the spread. The closer proximity of the tumor to the meninges leads to a higher incidence of NM. Medulloblastomas (tumors located in or near the fourth ventricle) and pineoblastoma (near the pineal gland) are notable examples of this principle.[11] Astrocytomas are not a significant cause of NM. Postoperative NM, presumably caused by intraoperative tumor cell seeding of the CSF, has been reported in 5% to 40% of patients after craniotomy. The risk of NM is higher in patients undergoing craniotomy for posterior fossa metastases than supratentorial metastases.[12]

CLINICAL FEATURES

Clinical diagnosis of NM is challenging, and sufficient suspicion is required to warrant diagnostic testing. A majority of patients present with multifocal neurologic symptoms that vary according to anatomic areas of the CNS: cerebrum (15% of patients), cranial nerve/brainstem (35%), and spinal cord (60%)[13,14] (**Table 1**). Cerebral symptoms include headache, dizziness/vertigo, confusion, fatigue, gait instability, aphasia, altered mental status, seizure, hemiparesis, and numbness. The most common of these manifestations are headache and mental status changes.[1,2,13–15] When

the posterior fossa is the primary site of the NM, most clinical symptoms are due to cerebellar dysfunction; these include unsteady gait, diplopia, ataxia, and falls. Cranial nerve lesions are reported in approximately 40% of patients.[1,2,13–15] The most common dysfunctions are of the oculomotor, facial, cochlear, and optic nerves. Cranial nerve and brainstem symptoms include loss of visual acuity, diplopia, facial muscle weakness, hearing loss, dysphagia and dysarthria, hoarseness, decreased hearing, and facial pain or numbness. Diplopia is the most common symptom of cranial nerve dysfunction, with cranial nerve VI the most frequently affected, followed by cranial nerves III and IV.[1,2,13–16] Symptoms involving the spinal cord may include lumbar pain, limb paresis or paralysis, bowel and bladder dysfunction, and loss of reflexes leading to cauda equine or cauda medullaris syndrome.

One of the most common complications of NM is communicating hydrocephalus due to blockage of the basal cisterns and obstruction to CSF absorption at the arachnoid granulation level.[9,17] Less common complications are basal ganglia or internal capsule infarctions due to vascular compression and development of vasculitis, with vasospasm and thrombosis from exudate surrounding small perforating vessels. These are seen more commonly in pediatric patients.

DIAGNOSIS

NM is diagnosed using the National Comprehensive Cancer Network guidelines.[18] Diagnosis is established on positive CSF cytology for malignant cells, and/or leptomeningeal and nodular enhancement on computed tomography (CT) or MR imaging in a patient with known malignancy. There are ongoing efforts by Response Assessment in Neuro-Oncology (the Leptomeningeal Assessment in Neuro-Oncology scorecard) and the European Association of Neuro-Oncology–European Society of Medical Oncology to standardize the diagnostic work-up and interpretation of NM.[19,20] These groups use clinical symptoms, imaging, and CSF analysis for diagnosis and assessment of treatment. Unfortunately, neither of the 2 systems has been validated.

In a suspected case of NM, work-up includes detailed clinical examination, MR imaging of the brain and entire spine with and without contrast, CSF analysis and pressure measurement, and systemic imaging, staging, and restaging of the primary tumor with PET-CT or MR imaging. Although positive CSF cytology provides the highest degree of certainty in an NM diagnosis, it is not

Table 1	
Major neurologic symptoms of neoplastic meningitis	
Cerebral symptoms	Headache
	Mental changes
	Nausea
	Vertigo
	Vomiting
	Seizures
	Communicating hydrocephalus
	Gait alterations
	Coordination disorders
Cranial nerve dysfunction	Diplopia
	Vision loss
	Hearing loss
	Facial paresis
	Hoarseness
	Hypoacusia
	Ocular motility deficits
	Dysphagia
Spinal symptoms	Bilateral/unilateral pain
	Loss of reflexes
	Paresthesia
	Motor deficits
	Weakness in extremities

essential for initiating treatment if the remainder of the evaluation is supportive of NM.

Diagnosis of NM largely depends on documenting circulating tumor cells in the CSF.[21] The site of the CSF tap and yield depend on the symptoms and type of the primary malignancy. Cytology of CSF obtained by lumbar puncture is more likely to be positive than CSF obtained from ventricles if spinal cord–related symptoms are present and vice versa if cranial-related symptoms are present.

CSF abnormalities include increased opening pressure (>200 mm of H_2O), increased leukocytes (>4/mm^3), elevated protein (>50 mg/dL), and decreased glucose (<60 mg/dL). These findings may be suggestive of NM but do not confirm a diagnosis.[14,19] CSF cytology may be positive in only 45% of the cases on the first lumbar puncture, with an increase in yield up to 80% with a second CSF examination. Each subsequent lumbar puncture has a poor yield of only 2%.[14,19]

Imaging plays a vital role and is the initial investigation of choice in a suspected case of NM. Contrast-enhanced (CE) MR imaging of brain (**Fig. 1**) and axial skeleton remains the most sensitive imaging modality for diagnosis, with sensitivity of 76% and specificity of 77% in patients with supportive clinical findings.[19,22] Bacterial, fungal, or viral meningeal inflammation, neurosarcoidosis, chronic meningitis, and Guillain-Barré syndrome may mimic NM; therefore, it is important to correlate the imaging findings with the appropriate clinical setting.

On MR imaging, noncontrast fluid-attenuated inversion recovery (FLAIR) images show hyperintensity within the sulci and cisterns due to increased CSF proteinaceous content (**Fig. 2A**). Contrast-enhanced T1-weighted imaging (T1WI) or magnetization-prepared rapid acquisition of gradient echo (MPRAGE) demonstrates subarachnoid, ventricular, or parenchymal enhancing nodules; focal or diffuse pial enhancement; and ependymal, sulcal, folial, or cranial nerve enhancement (**Fig. 2B**).[19,22,23] Postcontrast 3-dimensional T2-FLAIR images provide higher sensitivity in detecting leptomeningeal abnormalities than conventional postcontrast T1 images or postcontrast MPRAGE.[24] The most frequent brain MR imaging findings are subarachnoid nodules and pial enhancement. Due to dependency, enhancement commonly is appreciated around the basal cisterns and over the surface of the midbrain, pons, and over the cerebellar folia. Enlargement and enhancement of the cranial nerves are seen, most commonly within the oculomotor, facial, cochlear (**Fig. 3**), and optic nerves (**Fig. 4**). Most typically, enhancement is seen along the cisternal segments of the cranial nerves. Enhancement and dysfunction of cranial nerves III, IV, and VI are common causes of diplopia in patients with NM (**Fig. 5**).

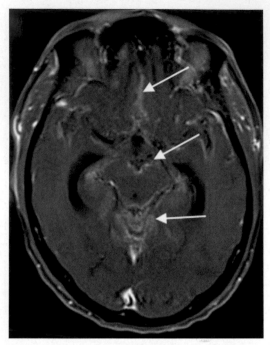

Fig. 1. Contrast-enhanced T1WI shows diffuse leptomeningeal enhancement (*arrows*) over the cerebral cortex, along the basal cisterns and cerebellar folia in a patient with breast cancer.

indicator of poor prognosis and could be used to identify responses to intrathecal chemotherapy. Microscopic metastases, however, are below the resolution of MR imaging; therefore, cytology has a higher rate of specificity but a lower rate of sensitivity.

In highly suspected cases of neoplastic meningitis with negative CSF and imaging examination, other tests, such as CSF immunohistochemical examinations, polymerase chain reactions, fluorescence in situ hybridization, and cytogenetic analysis, can improve the detection rate.[26,27] Tumor-specific markers—such as carcinoembryonic antigen for adenocarcinomas, α-fetoprotein, and β-human chorionic gonadotropin for germ cell tumors; 5-hydroxyindoleacetic acid for carcinoid tumors; and immunoglobulins for multiple myeloma—are employed very rarely for the NM diagnosis.[19,28] Nonspecific tumor markers, such as vascular endothelial growth factor, creatine kinase–BB isoenzyme, tissue polypeptide antigen, and lactate dehydrogenase isoenzyme-5, can be strong indirect indicators of NM. None is sensitive enough, however, to improve on the cytologic diagnosis. In certain malignancies like leukemia or lymphoma, the sensitivity of flow cytometry is several degrees higher than that of cytology for detecting CSF leukemia or lymphoma.

Hydrocephalus remains one of the most common complications of the NM due to blockage of the basal cisterns and obstruction to CSF absorption at the arachnoid granulation level (**Fig. 7**).[10,29] Placement of a ventriculoperitoneal shunt is an effective palliative approach in patients with symptomatic hydrocephalus. An Ommaya reservoir or similar devices, useful in administering intraventricular chemotherapy and CSF sampling, are employed routinely in NM patients. These devices are safer and more comfortable for the patient than

MR imaging also is sensitive for detecting metastatic deposits along the neuraxis. CE MR imaging of the spine shows smooth leptomeningeal enhancement or intradural extramedullary enhancing nodules, especially in the lumbar spine and over the cauda equine (**Fig. 6**).[25] Lumbosacral nerve root thickening and enhancement commonly is observed on CE MR imaging of the lumbar spine. Studies have suggested that MR imaging–proved leptomeningeal seeding is an

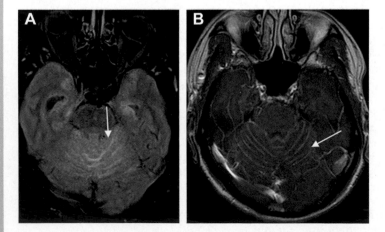

Fig. 2. Breast cancer with NM. Axial FLAIR image (*A*) shows hyperintensity within the cerebellar folia (*arrow*) due to increased CSF proteinaceous content. Axial postcontrast T1WI (*B*) shows leptomeningeal enhancement along the folia (*arrow*).

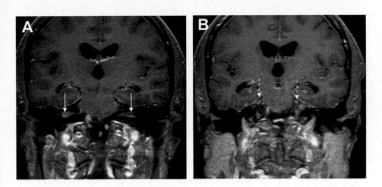

Fig. 3. Lung cancer patient presented with bilateral sensory-neural hearing loss. Contrast-enhanced coronal T1WIs show bilateral enhancement of the VII-VIII nerve complex (arrows [A]) and enhancement of the bilateral trigeminal nerves (dotted arrows [B]).

repeated lumbar punctures and help in the uniform distribution of the drug in the CSF.[10,29,30] It is crucial to ensure that the catheter's tip and side perforations are inserted entirely into the ventricle to avoid drug instillation into the brain parenchyma. This placement needs to be confirmed with a CT scan to avoid chemotherapy related leukoencephalopathy. Other complications include reservoir malfunction and infection. Underdiagnosis and assessing response to treatment remain significant problems in NM patients when the CSF and imaging tests are negative.

Early diagnosis and treatment of NM are vital because most untreated patients die within 1 week to 9 weeks (median 3 weeks) due to neurologic disease and tumor progression. The main aim of treatment is to extend survival and stabilize or improve neurologic symptoms. To date, brain and neuraxis imaging and CSF analysis remain the backbone of investigations in a suspected case of NM.

PARANEOPLASTIC SYNDROMES

Paraneoplastic syndromes (PNSs) are a group of disorders that present in patients with cancer. PNSs may involve any part of the nervous system (central and peripheral nervous disorders) and may affect multiple areas simultaneously. PNS is a rare neurologic disorder seen approximately in 0.01% of cancer patients.[31] PNS incidence largely depends on the tumor cell type. Approximately 30% of patients with thymoma have some form of neurologic autoimmunity, mostly myasthenia gravis, compared with pulmonary small cell carcinoma, which is associated with 1 or more PNSs in 3% of cases.[32,33] Other malignancies associated with PNSs include gynecologic malignancies arising from the breast, ovary, fallopian tube, and peritoneum; Hodgkin lymphoma and non-Hodgkin lymphoma; testicular cancer; and neuroblastoma. PNSs occur at a much lower rate in patients with larger cell lung, renal, uterine, and melanotic skin cancers.

PNSs encompass a variety of symptoms or syndromes, including limbic encephalitis, cerebellar degeneration, brainstem encephalitis, striatal encephalitis, and opsoclonus-myoclonus syndrome (Box 1).[31,34,35] Myelitis, motor neuron disease, stiff person syndrome, Lambert-Eaton myasthenic syndrome (LEMS), neuromyotonia, and Guillain-Barré syndrome also are included. Manifestations precede the diagnosis of cancer in many cases.

Paraneoplastic encephalopathy is an autoimmune-mediated disorder associated with various specific antibodies. Tumor-targeted immune responses are initiated by onconeuronal

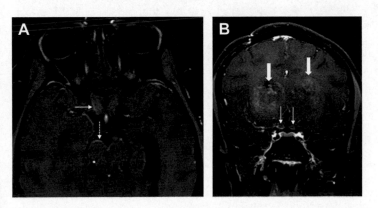

Fig. 4. Bilateral vision loss in a patient with CNS lymphoma. Axial (A) and coronal (B) postcontrast fat-saturated T1WIs show circumferential enhancement of the bilateral optic nerves (arrows) due to leptomeningeal metastasis (thin dash arrow). Note bilateral frontal lobe lymphoma across the corpus callosum (fat arrows [B]).

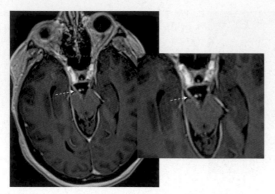

Fig. 5. A 21-year-old male patient with leukemia presented with a history of diplopia. Axial contrast-enhanced T1WI (*A*) and magnified view at the level of midbrain (*B*) show enhancement over the midbrain's surface and along the right third cranial nerve (*arrow*).

proteins expressed within the neoplasm (neoplastic cells) at the plasma membrane, nucleus, cytoplasm, or nucleolus. These antigens also are expressed in neurons or glia (coincidental targets). This leads to paraneoplastic neurologic syndrome by means of immune cross-reaction.

There are 2 main type antibodies: antibodies to intracellular antigens and antibodies to cell-surface antigens (**Table 2**).[34–38] The former includes Hu (antineuronal nuclear antibody type 1 [ANNA-1]), Ri (antineuronal nuclear antibody type 2 [ANNA-2]), antineuronal nuclear antibody type 3, anti-antiglial/neuronal nuclear antibody, Yo (Purkinje cell cytoplasmic antigen type 1 [PCA-1]), Purkinje cell cytoplasmic antigen type 2 (PCA-2), Ma1, Ma2, CV2/collapsing response mediator protein type 5 [CRMP-5], zinc finger transcription factor (Zic4), Tr, amphiphysin, and glutamic acid decarboxylase (GAD). The latter includes *N*-methyl-D-aspartate

receptor (NMDAR), voltage-gated potassium channel (VGKC), leucine-rich glioma inactivated 1 (LGI1) and contactin-associated protein 2, α-amino-3-hydroxy-5-methyl-4-isoxazolepropionicacid receptor (AMPAR), P/Q-types and N-type calcium channel, neuromyelitis optica, glycine receptor, acetylcholine (Ach) receptor, γ-aminobutyric acid B1 receptor (GABA$_B$R), and metabotropic glutamate receptor-5. Antibodies targeting intracellular antigens are targeted by cytotoxic T cells; histopathology is characterized by CD4 and CD8 lymphocyte T-cell infiltration. Histopathology of antibodies to the cell surface or synaptic antigens is characterized by B-lymphocyte and plasma cell infiltration, leading to antibody and complement deposition.

Clinical presentation of the PNSs largely depends on the primary target in the nervous system. Because some symptoms may precede the cancer diagnosis, imaging, especially when positive, plays an important role in PNS diagnosis. MR imaging brain remains the primary imaging of choice in a suspected case of PNS. In many suspected cases, the MR imaging can be normal, but image findings and clinical presentations help narrow the range of antibody tests to be ordered. Imaging appearance depends on the primary targets in the brain parenchyma. A typical pattern seen on MR imaging findings includes limbic encephalitis, cerebellar degeneration, brainstem encephalitis, striatal encephalitis, and myelitis/myelopathy.[35–38] Other commonly performed investigations are electroencephalogram (EEG) and CSF examination. EEG can show diffuse slowing of electrical activity with or without spikes indicative of heightened cortical irritability.[39] CSF examinations serve 2 primary purposes: to rule out infection, neoplasm, and other primary pathologies and to document the antibody.

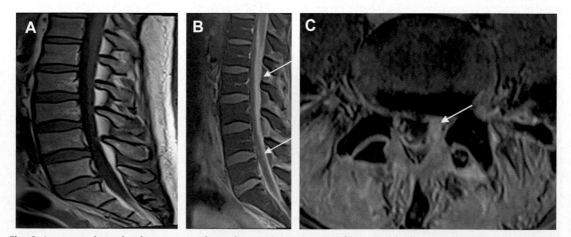

Fig. 6. Leptomeningeal enhancement along the cauda equine and filum terminale in a patient with breast cancer. Precontrast sagittal T1 (*A*), postcontrast sagittal T1 (*B*), and axial T1 (*C*) show diffuse enhancement along the filum terminale (*arrows* in *B*) and intraspinal nerve roots (*arrow* in *C*).

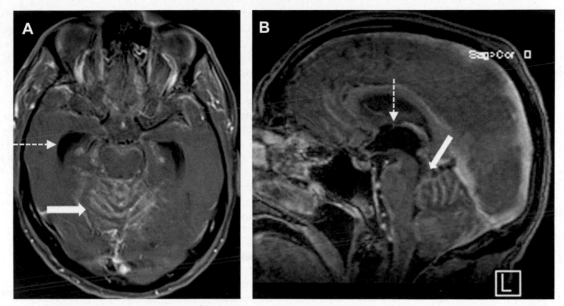

Fig. 7. Obstructive hydrocephalus due to NM in a patient with breast cancer. Postcontrast axial (*A*) and sagittal T1WIs (*B*) show diffuse, a thick enhancement (*thick arrow*) over the cerebellar folia, basal cisterns, and aqueduct, leading to dilatation of the temporal horns and third ventricle (*dash arrow*).

Paraneoplastic Cerebellar Degeneration

Paraneoplastic cerebellar degeneration (PCD) is a common PNS resulting from tumor induced autoimmunity against cerebellar antigens. There are more than 30 different antibodies associated with this condition with anti-Yo (PCA-1) antibody the most common.[40,41] In men, many reported tumors are adenocarcinomas of the gastrointestinal system and prostate. PNS has been seen with a variety of other antibodies, including Hu, Ri, Tr, Zic4, mGluR1, and voltage-gated calcium channels (VGCCs).[40,41] Patients present with nonspecific gait unsteadiness, which progresses to severe cerebellar ataxia over a few weeks or months. Other symptoms include cognitive and psychiatric morbidity, notably memory loss and emotional lability.

MR imaging of the brain often is normal in the early stages, but global volume loss in both the vermis and cerebellar hemispheres with relative sparing of the brainstem is seen in later stages (**Fig. 8**). A superior cerebellar hyperintense sign on FLAIR image also has been reported.[42] The underlying mechanism for this atrophy is believed to be an immunologic reaction to cerebellar degeneration-related protein 2, a protein found in the cerebellum that is produced ectopically by tumor cells.[40,41]

Autoimmune limbic encephalitis (ALE) is an inflammatory disease involving the limbic system, predominately in the medial temporal lobes. It commonly is associated with SCLC, breast cancer, and ovarian tumors, including teratoma, testicular tumor, and thymic tumor.[31,34,38] It also may be seen with colon cancer, pancreatic cancer, renal cell cancer, esophageal cancer, bladder cancer, prostate cancer, neuroblastoma, melanoma, and Hodgkin lymphoma and non-Hodgkin lymphoma. ALE involves intracellular antigen antibodies (anti-Ma2, Hu, and CV2/CRMP-5, GAD) and neuronal surface antibodies (NMDAR, VGKC, AMPAR, and GABA$_B$R) with or without tumor association.[31,34,38,39,43,44] The clinical picture of limbic encephalitis is characterized by rapid development of confusion, working memory deficit, mood changes, anxiety, depression, psychosis, and seizures. The subacute development of short-term memory loss is considered the hallmark of the disorder but is often overlooked because of other symptoms.

MR imaging remains the imaging modality of choice for ALE. It often shows increased signal on T2-weighted FLAIR imaging in the medial aspect of the temporal lobes (**Fig. 9**).[45,46] This abnormality more often is bilaterally asymmetric than unilateral. Involvement of the basal ganglia usually is noted whereas involvement of the lateral temporal lobe and insula is less common. In addition, there is lack of restricted diffusion and hemorrhages in ALE. Various other pathologies, such as herpes encephalitis, postictal edema, hypoglycemia, stroke, and tumors, may involve the medial temporal lobes. Early diagnosis and differentiation from viral encephalitis are vital for treatment. In herpes encephalitis, T2 hypersensitivity on MR imaging is seen involving the cortical and the

---

Box 1
Paraneoplastic disorders

Brain

    Paraneoplastic encephalomyelitis

    Limbic encephalitis

    Brainstem encephalitis

    Opsoclonus-myoclonus

    PCD

    Chorea

Eye

    Paraneoplastic optic neuritis

    Paraneoplastic retinal degeneration

Spinal cord

    Myelopathy

    Myelitis with rigidity and spasms

    Motor neuronopathy

    Acute necrotizing myelopathy

Nerves

    Sensory neuronopathy

    Sensorimotor peripheral neuropathy

    Autonomic neuropathy, gastrointestinal dysmotility

    Motor neuronopathy

Neuromuscular junction/muscle

    LEMS

    Myasthenia gravis

    Dermatomyositis

    Neuromyotonia

Muscle

    Polymyositis/dermatomyositis

    Acute necrotizing myopathy

Multifocal disorders

    Encephalomyeloneuropathies

---

subcortical regions of the bilateral temporal lobes, frontal lobes, and insula.[45,46] Restricted diffusion, gyral swelling, loss of gray-white matter interface, and mild or no enhancement also are associated. Petechial hemorrhages, when present, strongly favor herpes encephalitis over limbic encephalitis. Involvement of extratemporal regions, such as the cingulate gyrus and frontal lobes, are not uncommon. Postictal edema also can cause temporal lobe T2 hyperintensities and swelling. The lack of prodromal neuropsychiatric symptoms and the resolution of temporal lobe changes after cessation of seizure activity are supportive of seizure-related MR imaging changes rather than ALE. Ischemic stroke involving the medial temporal lobe usually presents acutely but sometimes causes only mild neurocognitive deficits.

CSF examination mainly is helpful to exclude mimics of ALE, in particular herpes encephalitis. Polymerase chain reaction testing for the herpes simplex virus in the CSF has high diagnostic sensitivity and specificity, but clinicians should be wary that it may be negative early in the disease course. The clinical presentation of acute herpes encephalitis is very different from that of ALE.

Brainstem Encephalitis

Paraneoplastic brainstem encephalitis can occur in association with limbic encephalitis, in isolation, or as the predominant clinical manifestation of paraneoplastic neuronal disorder (PND). This clinical syndrome is characterized by multiple cranial nerve palsies, long tract signs, and cerebellar ataxia. Less common features include movement disorders, such as parkinsonism, chorea, jaw opening dystonia, and myoclonus. Brainstem encephalitis commonly is seen in young men with testicular cancer (anti-Ma2).[31,47] Anti-Ri, anti-Hu, anti-Tr, and anti-NMDAR are less common causes of paraneoplastic brainstem encephalitis.[34–36,38,47] MR imaging shows patchy hyperintensity in the brainstem and/or basal ganglia on T2 or FLAIR images but rarely shows enhancing nodules on postcontrast scans (**Fig. 10**). Differential diagnoses include infectious brainstem encephalitis, tumor infiltration, vasculitis, and demyelinating disease.

Striatal Encephalitis/Paraneoplastic Chorea

Striatal encephalitis is a rare paraneoplastic encephalopathy. It is seen in anti-CV2/CRMP5 encephalitis cases associated with SCLC and thymoma.[48,49] The pattern can be seen in other paraneoplastic encephalopathies, including anti-VGKC, anti-NMDAR, and anti-Hu antibodies.[48,49] As the name suggests, MR imaging abnormality of the T2 hyperintensity is seen in the bilateral caudate nuclei and putamina; it also may be associated with limbic encephalitis and cerebellar degeneration. Differential diagnoses include infectious encephalitis, toxic and metabolic diseases, Sydenham chorea, Huntington disease, Wilson disease, and Creutzfeldt-Jakob disease.

OTHER PARANEOPLASTIC DISORDERS

Although some PND has unique features, others may be indistinguishable from common neurologic

Table 2
Neuronal paraneoplastic autoantibodies associated paraneoplastic neuronal disorders and tumors

Group I antibodies: autoimmune encephalitis with intracellular antigens		
Anti-Hu (ANNA1) anti-Hu	LE, sensory neuronopathy, autonomic and sensorimotor neuropathies	SCLC (may be seen with thymoma, or neuroblastoma)
Anti-Ma2	LE, BSE	Testicular seminoma (young patients) SCLC or breast cancer (older patients)
Anti-Ma1	BSE, PCD	Lung cancer
Anti-CV2/CRMP-5	Movement disorder (chorea) and ocular syndromes (uveitis, optic neuritis)	SCLC and thymoma
Anti-Ri antibody (ANNA-2)	Opsoclonus-myoclonus syndrome, BSE, PCD	Breast cancer, SCLC, and gynecologic malignancies
Anti-PCA 2	Encephalomyelitis, PCD,	SCLC
Anti-Yo antibody	PCD	Ovarian or breast malignancy
Anti-Tr	PCD	Hodgkin disease
Anti-amphiphysin	Stiff person syndrome,	SCLC
GAD	LE	Thymoma, SCLC
Group II antibodies: autoimmune encephalitis with cell-surface antigens or antibodies against synaptic receptors		
Anti-NMDAR	LE, hyperactivity, seizures, and memory change, psychiatric symptoms	Ovarian teratoma
Anti-VGKC	limbic encephalitis, neuromyotonia	SCLC, thymoma, prostatic cancer
Anti-VGCC	LEMS, PCD	SCLC
Anti-AMPAR	LE	Thymoma, SCLC
Anti- GABA$_B$R	LE	SCLC
Anti-mGluR1	PCD	Hodgkin lymphoma
LGI1	LE	Thymoma
Anti-ACh receptor	MG	Thymoma

Abbreviations: BSE, brainstem encephalitis; LE, limbic encephalitis; MG, myasthenia gravis.

disorders. Description of symptoms of PND depends on the site involved in the nervous system, commonly depending on multiple organelles. Neurologic presentations are classified depending on the anatomic site in.

Spinal cord presentations include myelopathy, myelitis with rigidity and spasms (stiff person syndrome), paraneoplastic sensory neuronopathy, and motor neuronopathy.[38,50] Spinal cord–related symptoms typically are in combination with other PND, such as limbic or brainstem encephalitis. Symptoms depend on the anatomic cells or area involved within the spinal cord. As the name suggests, stiff person syndrome is characterized by axial and proximal lower limb stiffness and spasms and is associated with anti-GAD antibodies or anti-amphiphysin antibodies in breast cancer.[38,50,51]

Rapidly progressive motor neuron disease is associated with anti-Hu antibodies whereas primary lateral sclerosis is seen in breast cancer patients.

The peripheral nervous system is involved far more commonly than the CNS and presents with neuropathies. Sensory neuronopathies are more common than motor neuropathies in PND. Malignancies may present either isolated or combined with other neuropathies. Hodgkin disease patients can present with acute inflammatory demyelinating polyradiculoneuropathy whereas non-Hodgkin lymphoma cases present with a subacute lower motor neuronopathy as a slowly progressive lower motor neuron syndrome affects the lower limbs. Neuromyotonia is an unusual manifestation of cancer characterized by muscle cramps, stiffness, twitching, sweating, and abnormal

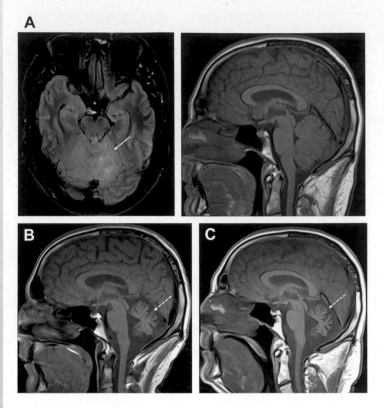

Fig. 8. PCD in a 56-year-old patient with adenocarcinomas of colon. Axial FLAIR and sagittal T1WIs (2014 [*A*]) show subtle superior cerebellar hyperintensity on FLAIR image (*arrow*) with normal volume. Sagittal T1WIs (MRI in 2017 [*B*] and MRI in 2019 [*C*]) show progressive global volume loss in both the vermis and cerebellar hemispheres (*arrows* in B and C).

relaxation after voluntary contraction. It is associated with thymomas and SCLC and involves antibodies against VGKCs.

LEMS is a paraneoplastic or primary autoimmune neuromuscular junction disorder characterized by proximal weakness and autonomic dysfunction.[52] It is caused by the presence of antibodies generated against the P/Q-type VGCCs on presynaptic nerve terminals that decrease the release of Ach.[52–54] A majority of LEMS cases are associated with SCLC, which expresses functional VGCCs. LEMS may be seen in other

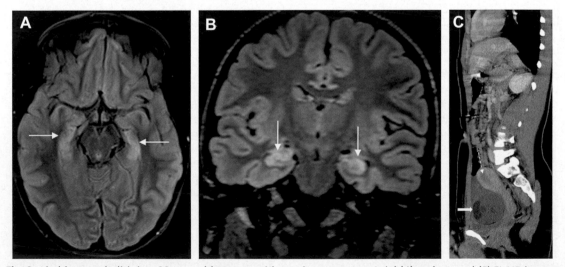

Fig. 9. Limbic encephalitis in a 28-year-old woman with ovarian teratoma. Axial (*A*) and coronal (*B*) FLAIR images show bilateral hyperintensity and mild enlargement of the hippocampus proper (*arrows*). Sagittal reconstructed image through the pelvis shows an ovarian mass with a fat signal (*arrow*). Note normal stretched uterus (*dash arrow*) due to mass effect.

malignancies, such as non–small cell and mixed lung carcinomas, prostate carcinoma, thymoma, and lymphoproliferative disorders.

Clinically, patients present with proximal muscle weakness, predominantly affecting lower limbs; areflexia; and autonomic disturbances, such as impotence, constipation, and dry mouth. Clinical presentation of LEMS may precede cancer diagnosis by months. The LEMS diagnosis is based on clinical features in patient with lung malignancies. The confirmation of a diagnosis is based on the detection of specific VGCC antibodies. P/Q VGCC antibodies are present in 80% to 90% of patients with LEMS.[55]

EVALUATION OF THE PARANEOPLASTIC NEURONAL DISORDER

PND diagnosis requires a multidimensional approach, high clinical suspicion, CSF and serum examination for routine and specific autoantibodies, and imaging.[34,36,38] Neuroimaging is an integral part in the evaluation of PND in the CNS but generally does not contribute to the diagnosis of PND in the peripheral nervous system. Besides MR imaging of brain and spinal cord, CT or MR imaging of the chest, abdomen, and pelvis are mandatory in suspected cases to determine the presence and location of underlying malignancies.[44] When the primary malignancy is unknown, the search initially may be focused on tumor types commonly associated with the patient's syndrome or type of antineuronal antibody. If the tumor found does not histologically match the syndrome or antibody, a search for a second neoplasm should be undertaken. Because PNS onset often precedes the cancer diagnosis or occurs when the tumor is small and difficult to detect, a multidisciplinary approach to a cancer diagnosis is warranted. In such cases, PET scans can be useful to locate the primary tumor. Mammograms, transvaginal ultrasounds, and, in rare instances, exploratory laparotomies may be performed in selected cases. In cases of an initial tumor screen that is negative, patients should be followed at regular intervals with scans (eg, every 6 months for the next 4 years). If there is a strong clinical suspicion of PNS, but imaging tests are negative, cancer screenings should be repeated periodically depending on the type of disorder. A patient with a confirmed diagnosis of LEMS with no malignancy documented on CT, MR imaging, or PET screening should continue to be screened every 3 months to 6 months for at least 2 years.[52,53] For classical PNSs with anti-Hu antibodies related to SCLC should be screened for every 6 months. For disorders with anti-NMDAR encephalitis, less frequent and shorter durations are reasonable (eg, evaluation for ovarian teratoma yearly for 2 years). In more than 90% of patients with solid tumors and PNS, the tumor is found within 1 year of PNS presentation.

ANTIBODY TESTING

The detection of specific autoantibodies remains crucial in establishing a diagnosis of autoimmune encephalitis. Documentation of these autoantibodies under the appropriate clinical findings helps to make the diagnosis of the immunologic subtypes of encephalitis. Onconeuronal and GAD antibodies are present in the serum and CSF; they are detectable with many techniques, including ELISA, immunoblotting, and immunohistochemistry.[34–36,38,44] It is advisable to include both CSF and serum for neuronal antibody testing in patients with suspected autoimmune encephalitis. Between the 2 tests, CSF examinations remain paramount because relevant antibodies may be found only in the CSF (anti-NMDAR encephalitis);

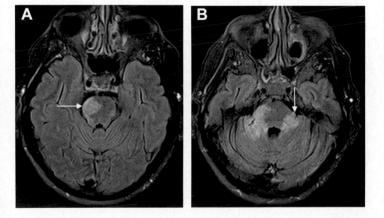

Fig. 10. Paraneoplastic brainstem encephalitis due to SCLC. Axial flair images (*A*, *B*) show patchy hyperintensity in the pons (*arrow* in *A*) and partly involving the middle cerebellar peduncles (*arrow* in *B*).

the antibody concentration in the CSF correlates better with the clinical course than antibody concentrations in the serum; the repertoire of antibodies in the CSF and serum can be different in the same patient (eg, NMDAR in CSF and serum and γ-aminobutyric acid type A (GABA$_A$) receptor only in serum); the types of antibodies in the CSF usually determine the clinical picture, and false-positive and false-negative results are less common with CSF analysis.

SPECIAL ANTIBODIES AND PARANEOPLASTIC ENCEPHALITIS

Group I Antibodies: Autoimmune Encephalitis with Intracellular Antigens

Group I antibodies that target intracellular neuronal antigens are associated closely with underlying malignancies. These antibodies employ the same mechanisms used by cytotoxic T cells to target intracellular neuronal antigens and onconeuronal antigens in the immune response to cancer. Group I antibodies have a decreased response to immunomodulatory therapy and an increased prevalence of irreversible neuronal damage, which leads to poor clinical outcomes. The most clinically relevant group I antibodies include anti-Hu, anti-Ma (Ta), anti-CV2/CRMP-5, anti-Ri, and anti-Yo.[34–36,38,44]

Anti-Hu antibody, also known as ANNA-1, is the most common paraneoplastic form of autoimmune encephalitis.[35–37] It is seen most commonly with SCLC and clinically presents with sensory neuropathy. Anti-Hu antibodies can be seen in patients with extrapulmonary small cell carcinoma, thymoma, or neuroblastoma.[56,57] A subset of patients with anti-Hu encephalitis can present with epilepsia partialis continua, motor seizures involving the face and distal extremities. MR imaging shows T2-FLAIR hyperintense lesions in the medial temporal lobes (**Fig. 11**) and variable involvement of the cerebellum and brainstem.

Anti-Ma (Ta) encephalitis is strongly associated with testicular tumors in young men and SCLC or breast cancer in older patients.[31,46] Neurologic symptoms are due to the involvement of the limbic, diencephalic, or brainstem dysfunction, which presents with limbic encephalitis and brainstem-related ophthalmoplegia (**Fig. 12**).

Anti-CV2/CRMP-5 is associated with SCLC and thymoma. Movement disorder (chorea) and ocular syndromes (uveitis and optic neuritis) are distinctive features.[44] On MR imaging T2-FLAIR, hyperintensity is seen in the striatum without restricted diffusion on diffusion-weighted imaging–apparent diffusion coefficient, differentiating it from Creutzfeldt-Jakob disease, which shows restricted diffusion.

The anti-Ri antibody is associated with breast cancer, SCLC, and gynecologic malignancies. Opsoclonus-myoclonus syndrome, brainstem encephalitis, and PCD have been described with this antibody.[44]

The anti-Yo antibody is the primary cause of PCD. It targets intracellular antigens in the Purkinje cells of the cerebellar cortex, leading to cerebellar degeneration.[44] It commonly is seen in women, associated with ovarian or breast malignancy, and clinically presents with subacute onset ataxia, nystagmus, and dysarthria. MR imaging shows diffuse cerebellar atrophy without brainstem atrophy.

Group II Antibodies: Autoimmune Encephalitis with Cell-surface Antigens

Group II antibodies target cell-surface neuronal antigens and are less likely to be associated with an underlying malignancy. Antibodies often target synaptic proteins and can result in the downregulation of receptors leading to altered synaptic transmission associated with epileptiform activity.

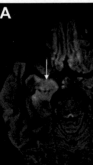
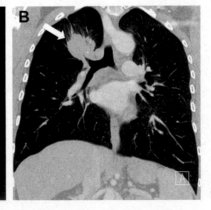

Fig. 11. Anti-Hu antibody limbic encephalitis due to SCLC. Axial FLAIR image (*A*) shows hyperintensity in the right medial temporal lobe (*arrow*). The coronal reconstructed image of the chest (*B*) shows a mass lesion (*arrow*) in the right upper lobe, biopsy-proved SCLC.

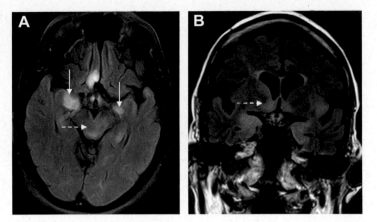

Fig. 12. Anti-Ma encephalitis from testicular tumors in a 29-year-old man. Axial (A) and coronal (B) FLAIR images show asymmetric hyperintensity in the medial temporal lobes (*arrows*), midbrain (*dash arrow* in A), nucleus accumbens (*dash arrow* in B), and paraterminal gyrus.

Anti-NMDAR encephalitis

NMDAR encephalitis is a common autoimmune encephalitis classically seen in young women and children with autoimmunity not associated with cancer.[44,58] A minority of NMDAR encephalitis cases, such as ovarian teratoma, can be associated with an underlying malignancy. This highlights the need to screen all patients with autoimmune encephalitis for an underlying malignancy regardless of the antibody profile. This form of the disease is associated with CSF IgG antibodies against the GluN1 subunit of the NMDAR.[44,58] Children usually present with irritability, hyperactivity, seizures, and memory change whereas the adults present with prodromal headache, psychiatric symptoms, fever, and gastrointestinal or upper respiratory symptoms. Motor or complex seizures develop at early stages, but their frequency decreases with disease evolution.

Diagnosis is obtained mostly through documentation of IgG antibodies against the GluN1 subunit of the NMDAR. The other commonly employed test is EEG, which shows a characteristic pattern, the extreme delta brush.[44,58,59] Even though a suspected patient routinely is neuroimaged, MR imaging brain remains normal in 80% to 90% of cases. When MR imaging is positive, a wide variation in the distribution and degree of T2-FLAIR hyperintense signal changes throughout the brain can be seen. Hyperintensities may involve the temporal lobe, insular cortex, and cingulate gyrus.[60,61] The classic patterns of limbic encephalitis, cerebellitis, brainstem encephalitis, and striatal encephalitis are rare.

VGKC encephalitis is another group II subtypes of autoimmune encephalitis and presents with classic features of limbic encephalitis and the development of medically intractable epilepsy.[34,36,37] These clinical features are explained by the high concentration of potassium channels in the limbic structures. Imaging features include T2-FLAIR hyperintensities in the medial temporal lobes, unilaterally or bilaterally, in the acute stages, with a propensity to develop chronic findings of mesial temporal sclerosis on follow-up imaging. Extralimbic involvement in VGKC encephalitis is rare. Although considered a nonparaneoplastic, 5% to 30% of cases have associated tumors (SCLC, thymoma, or prostatic cancer).[34,37,62,63]

Other antibodies associated with paraneoplastic disorders include anti-AMPAR (Glu R1 and GluR2) in patients with limbic encephalitis.[34,36,37] They are seen predominately in patients with lung, breast, or thymus tumors. Anti-GABA$_B$R encephalitis is seen with SCLC and usually exhibits the limbic encephalitis pattern.[34,36,37] Like other cell-surface antigen-mediated syndromes, such as anti-AMPAR and anti-GABA$_B$R encephalitis, respond to immunotherapy. The anti-Tr antibody is associated with Hodgkin lymphoma and may show features of limbic encephalopathy and cerebellar or brainstem syndrome.

DISCLOSURE

None.

REFERENCES

1. Gleissner B, Chamberlain MC. Neoplastic meningitis. Lancet Neurol 2006;5(5):443–52.
2. Chamberlain MC. Neoplastic meningitis. Oncologist 2008;13(9):967–77.
3. Kaplan JG, DeSouza TG, Farkash A, et al. Leptomeningeal metastases: Comparison of clinical features and laboratory data of solid tumors, lymphomas and leukemias. J Neurooncol 1990;9:225–9.
4. Siegal T, Lossos A, Pfeffer MR. Leptomeningeal metastases: Analysis of 31 patients with sustained off-therapy response following combined-modality therapy. Neurology 1994;44:1463–9.

5. Rosen ST, Aisner J, Makuch RW, et al. Carcinomatous leptomeningitis in small cell lung cancer: A clinicopathologic review of the National Cancer Institute experience. Medicine (Baltimore) 1982;61:45–53.

6. Amer MH, Al Sarraf M, Baker LH, et al. Malignant melanoma and central nervous system metastases: Incidence, diagnosis, treatment and survival. Cancer 1978;42:660–8.

7. Yap HY, Yap BS, Tashima CK, et al. Meningeal carcinomatosis in breast cancer. Cancer 1978;42:283–6.

8. Freilich RJ, Krol G, DeAngelis LM. Neuroimaging and cerebrospinal fl uid cytology in the diagnosis of leptomeningeal metastasis. Ann Neurol 1995;38:51–7.

9. Grossman SA, Krabak MJ. Leptomeningeal carcinomatosis. Cancer Treat Rev 1999;25:103–19.

10. Chamberlain MC. Radioisotope CSF flow studies in leptomeningeal metastases. J Neurooncol 1998;38: 135–40.

11. Balhuizen JC, Bots GT, Schaberg A. Value of cerebrospinal fluid cytology for the diagnosis of malignancies in the central nervous system. J Neurosurg 1978;48:747–53.

12. Lombardi G, Zustovich F, Farina P, et al. Blank for % Neoplastic meningitis from solid tumors: new diagnostic and therapeutic approaches. Oncologist 2011;16(8):1175–88.

13. Clarke JL, Perez HR, Jacks LM, et al. Leptomeningeal metastases in the MRI era. Neurology 2010; 74(18):1449–54.

14. Wasserstrom WR, Glass JP, Posner JB. Diagnosis and treatment of leptomeningeal metastases from solid tumors: experience with 90 patients. Cancer 1982;49(4):759–72.

15. Waki F, Ando M, Takashima A, et al. Prognostic factors and clinical outcomes in patients with leptomeningeal metastasis from solid tumors. J Neurooncol 2009;93(2):205–12.

16. Clarke JL. Leptomeningeal metastasis from systemic cancer. Continuum (Minneap Minn) 2012;18(2):328–42.

17. Hughes DC, Raghavan A, Mordekar SR, et al. Role of imaging in the diagnosis of acute bacterial meningitis and its complications. Postgrad Med J 2010;86: 478–85.

18. Brem SS, Bierman PJ, Brem H, et al. National Comprehensive Cancer Network, Central nervous system. J Natl Compr Canc Netw 2011;9:352–400.

19. Le Rhun E, Weller M, Brandsma D, et al. EANO-ESMO Clinical Practice Guidelines for diagnosis, treatment and follow-up of patients with leptomeningeal metastasis from solid tumours. Ann Oncol 2017;28(suppl_4):iv84–99.

20. Chamberlain M, Junck L, Brandsma D, et al. Leptomeningeal metastases: a RANO proposal for response criteria. Neurooncology 2017;19(4):484–92.

21. Thakkar JP, Kumthekar P, Dixit KS, et al. Leptomeningeal metastasis from solid tumors. J Neurol Sci 2020;411:116706.

22. Straathof CS, de Bruin HG, Dippel DW, et al. The diagnostic accuracy of magnetic resonance imaging and cerebrospinal fluid cytology in leptomeningeal metastasis. J Neurol 1999;246(9):810–4.

23. Singh SK, Leeds NE, Ginsberg LE. MR imaging of leptomeningeal metastases: comparison of three sequences. AJNR Am J Neuroradiol 2002;23:817–21.

24. Fukuoka H, Hirai T, Okuda T, et al. Comparison of the added value of contrast-enhanced 3D fluid-attenuated inversion recovery and magnetization-prepared rapid acquisition of gradient echo sequences in relation to conventional postcontrast T1-weighted images for the evaluation of leptomeningeal diseases at 3T. AJNR Am J Neuroradiol 2010;31:868–73.

25. Chamberlain MC. Neuraxis imaging in leptomeningeal metastasis: A retrospective case series. CNS Tumors 2046. J Clin Oncol 2012;30. abstr 2046.

26. Glantz MJ, Cole BF, Glantz LK, et al. Cerebrospinal fluid cytology in patients with cancer: minimizing false-negative results. Cancer 1998;82(4):733–9.

27. Hegde U, Filie A, Little RF, et al. High incidence of occult leptomeningeal disease detected by flow cytometry in newly diagnosed aggressive B-cell lymphomas at risk for central nervous system involvement: the role of flow cytometry versus cytology. Blood 2005;105(2):496–502.

28. Nakagawa H, Kubo S, Murasawa A, et al. Measurements of CSF biochemical tumor markers in patients with meningeal carcinomatosis and brain tumors. J Neuro-oncol 1992;12(2):111–20.

29. Glantz MJ, Hall WA, Cole BF, et al. Diagnosis, management, and survival of patients with leptomeningeal cancer based on cerebrospinal fluid-flow status. Cancer 1995;75:2919–31.

30. Glantz MJ, Van Horn A, Fisher R, et al. Route of intracerebrospinal fluid chemotherapy administration and efficacy of therapy in neoplastic meningitis. Cancer 2010;116:1947–52.

31. Dalmau J, Rosenfeld MR. Paraneoplastic syndromes of the CNS. Lancet Neurol 2008;7:327–40.

32. Vernino S, Lennon VA. Autoantibody profiles and neurological correlations of thymoma. Clin Cancer Res 2004;10:7270–5.

33. Elrington GM, Murray NM, Spiro SG, et al. Neurological paraneoplastic syndromes in patients with small cell lung cancer. A prospective survey of 150 patients. J Neurol Neurosurg Psychiatr 1991;54(9):764–7.

34. Saket RR, Geschwind MD, Josephson SA, et al. Autoimmune-Mediated Encephalopathy: Classification, Evaluation, and MR Imaging Patterns of Disease. Neurographics 2011;1:2–16.

35. Irani S, Lang B. Autoantibody-mediated disorders of the central nervous system. Autoimmunity 2008;41:55–65.

36. Pruitt AA. Immune-mediated encephalopathies with an emphasis on paraneoplastic encephalopathies. Semin Neurol 2011;31:158–68.

37. Rosenfeld MR, Titulaer MJ, Dalmau J. Paraneoplastic syndromes and autoimmune encephalitis: Five new things. Neurol Clin Pract 2012;2:215–23.

38. Graus F, Titulaer MJ, Balu R, et al. A clinical approach to diagnosis of autoimmune encephalitis. Lancet Neurol 2016;15(4):391–404.

39. Vernino S, Geschwind M, Boeve B. Autoimmune encephalopathies. Neurologist 2007;13:140–7.

40. Graus F, Delattre JY, Antoine JC, et al. Recommended diagnostic criteria for paraneoplastic neurological syndromes. J Neurol Neurosurg Psychiatry 2004;75:1135–40.

41. Sadeghian H, Vernino S. Progress in the management of paraneoplastic neurological disorders. Ther Adv Neurol Disord 2010;3:43–52.

42. Aragão Mde M, Pedroso JL, Albuquerque MV, et al. Superior cerebellar hyperintense sign on FLAIR-weighted magnetic resonance imaging in paraneoplastic cerebellar degeneration. Arq Neuropsiquiatr 2012;70:967.

43. Graus F, Saiz A. Limbic encephalitis: an expanding concept. Neurology 2008;70:500–1.

44. Kelley BP, Patel SC, Marin HL, et al. Autoimmune Encephalitis: Pathophysiology and Imaging Review of an Overlooked Diagnosis. AJNR Am J Neuroradiol 2017;38(6):1070–8.

45. Urbach H, Soeder BM, Jeub M, et al. Serial MRI of limbic encephalitis. Neuroradiology 2006;48:380–6.

46. Lawn ND, Westmoreland BF, Kiely MJ, et al. Clinical, magnetic resonance imaging, and electroencephalographic findings in paraneoplastic limbic encephalitis. Mayo Clin Proc 2003;78:1363–8.

47. Blaes F. Paraneoplastic brain stem encephalitis. Curr Treat Options Neurol 2013;15:201–9.

48. Vernino S, Tuite P, Adler CH, et al. Paraneoplastic chorea associated with CRMP-5 neuronal antibody and lung carcinoma. Ann Neurol 2002;51:625–30.

49. Hiraga A, Kuwabara S, Hayakawa S, et al. Voltage-gated potassium channel antibody-associated encephalitis with basal ganglia lesions. Neurology 2006;66:1780–1.

50. Alexopoulos H, Dalakas MC. Immunology of stiff person syndrome and other GAD-associated neurological disorders. Expert Rev Clin Immunol 2013;9: 1043–53.

51. Antoine JC, Mosnier JF, Absi L, et al. Carcinoma associated paraneoplastic peripheral neuropathies in patients with and without anti-onconeural antibodies. J Neurol Neurosurg Psychiatr 1999; 67(1):7–14.

52. Titulaer MJ, Verschuuren JJ. Lambert-Eaton myasthenic syndrome: tumor versus nontumor forms. Ann N Y Acad Sci 2008;1132:129–34.

53. Oguro-Okano M, Griesmann GE, Wieben ED, et al. Molecular diversity of neuronal-type calcium channels identified in small cell lung carcinoma. Mayo Clin Proc 1992;67:1150–9.

54. Katz E, Ferro PA, Weiss G, et al. Calcium channels involved in synaptic transmission at the mature and regenerating mouse neuromuscular junction. J Physiol 1996;497:687–9.

55. Motomura M, Lang B, Johnston I, et al. Incidence of serum anti-P/Q-type and anti-N-type calcium channel autoantibodies in the Lambert-Eaton myasthenic syndrome. J Neurol Sci 1997;147:35–42.

56. Graus F, Keime-Guibert F, Rene R, et al. Anti-Hu-associated paraneoplastic encephalomyelitis: analysis of 200 patients. Brain 2001;124:138–48.

57. Sillevis Smitt P, Grefkens J, de Leeuw B, et al. Survival and outcome in 73 anti-Hu positive patients with paraneoplastic encephalomyelitis/sensory neuronopathy. J Neurol 2002;249:745–53.

58. Dalmau J, Tüzün E, Wu H, et al. Paraneoplastic anti–N methyl-D-aspartate receptor encephalitis associated with ovarian teratoma. Ann Neurol 2007;61: 25–36.

59. Schmitt SE, Pargeon K, Frechette ES, et al. Extreme delta brush: a unique EEG pattern in adults with anti-NMDA receptor encephalitis. Neurology 2012;79: 1094–100.

60. Chan SH, Wong VC, Fung CW, et al. Anti-NMDA receptor encephalitis with atypical brain changes on MRI. Pediatr Neurol 2010;43:274–8.

61. Greiner H, Leach JL, Lee KH, et al. Anti-NMDA receptor encephalitis presenting with imaging findings and clinical features mimicking Rasmussen syndrome. Seizure 2011;20:266–70.

62. Vernino S, Lennon VA. Ion channel and striational antibodies define a continuum of autoimmune neuromuscular hyperexcitability. Muscle Nerve 2002;26:702–7.

63. Geschwind MD, Tan KM, Lennon VA, et al. Voltage-gated potassium channel autoimmunity mimicking Creutzfeldt-Jakob disease. Arch Neurol 2008;65: 1341–6.

Imaging of Neurologic Injury following Oncologic Therapy

Tao Ouyang, MD[a,b,*], Sangam Kanekar, MD[b,c,d]

KEYWORDS

- Radiation therapy • Radiation necrosis • Chemotherapy • Immunotherapy
- Immune check point inhibitor • CAR-T therapy • SMART syndrome • Methotrexate • Temozolimide

KEY POINTS

- Neurologic injury arise from treatment of central nervous system malignancies (primary and secondary) as result of direct toxic effects or indirect vascular, autoimmune, or infectious effects.
- Neuro-oncologists, radiation oncologists, and radiologists are likely to encounter an increase in number of patients with treatment-induced complications given increased survival rates and increased treatment options, including novel immunotherapies.
- Neurocognitive effects can occur in patients who live more than 6 months after radiation therapy and have been best described in children.
- Central nervous system complications of chemotherapy include aseptic meningitis, stroke-like syndromes, posterior reversible encephalopathy syndrome, dural sinus thrombosis, transverse myelopathy, and delayed leukoencephalopathy.
- Immunotherapy in neurologic tumors currently include check point inhibitors, vaccines, viral therapy and chimeric antigen receptor T-cell therapy.

INTRODUCTION

Primary and secondary central nervous system (CNS) malignancies present a treatment challenge owing to overall poor prognosis and presence of blood brain barrier. Glioblastoma (GBM) is the most aggressive primary brain tumor in adults, with a 2-year survival rate of approximately 17% and current median survival of 15 months. Close to 20,000 patients are diagnosed in the United States with GBM each year. Brain metastasis occurs in 8% to 10% of adult patients with cancer. The common primary malignancies that metastasize to the brain are lung, breast, and melanoma. Additional cancers with brain metastases include renal cell, colorectal cancer, and gynecologic cancers. Brain metastases are typically associated with advanced stage cancer. With improvement in the survival of patients with systemic cancers, it is expected that incidence of brain metastasis will only increase. Mainstream treatments for CNS malignancies include resection, radiation, chemotherapy, immunotherapy, and combination treatments.

In general, treatments have improved outcomes in some malignancies, especially lymphoma, leukemia, and melanoma.[1] Survival for malignant glioma has not significantly improved in the past 3 decades despite advances in treatment. Brain metastases are associated with a poor prognosis similar, to that of GBM, with a median survival of

[a] Department of Radiology, Penn State Health, Hershey, PA, USA; [b] Division of Neuroradiology, Penn State Milton Hershey Medical Center, Penn State College of Medicine, Mail Code H066 500 University Drive, Hershey, PA 17033, USA; [c] Department of Radiology, Penn State College of Medicine, Hershey, PA, USA; [d] Department of Neurology, Penn State College of Medicine, Hershey, PA, USA
* Corresponding author. Division of Neuroradiology, Penn State Milton Hershey Medical Center, Penn State College of Medicine, Mail Code H066 500 University Drive, Hershey, PA 17033.
E-mail address: touyang@pennstatehealth.psu.edu

Radiol Clin N Am 59 (2021) 425–440
https://doi.org/10.1016/j.rcl.2021.01.008
0033-8389/21/© 2021 Elsevier Inc. All rights reserved.

about 12 to 15 months. Despite major advances in oncologic diagnosis and treatment, the survival time for patients treated with radiation therapy remains at 3 to 6 months. Overall survival is often determined by the extent and activity of the primary tumor.

Unfortunately, all oncologic therapies are to some extent neurotoxic. Neurologic injury arise from treatment of CNS malignancies (primary and secondary) as result of direct toxic effects or indirect vascular, autoimmune, or infectious effects. Multimodality treatment may potentiate both therapeutic and toxic effects. Symptoms range from mild to severe and permanent and can be greatly debilitating to patients and their caregivers. Injuries can be immediate or delayed. Neuro-oncologists, radiation oncologists, and radiologists are likely to encounter an increase in the number of patients with treatment-induced complications given the increased survival rates and increased treatment options, including novel immunotherapies.

Many of the early complications are nonspecific and either do not require imaging for diagnosis or have no definite radiographic correlate. These complications include headache, nausea, vomiting, dizziness, confusion, dystonia, Parkinsonian symptoms, cerebellar syndrome, tremors, and seizures. Other early and delayed neurologic injuries, such as posterior reversible encephalopathy syndrome (PRES), dural sinus thrombosis, infarctions, myelopathy, leukoencephalopathy, and hypophysitis, have unique imaging features.

This article reviews the current treatment options for CNS malignancies and common and uncommon neurologic injuries that can result from treatment, with a focus on radiologic features.

RADIATION THERAPY

Radiation therapy remains mainstay of treatment for primary and secondary CNS malignancies. Approximately 200,000 patients per year receive radiation yearly in the United States.[2] Currently, photons, electrons, and protons are all used in particle-based radiation therapy. Cranial radiation therapy may be delivered externally or be injected or implanted. Treatment may be targeted or whole brain based, and administered as a single fraction or fractionated. Regardless, all radiation therapy relies on DNA breakage as the mechanism of cell death.

Whole brain radiation therapy is used for brain metastasis. It is administered to the entire brain, usually over multiple treatments. Local field external beam radiation is used for malignant gliomas because the overwhelming majority of recurrences occur at or immediately adjacent to the original tumor. Stereotactic radiosurgery delivers precisely targeted radiation to brain lesions and can be used for both metastases and primary brain tumors. For high-grade gliomas, adjuvant radiation therapy after maximal safe resection improves local control and survival. Involved field radiation therapy delivers radiation to the tumor or tumor bed plus a margin of radiographically normal tissue. The standard dose for GBM is 60 Gy given over 6 weeks in 2-Gy fractions, usually with concurrent chemotherapy. For anaplastic astrocytoma (World Health Organization grade III), usually a slightly lower total dose is used in slightly smaller fractions.

Particle radiation (neutrons, helium ions, and protons) have been studied as boosters to conventional radiation therapy. The theoretic advantage to these particles are finite path lengths and the ability to concentrate the majority of their dose at the end of their path length, with little exit dose. This feature potentially decrease radiation exposure of normal surrounding tissue. Proton radiation is commonly used to treat pediatric CNS tumors, such as medulloblastoma, but its superiority in other CNS malignancies is not established. Similarly, brachytherapy, which is the placement of radioisotope seeds in the tumor or surgical cavity, is of limited usefulness in malignant gliomas.[3,4] Malignant gliomas tend to be infiltrative tumors, and brachytherapy delivers high-dose radiation to areas located few millimeters from the seeds; therefore, it does not adequately reach the full extent of disease.

Sheline[5] was the first to classify the radiation-induced side effects according to their time of appearance after irradiation into acute disorders (days to weeks), early–delayed complications (1–6 months), and late–delayed complications (<6 months). The mechanism of radiation therapy-induced damage to the CNS seems to be complex and likely to include a combination of vascular injury, demyelination, neuronal damage, effects on the fibrinolytic enzyme pathway, and immune mediated.[6] The vascular injury is thought to be partly responsible for the abnormal vasculature, thrombosis, and fibrinoid necrosis eventually leading to radiation necrosis. Radiation therapy also causes cell depletion, especially oligodendrocytes, which in turn leads to demyelination and white matter necrosis. Other cells such as neurons, astrocytes, and microglia are also damaged. Other factors that increase the risk of radiation-induced toxicity are older age, concurrent diseases (such as diabetes and hypertension), vascular disease, concurrent chemotherapy, and genetic predisposition. In stereotactic radiosurgery, additional risk factors include dose, treatment volume, location of lesion(s), and concurrent systemic treatment.[7]

In the human body, different cell systems have different sensitivity to the radiation. Cells that are actively reproducing are more sensitive to radiation therapy than those that are not. Blood cells that are constantly regenerating are, therefore, most sensitive, whereas nerve and muscle cells are the slowest to regenerate and therefore are least sensitive to radiation. Although the vascular endothelial cells and oligodendrocytes have been regarded as direct primary targets of radiation, the overall effect is thought to be multifactorial and attributed to more than 1 cell lineage.

Early Complications of Radiation Therapy

Many of the early complications are nonspecific and without radiographic features, including fatigue, headache, local skin reaction, alopecia, nausea and vomiting, dizziness and vertigo, and anorexia. Some patients present with acute encephalopathy and seizures without imaging correlates. Focal neurologic deficits and seizure in some cases can worsen owing to cerebral edema can be seen in some cases, especially when the treated lesion is larger in size and after stereotactic radiosurgery, and can account for symptoms within 2 weeks of treatment. Other complications include serous otitis and parotitis.

Delayed Complications of Radiation Therapy

Pseudoprogression refers to treatment effects that mimic the appearance of tumor progression, often occurring in the first 3 months after treatment. Pseudoprogression is more common in patients with *MGMT*-methylated GBM. Differentiating psuedoprogression from true progression is a particular challenge in the interpretation of surveillance MR imaging. Radiation necrosis (RN) is the delayed effect of radiation therapy that can occur anywhere from 1 to 10 years after treatment, with the peak period between 1 and 3 years. On MR imaging, RN can have a confusing and bizarre appearance with hyperintensity on T2-weighted (T2W) imaging and fluid attenuation inversion recovery (FLAIR) imaging, edema, and marked enhancement. Knowledge of the radiation therapy history and plan is helpful to differentiate RN from true progression. Advanced MR techniques are also helpful, especially perfusion and spectroscopy, because the cerebral blood volume will be low in RN and spectroscopy will demonstrate elevated lactate without elevation of choline (**Fig. 1**). Necrosis seems to be dose dependent and tends to occur at or near the site of treatment.

RN can occur in more distant sites, such as the inferior frontal lobes and brain stem in patients treated for nasopharyngeal carcinoma. Pseudoprogression and RN are discussed in detail elsewhere in this issue.

Stroke, cavernous malformations, and hemorrhage can occur as a delayed complications of radiation therapy, especially in patients who received radiation therapy at a younger age or received high doses, with irradiation of the circle of Willis region. Stroke has been noted in both pediatric and adult patients and seems to be associated with dose to the circle of Willis.[8] Moya moya–like disease has been reported approximately 3 to 4 years after radiation therapy and is found in higher rates in children and those with neurofibromatosis type 1.[9] Cavernoma develops approximately 3 to 6 years after radiation therapy and may grow over time; occasionally, they can hemorrhage and cause edema. The typical MR imaging appearance of cavernoma is of a relatively well-defined lesion with heterogeneous T1-weighted (T1W) signal owing to subacute blood products and a T2W hypointense rim. There is exuberant blooming on susceptibility weighted imaging sequences (**Fig. 2**). Usually, there is little or no surrounding edema, unless there is a recent hemorrhage.

Stroke-like migraine attacks after radiation therapy syndrome is a delayed complication characterized by complex neurologic signs and symptoms in patients with history of chemoradiotherapy, usually whole brain radiation. It has been reported in patients ranging from 6 to 30 years after radiation treatment. Patients present with subacute onset of stroke-like symptoms, such as homonymous hemianopsia, hemiplegia, aphasia, and/or seizures. MR imaging reveals cortical edema and gadolinium enhancement, often leptomeningeal, not following any particular vascular distribution (**Fig. 3**).[10] Findings are potentially confusing for tumor progression or recurrence. It is still a poorly understood entity. The majority of patients have resolution of symptoms over the course of several weeks, with resolution of radiographic abnormalities, but up to 45% can have residual deficits.[11] Stroke-like migraine attacks after radiation therapy syndrome can also recur.

Pituitary and hypothalamic dysfunction are common after radiation therapy and may occur in up to 80% of patients, with grown hormone deficiency being the most commonly encountered complication in children.[12] Young and pediatric patients with sellar and/or suprasellar disease may experience hypothalamic hyperphagia and obesity after treatment.

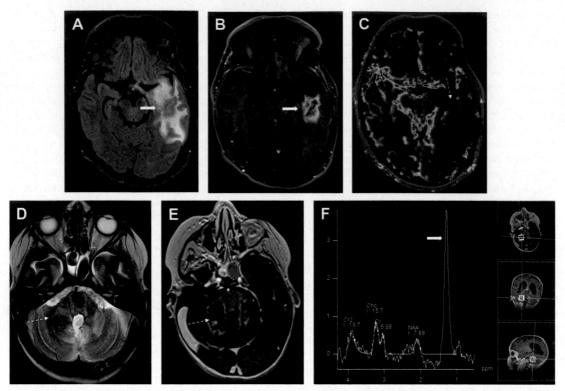

Fig. 1. Two cases of RN. Axial FLAIR (*A*) and T1 post-contrast (*B*) shows edema surrounding an enhancing lesion in the left temporal lobe (*solid arrows*). Enhancement pattern is peripheral and feathery. MR perfusion with overlay (*C*) shows low CBV (*dotted arrow*). Axial T2W (*D*) and T1 post-contrast (*E*) images from another patient shows faint irregular peripheral enhancement in the right cerebellum and brachium pontis (*dotted arrows*), MR spectroscopy (*F*) of the same region reveals a large lactate peak at 1.3 ppm (*solid arrow*) without choline elevation.

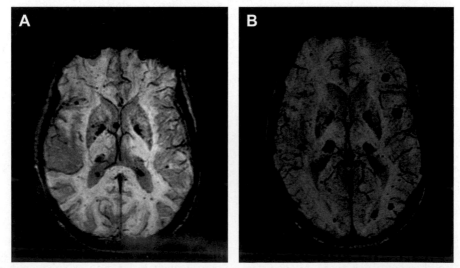

Fig. 2. Radiation-induced cavernomas. A 51-year-old male patient was treated with whole brain radiation therapy for a pineal tumor in 2014. Postradiation axial susceptibility weighted imaging (in 2019) (*B*) shows interval development of multiple cavenomas. Preradiation axial susceptibility weighted image from 2014 (*A*) for comparison.

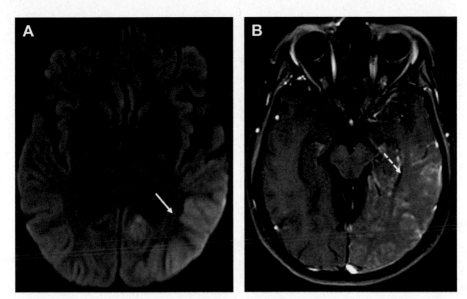

Fig. 3. Stroke-like migraine attacks after radiation therapy (SMART) syndrome. A 28-year-old woman with a history of medulloblastoma presented with headache and stroke-like migraine. Axial FLAIR image (A) shows left posterior temporal and occipital cortical hyperintensity and mild swelling (*arrow*) with corresponding cortical enhancement (*dotted arrow*) on the postcontrast T1WI (B).

Delayed radiation effects on the spinal cord can present as a myelopathy syndrome or a lower motor neuron syndrome. Imaging shows T2W hyperintensity of the spinal cord with or without enhancement and follow-up imaging shows volume loss indicating myelomalacia.[13] Rarely, patients can present with cord hemorrhage, thought to be from an underlying radiation-induced vascular malformation (**Fig. 4**).

Radiation-induced malignancy is a dreaded late complication of wide field radiation. Malignancies that can develop include meningioma, glioma, sarcoma, and nerve sheath tumor (**Fig. 5**). These may occur anywhere from 5 years to decades after treatment and are a serious concern for patients with long expected survival after primary malignancy. This entity is less of a concern in patients with metastatic CNS disease or GBM, whose

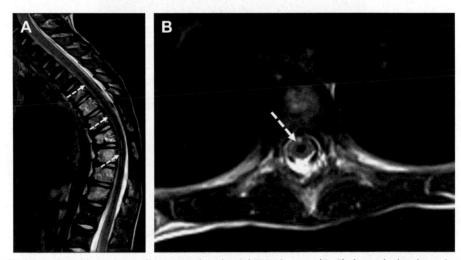

Fig. 4. Radiation-induced hematomyelia. Sagittal and axial T2W images (A, B) through the thoracic cord shows mild expansion of the cord and low signal owing to hemorrhage within the central portion (*arrows*) along with syrinx.

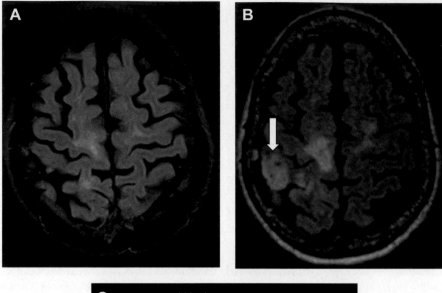

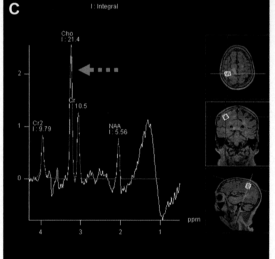

Fig. 5. Presumed post radiation secondary glioma in a patient treated with whole brain radiation for cerebral metastasis. Axial FLAIR (A) shows no mass lesion in the bilateral cerebral parenchyma. Four years follow up MRI, axial FLAIR (B) shows mass lesion in the right post central gyrus, with elevated choline peak (dotted arrow) on MR spectroscopy (C).

expected survival is often (much) shorter than 5 years. It is possible that narrow field radiation such as stereotactic radiosurgery may be associated with a lower incidence of secondary malignancy. Outcomes comparing photon versus proton based therapies are lacking.

Neurocognitive effects can occur in patients who live more than 6 months after radiation therapy and have been best described in children who survived brain tumors or acute lymphocytic leukemia.[14,15] Children, especially those who were treated with high-dose chemoradiotherapy before age 6, showed lower scholastic achievement and lower IQ. This effect seems to be dose dependent based on research with children with high- versus low-risk medulloblastoma.[16] In adults, whole brain radiation therapy has also been linked to decline in memory and learning functions in patients with non-small cell lung cancer.[17] Radiographic findings include nonspecific white matter FLAIR hyperintensity and brain atrophy (Fig. 6). The relationship between partial brain radiation and neurocognitive decline is less well-established, and targeted radiotherapies may decrease the effect on cognition.

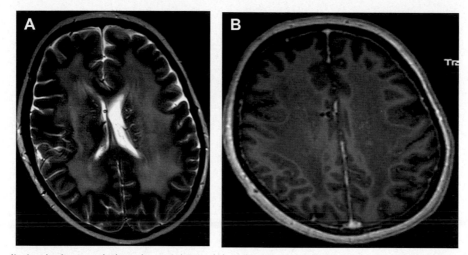

Fig. 6. Radiation leukoencephalopathy. Axial T2W (*A*) and axial T1W (*B*) images show diffuse hyperintensity and hypointensity respectively of the cerebral white matter owing to radiation-induced demyelination.

CHEMOTHERAPY

Chemotherapy, both systemic and intrathecal, and often in combination, remains some of the most effective and widely used treatments for cancer. There are many classes of chemotherapy agents based on their mechanism of action, and many are known to cause neurologic complications. Complications can be acute (during treatment or within 50 days from end of therapy), subacute or delayed (within 3 months of therapy), and late (beyond 3 months). Peripheral neuropathy is most common chemotherapy associated neurotoxicity, especially with platinum based agents. Taxanes and vinca alkaloid agents are also associated with sensory neuropathy, and vincristine has been associated with autonomic and cranial neuropathies.[18]

CNS complications include aseptic meningitis, stroke-like syndromes, PRES, dural sinus thrombosis, transverse myelopathy, and delayed leukoencephalopathy (**Fig. 7**). Methotrexate (MTX) CNS toxicity is best described, but other antimetabolites can cause optic neuropathy, cerebellar syndrome, acute encephalopathy, and cerebral venous thrombosis and venous infarction or hemorrhage in the brain.

Methotrexate

MTX is a frequently used chemotherapy agent and is one of the few approved for intrathecal injection. It works by reducing the amount of tetrahydrofolate available for DNA synthesis, ultimately leading to cell death. There are several well-described MTX-related neurologic complications, including aseptic meningitis, transverse myelopathy, and

toxic and necrotic encephalopathy syndromes. Aseptic meningitis is the most common acute CNS toxicity from MTX after intrathecal administration. Symptoms develop as soon as 2 to 4 hours after receiving MTX and usually resolve after 72 hours. Cerebrospinal fluid analysis and MR imaging are usually unrevealing and not required for diagnosis.

Acute toxic encephalopathy after MTX administration has characteristic radiologic findings of restricted diffusion in the white matter, usually affecting the periventricular white matter or centrum semiovale. Usually there is little edema or enhancement. These areas maybe hyperintense on T2W and FLAIR imaging, but sometimes may have little signal change on these sequences. Abnormalities on diffusion-weighted imaging are the hallmark for this diagnosis (**Fig. 8**). Imaging findings may be seen shortly after administration of systemic or intrathecal MTX and is usually reversible.

An acute transverse myelopathy has also been described with MTX, with resemblance radiologically to subacute combined degeneration. Hyperintense T2W and short T1 inversion recovery signal is seen in the spinal cord, predominantly affecting the dorsal columns. There can be variable enhancement, if any (**Fig. 9**). Acute myelopathy is variably reversible. It does not seem dose dependent, suggesting that patient factors maybe at play, and seem to be associated with advanced or young age and prior spinal radiation.[19,20]

A much more debilitating delayed complication of systemic and intrathecal MTX therapy is delayed multifocal necrotizing leukoencephalopathy, which can occur months to years after

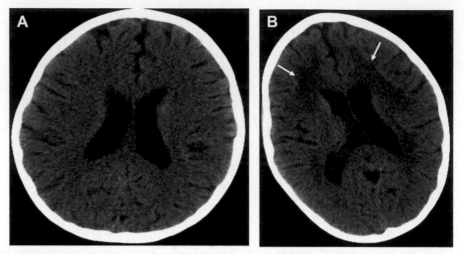

Fig. 7. Postchemotherapy leukoencephalopathy. Prechemotherapy CT scan of the 35-year-old male patient with acute lymphocytic leukemia (ALL) treated with chemotherapy. A follow-up scan at 2 years shows diffuse hypo-density of the cerebral white matter owing to chemotherapy-induced demyelination.

treatment.[19] The patient presents with severe dementia with personality changes. MR imaging shows brain atrophy, confluent white matter, FLAIR hyperintensity, necrosis, and patchy areas of enhancement. Usually, this complication occurs after repeated high-dose MTX or combined MTX and radiation therapy.

Temozolimide

Temozolimide, an alkylating agent, deserves special discussion because it is now part of the standard therapy for malignant gliomas and is also sometimes used in low-grade gliomas. Its mechanism of action seems to be methylation of DNA, leading ultimately to the apoptosis of tumor cells. The standard treatment for malignant glioma is concurrent radiation with temozolomide, followed by at least 6 months of adjuvant temozolimide.[21] Longer term low-dose temozolimide as maintenance therapy is often used. Acute toxicity includes nausea, thrombocytopenia, and leukopenia.[22] The primary radiographic complication of temozolimide is potentiation of pseudoprogression in the setting of concurrent chemoradiation. Some studies have shown that MGMT promoter methylation in gliomas is a predictor of response to temozolimide.[23]

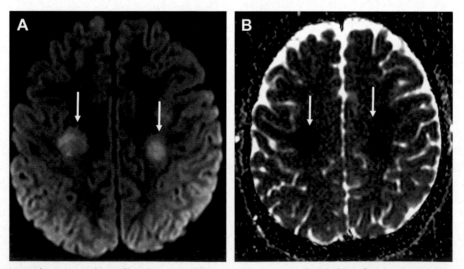

Fig. 8. Acute methotrexate demyelination. Axial DWI and ADC images (*A, B*) show focal areas of restricted diffusion in the centrum semiovale bilaterally (*arrows*) in a patient treated with intrathecal methotrexate for ALL four days prior to MRI. Patient presented with sudden onset of transient paresis.

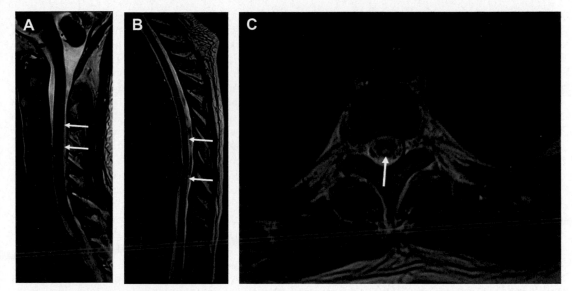

Fig. 9. Acute MTX-induced myelitis. Acute onset paraparesis in a patient within 48 hours of intrathecal instillation of methotrexate. Sagittal and axial T2 image of the cervical (*A*), and thoracic spine (*B, C*) shows linear T2 hyperintensity in the dorsal columns of the cervical cord and the central thoracic cord (*arrows*).

There is also interest in the combination chemotherapies with temozolimide for GBM and anaplastic astrocytoma, as well as for recurrent GBM with MGMT promoter methylation.[24] Additional agents being investigated include vincristine, CCNU, and procabazine. CCNU is also being studied as combination therapy with bevazimumab in recurrent GBM.[25]

Targeted Agents

Targeted agents are the newest frontier in chemotherapeutics and more than 100 new agents have been approved in the last decade.[26] These include 20 classes of tyrosine kinase inhibitors (eg, imatinib, sunitinib, and sorafenib) and monoclonal antibodies (bevacizumab, rituzimab, and alemtuzumab). These newer agents also cause neurologic side effects, some similar to conventional chemotherapy agents, including headache, fatigue, cranial and peripheral neuropathies. In addition, tyrosine kinase inhibitors are associated with a small risk of spontaneous subdural hematomas. Both rituzimab and alemtuzumab, which are antibodies against CD20 and CD25, respectively, have been associated with progressive multifocal leukoencephalopathy with JC virus reactivation.[27,28] The vascular endothelial growth factor targeting agents can cause hypertension and PRES as well as an increase the risk of ischemic stroke.[27]

Bevacizumab is a humanized monoclonal antibody that targets vascular endothelial growth factor-A, a highly expressed proangiogenic factor in gliomas. Targeting vascular endothelial growth factor decreases tumor vascularity. Bevacizumab is now often used in patients with malignant glioma with radiographic disease progression after completing standard concurrent chemoradiation. Decreased contrast enhancement, edema, and permeability can be seen as early as 1 day after initiation of bevacizumab therapy. Radiologic response rates are high, ranging from 25% to 60%. Despite remarkable imaging response after bevacizumab, there has been no proven substantial benefit in overall survival.[29] Bevacizumab is associated with PRES as well as a phenomenon called pseudoresponse, where tumoral enhancement improves significantly but progression ultimately manifests as nonenhancing, FLAIR hyperintense disease. Development of nonenhancing restricted diffusion within the tumor and vicinity has been termed coagulative necrosis and has been associated with a poorer prognosis.[30]

PRES is thought to be related to failure of autoregulation of cerebral blood pressure and local CNS inflammation. PRES was originally described in uncontrolled hypertension, eclampsia, and patients undergoing immunosuppression for organ transplantation.[31] Patients present with headache, confusion, visual changes, or seizures. MR imaging typically demonstrates focal regions of symmetric hemispheric white matter edema. The parietal and occipital lobes are most commonly affected, followed by the frontal lobes, the inferior temporal–occipital junction, and the cerebellum. These areas are usually hypointense on T1W imaging and hyperintense on T2W and FLAIR imaging. The subcortical U fibers are often affected. There may be associated restricted diffusion and/or hemorrhage (**Fig. 10**). PRES is seen more commonly in patients receiving cyclosporine and cyclophosphamide and targeted gents such as bevacizumab, ipilimumab, sunitinib, and rituximab. Treatment is symptom based, as well as removal of the suspected causative agent. The clinical and radiographic changes of this syndrome are usually reversible unless cerebral infarction has occurred.

Cerebral venous sinus thrombosis is a potentially devastating entity that can lead to venous infarction and hemorrhage. It has been associated with chemotherapy regimens including platinum based agents and L-asparaginase. On computed tomography scans, the dural sinus or cerebral vein will appear abnormally hyperdense. On MR imaging, a thrombus in the affected vessel will appear hyperintense on T1W imaging and of varying signal intensity on T2W imaging. A thrombosed vein will appear abnormally hyperintense on FLAIR imaging and drop out on susceptibility weighted imaging, which is classic. Postcontrast T1W images may show a nonenhancing clot within the affected vessel. The brain parenchyma may appear normal or be edematous/ischemic, and in some cases parenchymal hemorrhage will be present (**Fig. 11**).

Progressive multifocal leukoencephalopathy is an infectious process that affects the white matter, caused by reactivation of the JC virus. This virus is present usually in asymptomatic individuals, but in the context of immunosuppression, circulates in B cells and infects and destroys oligodendrocytes. On MR imaging, there are confluent asymmetrical white matter lesions which are hyperintense on T2W and FLAIR imaging, and may not enhance (**Fig. 12**). There is often subcortical U fiber involvement. Appearance is different from PRES in its asymmetry and distribution, with no predilection for the parietal or occipital lobes. Lesions can progress fairly rapidly. Diagnosis is made by cerebrospinal fluid testing and there is no effective treatment.

Many patients who received chemotherapy describe more global neurocognitive impairment that is less dramatic than the multifocal leukoencephalopathy of MTX. This complication is often colloquially termed "chemo brain" and mostly affects short-term memory and executive function. There may be little or subtle radiologic findings, such as diffuse white matter T2W and FLAIR hyperintensity and volume loss. However, there is some overlap between treatment effects and the effect of cancer itself on the brain.

COMBINATION THERAPIES

The use of chemotherapy potentiated effectiveness of radiation by introducing unique and increased DNA aberrations that differ from those induced by either radiation or chemotherapy alone. Unlike conventional chemotherapy, which exerts its cytotoxic effects on all replicating cells, conformal radiation is particularly effective at producing DNA damage specifically in tumor cells.[32] Commonly used chemoradiation regimens include antimetabolites, platinum-based agents, alkylating agents, and, more recently, novel agents such as antibodies and immunotherapy. Antimetabolites

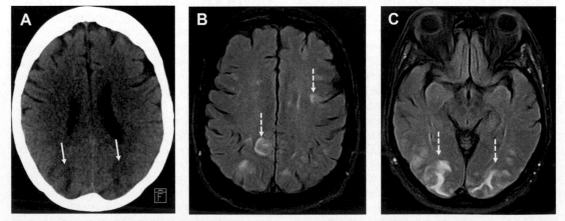

Fig. 10. PRES in patient who was undergoing chemotherapy treatment for leukemia. Axial CT scan (*A*) shows symmetrical hypodensities (*solid arrows*) in the posterior parietal lobe cortex bilaterally. Axial FLAIR (*B, C*) images show bilateral symmetrical hyperintensity in the cortex and subjacent white matter of occipital and frontal lobes (*dotted arrows*).

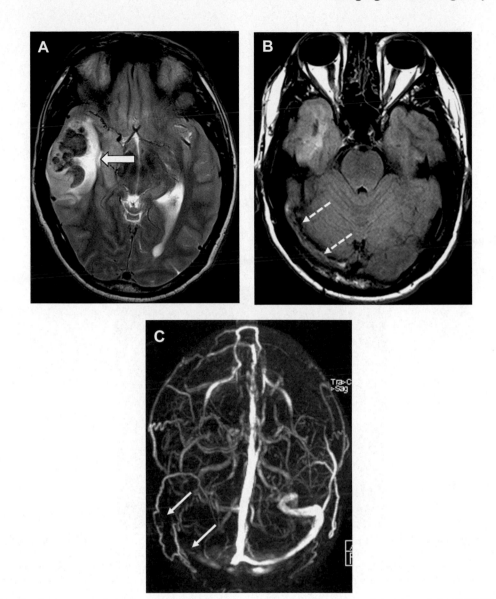

Fig. 11. Cerebral venous thrombosis in patient treated with cisplastin for neuroblastoma. Axial T2W (*A*) shows hemorrhagic stroke in the right temporal lobe (*thick arrow*). Axial FLAIR image (*B*) and MR venogram (*C*) shows thrombosis of the right lateral and sigmoid sinuses, appearing as abnormal FLAIR hyperintense signal (*dotted arrows*) and absence of flow related signal (*solid arrows*) respectively.

are commonly used in combination with radiation. The combination of these agents with radiation leads to the production of complex, slowly repaired radiation-induced DNA damage. Platinum-based agents such as cisplatin are the most widely used chemotherapeutic agents in combination with radiation, especially in lung and head and neck cancers. The standard therapy for GBMs is concurrent temozolomide radiation. Radiosensitization by temozolomide involves inhibition of DNA repair and/or an increase in radiation-induced double-stranded breaks. Other novel agents sensitize tumor cells to radiation by

inhibition of the ubiquitin proteosome system (bortezomib) or modulation of tumor oxygen levels and aberrant tumor vasculature (bevacizumab).

IMMUNOTHERAPY

Immunotherapy has become a successful treatment option for many advance cancers, and can be used as stand alone or in combination with other modalities.[33] There are currently more than 500 open immunotherapy clinical trials at the time of this review. The brain is not as immune-privileged organ as previously thought, and

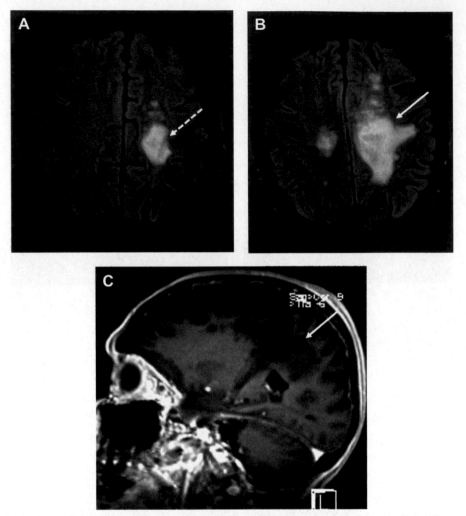

Fig. 12. Progressive multifocal leukoencephalopathy (PML) in 69-year-old male patient on chemotherapy for multiple myeloma. Axial FLAIR image in Aug 2017 (*A*) show a hyperintense PML lesion in the juxtacortical and centrum semiovale of the left frontal lobe (*dotted arrow*). Axial FLAIR and sagittal T1W images in Oct 2017 (*B, C*) show significant increase in the size of the lesions (*solid arrows*) with deterioration of the patient's symptoms.

immune checkpoint inhibitors have been successful for brain metastasis from melanoma and non-small cell lung cancer. Immunotherapy in CNS tumors currently include check point inhibitors, vaccines, viral therapy and chimeric antigen receptor T-cell (CAR-T) therapy.

Immune Check Point Inhibitors

Immune check point inhibition first emerged as a viable option in 2010, with CTLA-4 inhibitor (ipilimumab) in advanced melanoma resulting in improved overall survival.[34] Immune check points are signals (stimulatory or inhibitory) between tumor cells, T cells, dendritic cells, and macrophages in the tumor microenvironment. These checkpoints regulate T-cell activation to

tumor cells. It is known that tumors cause immune suppression and "escape" from T-cell–mediated immune responses so they can proliferate within the host.[35] Immune checkpoint inhibitors, including CTLA-4 inhibitor (ipilimumab), programmed death (PD)-1 inhibitors (nivolumab and pembrolizumab), and PD ligand 1 (L1) inhibitors (atezolizumab and durvalumab), counteract against tumor cells and activate the host's immune response against cancer. Currently, these agents are approved for use in the United States for numerous malignancies including melanoma, non-small cell lung cancer, renal cell carcinoma, Hodgkin lymphoma, head and neck squamous cell carcinoma, urothelial cell carcinoma, cervical cancer, colorectal cancers, and breast cancer.

Unique complications associated with use of immunotherapies have been collectively termed immune-related adverse events and can arise in almost any organ system. The mechanism is thought to be immune system activation with misdirection or overactivation. Organ-specific adverse events include hypophysitis, encephalitis, pneumonitis, hepatitis, myocarditis, colitis, and sarcoid-like lymphadenopathy. Neurologic adverse events are uncommon, occurring in 1% to 3% of patients and are mostly nonspecific such as headache, dizziness, and lethargy.[36] Other complications are similar to those from conventional chemotherapy agents and can include aseptic meningitis, acute and subacute encephalopathy, transverse myelopathy, PRES, demyelination, and polyneuropathies.[37] A well-described complication specific to immune checkpoint inhibitors is hypophysitis, with up to 17% of patients receiving ipilimumab developing hypophysitis.[38] On MR imaging, this appears as enlarged and enhancing pituitary gland and stalk that is either new from prior imaging studies and/or abnormal for age (**Fig. 13**).

Chimeric Antigen Receptor T-cell Therapy

CAR-T therapy is currently approved in leukemia and B-cell lymphoma. Essentially, CAR-T cells are genetically modified T cells that recognize a tumor-specific antigen and contains a T-cell activation signal inside the cell. When these modified T cells are introduced to the patient, they initiate lysis of the tumor cells bearing the tumor-specific antigen. The most common toxicity from CAR-T therapy is cytokine release syndrome, which is a systemic inflammatory response. Incidence of neurotoxicity varies greatly in reports, ranging

from 0% to 50%,[39] and may occur with and without systemic cytokine release. Neurotoxicity ranges from headaches and delirium to encephalopathy and seizures. Severe cases may require intensive care and dexamethasone treatment. Neuroimaging and cerebrospinal fluid analysis is recommended to exclude an underlying infection.

Immunotherapies in Glioblastoma

The low mutation burden in GBM, local and systemic immunosuppression of GBM, and its infiltrative nature likely account for difficulties in effective treatment of GBM with immune checkpoint inhibitors. GBM is a highly immunosuppressive solid tumor, even though it is confined to the brain. GBM is also highly infiltrative in a way that brain metastases are not. Immune checkpoint inhibitors tend to accumulate in the necrotic center of the tumor there where is more blood–brain barrier breakdown rather the infiltrative margins. The disease is also highly likely to recur. At this time, there are no immunotherapies approved by the US Food and Drug Administration for the treatment GBM, and GBM is notoriously immunosuppressive and immunologically quiet.[40] Checkpoint inhibitors are being studied in combination with other therapies. At the time of this writing, there were 8 published studies of immune checkpoint inhibitor alone and in conjunction with other agents for GBM and 3 yet unpublished studies, none of which found significant benefit in the immune checkpoint inhibitor group.[41] PD-1 and PD-L1 axis inhibitors, such as nivolumab and pembraolizumab, are the best studied immune checkpoint inhibitors in GBM. CTLA-4 and PD-1/PD-L1 dual blockade is also being studied. Another immunotherapy currently being studied is the proteasome inhibitor

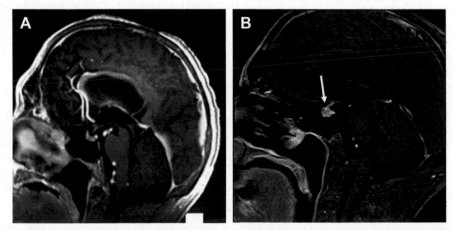

Fig. 13. Ipilimumab hypophysitis in patient with melanoma. Contrast enhanced sagittal T1W image before immunotherapy (*A*) shows normal appearance of the pituitary and infundibulum. There is mild hyperplasia of the pituitary gland (*arrow*) and thickening of the infundibulum after immunotherapy (*B*).

marizomib, which has demonstrated activity against CNS multiple myeloma. Several clinical trial with marizomib for GBM and recurrent GBM are underway.[42]

Other immunotherapies for GBM include vaccine therapy, which is designed to elicit an immune response to the cancer. Vaccines include direct antigen exposure as well as antigen-presenting cells (dendritic cells). The best studied tumor specific antigen is a mutation of epidermal growth factor, epidermal growth factor variant III. The epidermal growth factor mutation is seen in 2% to 25% of GBM. An epidermal growth factor variant III–specific peptide was developed by Celldex therapeutics, rindopepimut. A phase III trial of rindopepimut showed no significant improvement in survival in wither the treatment or the control arms, however.[43] A number of tumor-associated antigens are being studied, including single antigen vaccine called SurVaxM and vaccines targeting multiple antigens such as Sl701 and ICT-101. These are currently in phase II and I trials, respectively.[44]

Customized vaccines are also promising. These vaccines are limited to patients with surgically accessible GBM, because a volume of the tumor is required to produce the vaccine, which is then reintroduced to the patient. Two such agents under study are DC-Vax-L and HSPPC-96. Dc-Vax-L, which uses tumor lysate to generate dendritic cells, was first studied 10 years ago with reports of durable responders surviving more than 7 years.[45] Phase III of this vaccine for newly diagnosed GBM is still underway. HSPPPC-96 is in phase II trials.[46] Viral therapy is a form of immunotherapy that virus vectors introduce genes into tumor cells to attract host immune response, ideally leading to tumor lysis. Two of these, ASPECT and Toca5, have made it to phase III trials.[47,48]

CAR-T therapy has been most effective against hematologic malignancies owing to their highly clonal nature and location (peripheral blood). The main challenges in the development of cell therapy in GBM are the location of the tumor, determining the most efficacious route of cell delivery (intravenous vs intrathecal), and the identification of a universal cell surface antigen to target. Tumor antigens that are potential CAR targets in GBM include IL-13Ra2, epidermal growth factor version III, Her2, and EphA2. Several factors contribute to lack of response to CAR T-cells in GBM, including a lack of stably expressed antigens, intratumoral heterogeneity, impaired CAR T-cell proliferation in a hypoxic environment, and an immunosuppressive microenvironment that leads to antigen escape.[49]

PEDIATRIC BRAIN

More than 10,000 children under the age of 14 are diagnosed with malignancy each year. More than 80% of these children are expected to be long-term survivors thanks to advances in modern cancer treatment. Although early neurologic toxicities and complications in children receiving treatment for cancer are similar to adults, higher survival rates and longer post-treatment lifespans mean that neurologic injury is even more impactful in survivors of childhood cancer. Moreover, the developing CNS system of a child is potentially more susceptible to the effects of radiation and chemotherapy, for reasons that have been details elsewhere in this article.

Cranial radiation therapy in pediatric patients with cancer has been associated with serious adverse effects that can lead to poor educational attainment and unemployment in long-term survivors. This has been well-studied in childhood survivors of acute lymphocytic leukemia. Contemporary protocols have now replaced chemoradiotherapy with systemic and intrathecal chemotherapy for acute lymphocytic leukemia, which has decreased the degree of survivors' cognitive impairment. Nevertheless, survivors of childhood acute lymphocytic leukemia displayed more neurocognitive and parent-rated neurobehavioral problems than population norms.[50] Survivors who developed acute leukoencephalopathy during therapy demonstrated more neurobehavioral problems than those who did not.[51]

Survivors of childhood cancer also have significantly higher incidence of secondary CNS neoplasms, primarily glioma and meningioma, compared with the general population. The imaging appearance of these malignancies as same as those occurring in patients without prior cancer treatment. Nearly all cancer survivors who developed a CNS neoplasm had been exposed to cranial radiation, and some studies showed a correlation between radiation dose and risk of subsequent CNS tumors.[52]

SUMMARY

The arsenal of treatments for CNS primary and secondary malignancies continue to grow, even though the mainstay of treatment remains radiation and chemotherapy, especially for malignant gliomas. Targeted and immune therapies are clearly the future of cancer care. All oncologic treatments carry inherent toxicities to the CNS, and many are associated with specific imaging appearances. The job of the neuroradiologist is made more complicated by treatment effects that mimic tumor progression or response. Moreover, additional neurologic toxicities of newer immunotherapies may yet be discovered as their use becomes widespread. Recognizing these complications and differentiating treatment effects from effects of the cancer itself are priorities for the treating team and can significantly impact the course of treatment and outcome.

DISCLOSURE

None.

REFERENCES

1. National Cancer Institute Surveillance. Epidemiology, and End Results (SFFR) Program. Available at. www.seer.cancer.gov. Accessed August 14, 2020.
2. Nolan CP, Lisa M, DeAngelis LM. Neurologic complications of chemotherapy and radiation therapy. Neurooncology 2015;21(2):429–51.
3. Laperriere NJ, Leung PM, McKenzie S, et al. Randomized study of brachytherapy in the initial management of patients with malignant astrocytoma. Int J Radiat Oncol Biol Phys 1998;41:1005–11.
4. Green SB, Shapiro WR, Burger PC, et al. A randomized trial of interstitial radiotherapy (RT) boost for newly diagnosed malignant glioma: Brain Tumor Cooperative Group (BTCG) trial 8701 (abstract). Proc Annu Meet Am Soc Clin Onco 1994; 13:174.
5. Sheline G. Radiation therapy of brain tumors. Cancer 1977;39:873–81.
6. Kumar AJ, Leeds NE, Fuller GN, et al. Malignant gliomas: MR imaging spectrum of radiation therapy- and chemotherapy-induced necrosis of the brain after treatment. Radiology 2000;217(2):377–84.
7. Tanguturi SK, Alexander BM. Neurologic Complications of Radiation Therapy. Neurol Clin 2018;36(3): 599–625.
8. El-Fayech C, Haddy N, Allodji RS, et al. Cerebrovascular diseases in childhood cancer survivors: role of the radiation dose to Willis circle arteries. Int J Radiat Oncol Biol Phys 2017;97(2):278–86.
9. Ullrich NJ, Robertson R, Kinnamon DD, et al. Moyamoya following cranial irradiation for primary brain tumors in children. Neurology 2007;68(12):932–8.
10. Kerklaan JP, Lycklama Nijeholt GJ, Wiggenraad RG, et al. SMART syndrome: a late reversible complication after radiation therapy for brain tumours. J Neurol 2011;258(6):1098–104.
11. Black DF, Morris JM, Lindell EP, et al. Stroke-like migraine attacks after radiation therapy (SMART) syndrome is not always completely reversible: a case series. AJNR Am J Neuroradiol 2013;34(12): 2298–303.
12. Constine LS, Woolf PD, Cann D, et al. Hypothalamic-pituitary dysfunction after radiation for brain tumors. N Engl J Med 1993;328(2):87–94.
13. Gibbs IC, Patil C, Gerszten PC, et al. Delayed radiation-induced myelopathy after spinal radiosurgery. Neurosurgery 2009;(64):a67–72.
14. Lahteenmaki PM, Harila-Saari A, Pukkala EI, et al. Scholastic achievements of children with brain tumors at the end of comprehensive education: a nationwide, register-based study. Neurology 2007; 69(3):296–305.
15. Harila-Saari AH, Lahteenmaki PM, Pukkala E, et al. Scholastic achievements of childhood leukemia patients: a nationwide, register-based study. J Clin Oncol 2007;25(23):3518–24.
16. Palmer SL, Armstrong C, Onar-Thomas A, et al. Processing speed, attention, and working memory after treatment for medulloblastoma: an international, prospective, and longitudinal study. J Clin Oncol 2013; 31(28):3494–500.
17. Sun A, Bae K, Gore EM, et al. Phase III trial of prophylactic cranial irradiation compared with observation in patients with locally advanced non-small-cell lung cancer: neurocognitive and quality-of-life analysis. J Clin Oncol 2011;29(3):279–86.
18. Legha SS. Vincristine neurotoxicity. Pathophysiology and management. Mcd Toxicol 1986;1(6):421–7.
19. Cachia D, Kamiya-Matsuoka C, Pinnix CC, et al. Myelopathy following intrathecal chemotherapy in adults: a single institution experience. J Neurooncol 2015;122(2):391–8.
20. Oka M, Terae S, Kobayashi R, et al. MRI in methotrexate-related leukoencephalopathy: disseminated necrotising leukoencephalopathy in comparison with mild leukoencephalopathy. Neuroradiology 2003;45(7):493–7.
21. Stupp R, Mason WP, van den Bent MJ, et al. Radiotherapy plus concomitant and adjuvant temozolomide for glioblastoma. N Engl J Med 2005;352(10): 987–96.
22. Mannas JP, Lightner DD, Defrates SR, et al. Long-term treatment with temozolomide in malignant glioma. J Clin Neurosci 2014;21(1):121–3.
23. Esteller M. Epigenetics in Cancer. N Engl J Med 2008;358:1148–59.
24. Kyritsis AP, Levin VA. An algorithm for chemotherapy treatment of recurrent glioma patients after temozolomide failure in the general oncology setting. Cancer Chemother Pharmacol 2011;67(5):971–83.
25. Erdem-Eraslan L, van den Bent MJ, Hoogstrate Y, et al. Identification of patients with recurrent glioblastoma who may benefit from combined bevacizumab and CCNU therapy: a report from the BELOB Trial. Cancer Res 2016;76(3):525–34.
26. Zukas AM, Schiff D. Neurological complications of new chemotherapy agents. Neurooncology 2018; 20(1):24–36.

27. Piccinni C, Sacripanti C, Poluzzi E, et al. Stronger association of drug-induced progressive multifocal leukoencephalopathy (PML) with biological immuno-modulating agents. Eur J Clin Pharmacol 2010; 66(2):199–206.

28. Glusker P, Recht L, Lane B. Reversible posterior leukoencephalopathy syndrome and bevacizumab. N Engl J Med 2006;354(9):980–2.

29. Kim MM, Umemura Y, Leung D. Bevacizumab and glioblastoma: past, present, and future directions. Cancer J 2018;24(4):180–6.

30. Nguyen HS, Milbach N, Hurrell SL, et al. Progressing bevacizumab-induced diffusion restriction is associated with coagulative necrosis surrounded by viable tumor and decreased overall survival in patients with recurrent glioblastoma. AJNR Am J Neuroradiol 2016;37(12):2201–8.

31. Bartynski WS. Posterior reversible encephalopathy syndrome, part 1: fundamental imaging and clinical features. AJNR Am J Neuroradiol 2008;29(6): 1036–42.

32. Morgan MA, Parsels LA, Maybaum J, et al. Improving the efficacy of chemoradiation with targeted agents. Cancer Discov 2014;4(3):280–91.

33. Nishino M, Hatabu H, Hodi FS. Imaging of cancer immunotherapy: current approaches and future directions. Radiology 2019;290(1):9–22.

34. Hodi FS, O'Day SJ, McDermott DF, et al. Improved survival with ipilimumab in patients with metastatic melanoma. N Engl J Med 2010;363(8):711–23.

35. Pardoll DM. The blockade of immune checkpoints in cancer immunotherapy. Nat Rev Cancer 2012;12(4): 252–64.

36. Spain L, Walls G, Julve M, et al. Neurotoxicity from immune-checkpoint inhibition in the treatment of melanoma: a single centre experience and review of the literature. Ann Oncol 2017;28(2):377–85.

37. Ly KI, Arrillaga-Romany IC. Neurologic complications of systemic anticancer therapy. Neurol Clin 2018;36(3):627–51.

38. Bot I, Blank CU, Boogerd W, et al. Neurological immune-related adverse events of ipilimumab. Pract Neurol 2013;13(4):278–80.

39. Brudno JN, Kochenderfer JN. Toxicities of chimeric antigen receptor T cells: recognition and management. Blood 2016;127(26):3321–30.

40. McGranahan T, Therkelsen KE, Ahmad S, et al. Current state of immunotherapy for treatment of glioblastoma. Curr Treat Options Oncol 2019;20(3):24.

41. Brahm CG, van Linde ME, Enting RH, et al. The current status of immune checkpoint inhibitors in neuro-oncology: a systematic review. Cancers (Basel) 2020;12(3):586.

42. Bota DA, Kesari S, Piccioni DE, et al. A phase 1, multicenter, open-label study of marizomib (MRZ) with temozolomide (TMZ) and radiotherapy (RT) in newly diagnosed WHO grade IV malignant glioma (glioblastoma, ndGBM): dose-escalation results. J Clin Oncol 2018;36(15 suppl):e14083.

43. Weller M, Butowski N, Tran DD, et al. Rindopepimut with temozolomide for patients with newly diagnosed, EGFRvIII-expressing glioblastoma (ACT IV): a randomised, double-blind, international phase 3 trial. Lancet Oncol 2017;18:1373–85.

44. Lim M, Xia Y, Bettegowda C, et al. Current state of immunotherapy for glioblastoma. Nat Rev Clin Oncol 2018;15:422–42.

45. Liau LM, Ashkan K, Tran DD, et al. First results on survival from a large Phase 3 clinical trial of an autologous dendritic cell vaccine in newly diagnosed glioblastoma. J Transl Med 2018;16:142.

46. Bloch O, Crane CA, Fuks Y, et al. Heat-shock protein peptide complex-96 vaccination for recurrent glioblastoma: a phase II, singlearm trial. Neurooncology 2014;16:274–9.

47. Westphal M, Ylä-Herttuala S, Martin J, et al. Adenovirus-mediated gene therapy with sitimagene ceradenovec followed by intravenous ganciclovir for patients with operable high grade glioma (ASPECT): a randomised, open-label, phase 3 trial. Lancet Oncol 2013;14:823–33.

48. Cloughesy TF, Landolfi J, Vogelbaum MA, et al. Durable complete responses in some recurrent high-grade glioma patients treated with Toca 511 + Toca FC. Neurooncology 2018;20:1383–92.

49. Majd N, Dasgupta P, de Groot J. Immunotherapy for neuro-oncology. Adv Exp Med Biol 2020;1244: 183–203.

50. Cheung YT, Sabin ND, Reddick WE, et al. Leukoencephalopathy and long-term neurobehavioural, neurocognitive, and brain imaging outcomes in survivors of childhood acute lymphoblastic leukaemia treated with chemotherapy: a longitudinal analysis. Lancet Haematol 2016;3(10):e456–66.

51. Schroyen G, Meylaers M, Deprez S, et al. Prevalence of leukoencephalopathy and its potential cognitive sequelae in cancer patients. J Chemother 2020;32:327–43.

52. Bowers DC, Nathan PC, Constine L, et al. Subsequent neoplasms of the CNS among survivors of childhood cancer: a systematic review. Lancet Oncol 2013;14(8):e321–8.

Radiogenomics of Gliomas

Chaitra Badve, MBBS, MD[a],*, Sangam Kanekar, MD[b]

KEYWORDS

- Radiogenomics • Radiomics • Gliomagenesis
- Visually accessible rembrandt imaging (VASARI) feature set • The cancer genome atlas (TCGA)
- Isocitrate dehydrogenase (IDH) • 1p/19q codeletion
- Epidermal growth factor receptor (EGFR) and vascular endothelial growth factor (VEGF)

KEY POINTS

- Current research in brain tumors is focused on tumor genomics to identify novel therapeutic targets, devise personalized treatment options, and thereby improve individual patient outcomes.
- Radiogenomics is the study of relationship between imaging features (radiophenotypes) and genetic/molecular profile of disease state, typically neoplasms.
- Primary de novo tumors account for more than 80% of glioblastomas (GBs), occur in older patients, and typically show epidermal growth factor receptor gene amplification and mutation, loss of heterozygosity (LOH) of chromosome 10q containing phosphatase and tensin (PTEN) homolog, deletion of p16, and less frequently murine double minute 2 (MDM2) amplification.
- Secondary GBs develop from lower-grade astrocytomas or oligodendrogliomas, occur in younger patients, and often include mutations of TP53, retinoblastoma, and LOH of chromosome 19q.
- The radiomic features derived from clinical sequences, such as T2, fluid-attenuated inversion recovery (FLAIR), T1, and T1 with contrast, as well as from advanced imaging techniques, such as diffusion, perfusion, and diffusion tensor imaging, can give a detailed overview of the local and global genomic heterogeneity of the tumor environment.

INTRODUCTION

The 2003 Human Genome Project and the 2016 World Health Organization (WHO) classification have made significant impact on understanding of brain tumors.[1,2] Current brain tumor classification is based on genomic and molecular profile of tumor tissue, and these characteristics play an important role in treatment planning and prognostication. Current research in brain tumors is focused on tumor genomics to identify novel therapeutic targets, devise personalized treatment options, and thereby improve individual patient outcomes.[3] In parallel, MR imaging of brain tumors also has seen rapid growth, with development of advanced imaging techniques that provide insight into tissue characteristics at cellular and molecular levels. MR image processing and analysis have made remarkable progress, with development of niche areas of texture analysis/radiomics and applications of machine learning techniques and artificial intelligence.[4] Because MR imaging offers a unique noninvasive way of comprehensively evaluating tumor milieu, it is no surprise that a new field of radiogenomics has made significant strides in merging imaging with genomic mapping. One of the earliest initiatives to encourage interest in this area was The Cancer Genome Atlas (TCGA) program, which was a joint effort between the National Cancer Institute and the National Human Genome Research Institute. The Cancer Imaging Program has made radiological imaging data for glioblastoma (GB) patients enrolled in TCGA publicly available via the Cancer Imaging Archive (TCIA).[5] This large-scale effort has paved the way for numerous impactful studies exploring potential

[a] Department of Radiology, Division of Neuroradiology, University Hospitals Cleveland Medical Center, BSH 5056, 11100 Euclid Avenue, Cleveland, OH 44106, USA; [b] Department of Radiology and Neurology, Division of Neuroradiology, Penn State College of Medicine, Penn State Milton Hershey Medical Center, Mail Code H066 500, University Drive, Hershey, PA 17033, USA
* Corresponding author.
E-mail address: Chaitra.Badve@UHhospitals.org

Radiol Clin N Am 59 (2021) 441–455
https://doi.org/10.1016/j.rcl.2021.02.002
0033-8389/21/© 2021 Elsevier Inc. All rights reserved.

correlations between tumor imaging features, histologic patterns, and genetic profiles and firmly established the field of radiogenomics.

OVERVIEW OF GLIOMA BIOLOGY

Human gliomas can be classified into low-grade gliomas (LGGs) and high-grade gliomas based on their histopathology.[2] LGGs are treated with maximal safe resection and eventual reoperation with adjuvant radiation and/or chemotherapy, and typically have a life expectancy of 10 years to 15 years after diagnosis.[6] High-grade gliomas comprise anaplastic astrocytomas (grade III) and GBs (grade IV). Treatment of GB remains a challenge, with median overall survival of 14 months despite aggressive therapy. The GB treatment regimen consists of a combination of maximally safe surgical resection followed by radiation therapy and concurrent chemotherapy.[7] Tumor heterogeneity, one of the hallmarks of GB, is the presence of multiple different cell subpopulations within a single tumor. It is caused by cancer stem cells that possess varying degrees of ability to self-renew and differentiate into different tumor cell types and also the ability for clonal evolution that may enhance genetic diversity within the affected tissues. Because tumor fragments from the same patient may have different molecular subtypes in different tumor regions, GB grading can be complex. GBs also show epithelial to mesenchymal transitions, thought to be due to signaling pathways of Wnt, transforming growth factor β, and NOTCH. This transition is partly responsible for the migration, diffusion invasion, and angiogenesis of GB. By virtue of the inherent heterogeneity of these tumors, not all of the cells within a glioma respond to chemotherapy and radiation equally and effectively, resulting in tumor progression/recurrence.[8]

Gliomagenesis is a multifactorial process involving more than 60 genetic alterations. Primary de novo tumors accounts for more than 80% of GBs, occur in older patients and typically show epidermal growth factor receptor (EGFR) gene amplification and mutation, loss of heterozygosity (LOH) of chromosome 10q containing phosphatase and tensin homolog (PTEN), and deletion of p16, and less frequently murine double minute 2 (MDM2) amplification. Secondary GBs develop from lower-grade astrocytomas or oligodendrogliomas, occur in younger patients, and often include mutations of TP53, retinoblastoma (RB), and LOH of chromosome 19q.[9] Because it is well-established that treatment response and overall survival depend on the molecular and genomic characteristics, identifying the radiogenomic links becomes vitally important for the radiologist and the oncologist.

DEFINITIONS AND TERMINOLOGY

Radiogenomics is the study of relationship between imaging features (radiophenotypes) and genetic/molecular profile of disease state, typically neoplasms. In a broader sense, radiogenomics also may encompass study of genomic changes induced by radiation therapy, but a more focused definition used commonly by cancer imaging community refers to the earlier description alone.[10] The radiophenotypes used for radiogenomics can be derived from conventional clinical imaging data or from advanced imaging techniques, such as permeability imaging, perfusion imaging, diffusion tensor imaging (DTI), and MR spectroscopy. The radiophenotypes can be radiologist derived, also known as semantic, and harvested with minimal data processing, or they can be computer-derived radiomic parameters, which quantitatively measure texture features that are not visible to human eye. The genomic profile of tumors can be determined by analysis of DNA, RNA, or protein, with emphasis on presence, absence, overexpression, or suppression of these markers. The commonly used techniques can identify targeted gene mutations or their downstream effects or provide whole-genome sequencing.

MOLECULAR CHARACTERISTICS OF GLIOMAS

The 2016 WHO classification of brain tumors outlined specific molecular parameters for diagnosis of brain tumors in combination with the more traditionally used histologic features.[2] This has significantly altered the overall clinical approach to diagnosis and classification of glioma subtypes.

Isocitrate Dehydrogenase Gene 1/Isocitrate Dehydrogenase Gene 2

Isocitrate dehydrogenase gene (IDH) mutation is one of the key molecular markers described in relation to gliomas. IDH is a key enzyme in the cell citric acid cycle and a mutation in IDH1 or IDH2 gene results in altered enzyme activity with accumulation of 2-hydroxyglutarate (2-HG). Accumulation of 2-HG, in turn, causes a cascade of events that results in DNA hypermethylation to affect cell differentiation and neoplasia. This mutation can be detected in clinical setting by immunohistochemistry and whole-genome sequencing. Detection of IDH1/2 has significant implications for diagnosis and prognosis of gliomas. GBs are classified as primary (wild-type) or secondary (IDH-mutant) based on IDH mutational status.[11]

IDH mutation is also indicative of a diffuse glioma (grade II and grade III) and is useful to distinguish these tumors from reactive gliosis or discrete grade I gliomas, such as pilocytic astrocytoma. Presence of IDH mutation is a favorable prognostic indicator with better overall survival and progression-free survival. More importantly, patients with a LGG (grade II or III) with a wild-type IDH have worse outcomes that are similar to grade IV tumors.[12]

1p/19q Codeletion

1p/19q codeletion was one of the earliest chromosomal abnormalities described in patients with oligodendroglial tumors and is detected in clinical setting using fluorescence in situ hybridization.[13] Only recently has it been shown that the codeleted tumors have key physical and chemical attributes that have an impact on migration, apoptosis, and cell-cycle regulations. Presence of 1p/19q codeletion is indicative of LGGs, supports the diagnosis of an oligodendroglial tumor, and is seen in more than 70% tumors with oligodendroglial origin.[14] Presence of this codeletion is associated strongly with excellent response to chemotherapy with alkylating agents and remains a strong favorable prognostic factor associated with improved survival. A key study based on TCGA database found that LGGs with 1p/19q codeletion and IDH mutations had significantly higher survival (median survival of 8 years) compared with patients with IDH mutations without codeletion (median survival of 6.3 years) and patients with IDH wild-type tumors (median survival of 1.7 years).[15–17] In another study, grade II and grade III gliomas were classified into 5 different subtypes based on IDH, 1p/19q, and telomerase reverse transcriptase (TERT) mutational status with distinct clinical outcomes.[18]

O6-methylguanine-DNA Methyltransferase

O6-methylguanine-DNA methyltransferase (MGMT) is a DNA repair enzyme located on chromosome 10q, and methylation of the promoter region of the gene results in lower levels of this enzyme, resulting in less efficient DNA repair in tumor cells damaged due to cytotoxicity.[19] MGMT methylation status is detected with pyrosequencing or by a quantitative polymerase chain reaction test. It is a positive prognostic factor and is a strong predictor of positive therapeutic response to temozolomide in new and recurrent high-grade gliomas.[20,21] MGMT methylation also frequently is seen in IDH-mutant LGGs and is associated with favorable survival.[22] In patients with GBs treated with standard therapy, the incidence of pseudoprogression is significantly higher in tumors with methylated MGMT.[23]

Epidermal Growth Factor Receptor and Vascular Endothelial Growth Factor

High-grade gliomas are associated with abundant and disorderly cellular and vascular proliferation. Amplification and mutation of the EGFR gene located on chromosome 7q12 induce rapid cellular growth, resulting in an aggressive proliferative neoplasm. EGFR amplification is commonly associated with classical subtype and is seen more frequently in primary GBs compared to secondary GBs. The EGFR mutated cell lines can be suppressed by EGFR inhibitors, such as erlotinib and gefitinib, raising the possibility of targeted therapeutics. Clinically, EGFR abnormalities can be detected by immunohistochemistry or EGFR staining.[24–28] High-grade gliomas also are characterized by overexpression of vascular endothelial growth factor (VEGF), which is responsible for neo-angiogenesis.[29] Hypoxia in the tumor microenvironment acts as a stimulus for angiogenesis by activation of hypoxia inducible factor 1 subunit alpha. Other factors that drive hypervascularization such as angiopoietin-1 and angiopoietin-2, hepatocyte growth factor, and platelet-derived growth factor (PDGF) are also activated by hypoxia. The ultimate result of this process is a neoplasm with profuse leaky aberrant vasculature with deficient blood-brain barrier. Bevacizumab is an anti-angiogenic agent that targets VEGF overexpression and often is used in treatment of recurrent GBs.[30]

Other Key Mutations

Other key molecular aberrations and genetic mutations in gliomas include alpha-thalassemia mental retardation (ATRX), TERT, TP53, and neurofibromatosis type 1 (NF1) histone H3 K27M, among several others.[9,31–34] X-linked gene of ATRX mutations affect DNA repair and are found in low-grade astrocytomas. TERT mutations result in intact length of telomeres, which confers the ability to divide ad infinitum. These often are seen in gliomas in combination with ATRX mutations. Based on the findings from TCGA study, the key signaling pathways that drive tumor growth in GBs are the RB pathway, the TP53 pathway, and the PTEN/NF1/RTK (receptor tyrosine kinase) pathway. The RB and TP53 are known tumor suppressor genes, and mutations in this pathway result in increased mitotic activity and suppressed apoptosis, respectively. The PTEN/NF1/RTK pathway abnormalities simultaneously cause increased cell growth, modulate cell cycle, and affect tumor suppression. Lastly, histone H3 gene mutations cause abnormalities of DNA packing and are seen in pediatric diffuse intrinsic pontine gliomas and pediatric GBs. Recent WHO classification has defined a new entity called diffuse midline glioma with H3 K27M-mutant. Although these tumors demonstrate low grade on histology, they are considered grade IV due to their aggressive behavior.[2]

Transcriptomic Subtypes

Depending on the molecular and genomic characteristics, GBs can be classified into classical, mesenchymal, neural, and proneural. Each subtype is associated with a distinct set of molecular features with distinct clinical behaviors. For example, the proneural subtype is associated with IDH mutations, includes a majority of secondary GBs, and is associated with best prognosis. The mesenchymal type, on the other hand, is associated with increased mutations of PTEN, TP53, and NF1 genes and correlates with poor radiation response and shorter survival. The neural subtype is characterized histologically by higher astrocyte and oligodendroglial differentiation and is highly infiltrated by healthy brain cells.[25,27] **Fig. 1** provides an overview of current classification of adult and pediatric gliomas.

APPROACH TO RADIOGENOMIC ANALYSIS

Simply put, a radiogenomic study allows for assessment of relationship between imaging patterns and genomic signatures in disease states, typically cancer. These studies are focused primarily either on identifying the possible molecular associate with the specific radiographic correlate or studying how a particular genomic variation might have an impact on the tumors' imaging characteristics. The first category of studies can be classified as exploratory, whereas the second category of studies can be classified as hypothesis driven. Early radiogenomic literature focused primarily on a single imaging characteristic (for example, presence of necrosis) and correlated the presence or absence of this feature with the corresponding tissue molecular and genomic features. These studies predominantly used semantic features to harvest tumor radiophenotypes (for example, the Visually Accessible Rembrandt Imaging [VASARI] feature set) and incorporated targeted tissue sampling using neuronavigational techniques to sample areas with specific imaging features. Subsequent radiogenomic studies using semantic features explored associations between imaging phenotypes and more targeted genomic characteristics with direct implications for treatment planning and outcome. More recent studies have focused on exploring correlations between

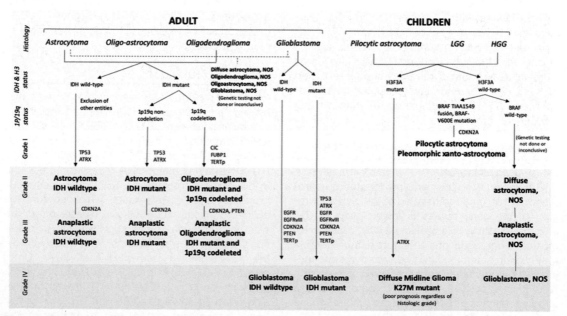

Fig. 1. Schematic classification of adult and pediatric diffuse gliomas according to status of relevant biomarkers. HGG, high grade glioma; NOS, not otherwise specified. (*From* Delgado-López PD, Saiz-López P, Gargini R, Sola-Vendrell E, Tejada S. A comprehensive overview on the molecular biology of human glioma: what the clinician needs to know. Clin Transl Oncol. 2020.)

computer-derived radiomic features and large-scale gene expression patterns. A smaller subset of these studies falls under the category of a directed or hypothesis-driven approach, where more specific gene expression profiles or genetic pathways are targeted for analysis using quantitative metrics derived from conventional and advanced imaging sequences.

RADIOGENOMIC STUDIES USING SEMANTIC FEATURES

TCGA initiative led to the development of the VASARI feature set, which consisted of 24 common MR imaging observations routinely made during clinical interpretations (https://www.cancerimagingarchive.net/). These observations were made using standard contrast-enhanced MR imaging acquisitions and included features, such as location, laterality, proportion and quality of enhancement, proportion of necrosis, cysts, diffusion, and so forth. These feature sets were utilized to create subjective and objective markups of baseline MR imaging–GB studies stored in TCIA for TCGA and linked to the Repository of Molecular Brain Neoplasia Data (REMBRANDT) set.[35] These imaging data sets were utilized mainly to understand the correlation of imaging phenotypes with survival, molecular subtypes, mutation status, and copy number expression. Some of the key VASARI imaging features that have demonstrated correlation with brain tumor genomics are location, tumor volume, edema, and necrosis, enhancing versus nonenhancing areas, and diffusion characteristics. Although perfusion imaging was not included in the VASARI data set, perfusion characteristics of tumor have also emerged as key semantic feature for radiogenomic correlation.

Location and Volume

Tumor volume and location of tumor are shown to be robust imaging phenotypes that have strong correlation with genomic features.[36–42] For tumor volume analysis, fluid-attenuated inversion recovery (FLAIR) and postcontrast T1-weighted images are used most commonly to segment out enhancing tumor volume, nonenhancing tumor volume, and necrosis with manual or automated techniques and then correlated with genomic profile. For studies based on tumor location, features, such as location, laterality, involvement of eloquent cortex, multifocality, periventricular involvement, and extension across midline, have been used to explore genomic correlations. For example, MGMT methylated IDH-mutant tumors are located primarily in the frontal lobe or subventricular region of the frontal horns of the lateral ventricles and are less likely to invade eloquent areas of the brain, whereas amplified and variant EGFR-expressing tumors occurred most frequently in the left temporal lobe.[36,42]

In 2012, Zinn and colleagues[43] studied 78 GB patients from TCIA data set and generated a prognostic model for patient survival based on the volume of enhancing tumor (including the necrotic core), patient age, and Karnofsky performance scale status (VAK). Larger volume tumor, age of 60 years or more, and Karnofsky performance scale status less than 100 were noted and patients with none or only 1 feature were categorized as VAK-A, whereas patients with 2 or all 3 features were categorized as VAK-B. The investigators also identified differences in gene and mRNA expression profile between these 2 groups. They found class VAK-A was associated with P53 activation whereas class VAK-B was associated with P53 inhibition. Adding MGMT-promoter methylation status to VAK-A stratified the data further, such that the MGMT methylated VAK-A cohort was found to have significantly longer survival compared with other 3 groups (**Fig. 2**).[43]

Enhancement Characteristics

Enhancing and nonenhancing components of GB have been extensively studied in relation to gene expression. In one of the earliest efforts, Pope and colleagues[44] compared the imaging findings of 52 GBs with microarray analysis of tissue derived from areas with different enhancement characteristics. They specifically analyzed the gene expression between lesions with complete enhancement and lesions with incomplete ring enhancement and confirmed that interleukin-8 and VEGF gene expression were higher in the former subset compared with the later.[44] Barajas and colleagues[45] also had similar results demonstrating the intertumoral and intratumoral regional differences in genetic and cellular expression patterns. They further confirmed that the contrast enhancing regions had more complex vascular hyperplasia as well as increased hypoxia and tumor cell density and up-regulation of VEGF and various collagen genes.[45]

Peritumoral Edematous/Tumor-Infiltrated Tissue

The nonenhancing T2-FLAIR hyperintensity surrounding the enhancing tumor core often represents a mixture of edema and tumor infiltration, particularly in GBs. This region is of particular interest because it often includes the site of future recurrence, which invariably occurs in GBs. Various studies have explored the radiogenomic

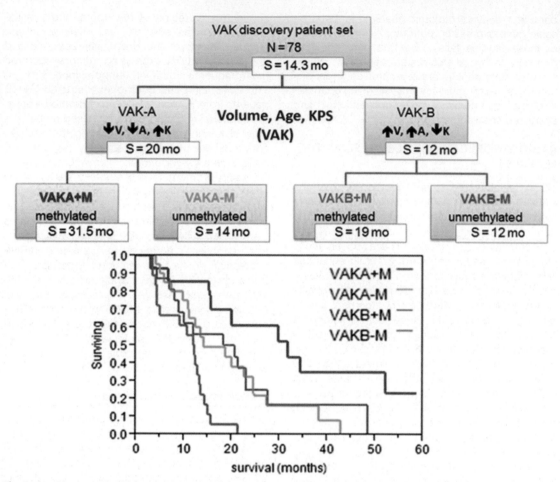

Fig. 2. VAK MGMT model for survival stratification. (*From* Zinn PO, Sathyan P, Mahajan B, Bruyere J, Hegi M, Majumder S, et al. A novel volume-age-KPS (VAK) glioblastoma classification identifies a prognostic cognate microRNA-gene signature. PLoS One. 2012;7(8):e41522.)

characteristics of this region. Zinn and colleagues[46] demonstrated that there was up-regulation of PERIOSTIN (POSTN) gene set and down-regulated microRNA-219 in the T2-FLAIR hyperintensity. PERIOSTIN was found to be promoting mesenchymal transition and invasion in GB and POSTN expression was up-regulated significantly in the mesenchymal subtype of GB.[46] Pope and colleagues[44] found that the incompletely enhancing tumor regions (regions defined as nonenhancing FLAIR hyperintense areas with suspicion of tumor infiltration) had distinct genetic profile compared with the enhancing tumor regions and demonstrated higher expression levels of the stem cell and oligodendrocyte lineage marker OLIG-2[46] as well as genes associated with secondary GB.

Necrosis

Necrosis is a hallmark of GB and is closely associated with shortened patient survival in high-grade gliomas.[47,48] Colen and colleagues[49] studied the phenomenon of cell death in GBs with respect to sex-specific differences and found overall lower volumes of necrosis on imaging in women compared with men. Women with higher volumes of necrosis had poor outcomes compared with men (6.5 months vs 14.5 months, respectively; $P = .01$). Larger area of necrosis in women was associated with MYC, an oncogenic transcription factor (via an oncogenic pathway), whereas in men it was associated with Tp53 (via an apoptotic pathway).[49] Van Meter and colleagues[50] explored intratumor genetic variations between the enhancing peripheral mass and a poorly enhancing central tumor core on contrast-enhanced T1-weighted MR imaging and found increased expression of genes associated with cell migration, angiogenesis, cell survival, and integrin signaling in the enhancing core, with the poorly enhancing and low perfused core having an elevated rate of expression for hypoxia-induced gene. Yamashita and colleagues[51] found correlation between IDH1 status and area of necrosis. Barajas and colleagues[45] confirmed these findings by reporting the increased expression of genes associated with mitosis, angiogenesis, and apoptosis.

Restricted Diffusion on Diffusion-Weighted Imaging–Apparent Diffusion Coefficient

In tumor imaging, lower apparent diffusion coefficient (ADC) values are known to reflect areas of hypercellularity. Zinn and colleagues[52] studied ADC values in the nonenhancing, FLAIR hyperintense lesions of the tumor in 35 GB patients and found that lower ADC values (restricted diffusion) were seen in the peritumoral edematous/tumor-infiltrated tissue. These lower ADC values were correlated further with distinct genomic networks and differentially expressed genes that play a role in invasion.[52] ADC measurements have shown promise in predicting MGMT methylation status and patient survival.[53–55] Heiland and colleagues[56] studied the role of DTI-derived parameters in identification of gene expression pathways in 21 patients, which were correlated with biopsy tissue. They documented that GB with high fractional anisotropy had a worse prognosis and was associated with activation of the epithelial mesenchymal pathway, whereas higher mean diffusivity was suggestive of more favorable prognosis.[56] Hong and colleagues[41] were able to demonstrate ADC differences based on IDH1 and ATRX profiles of GBs.

Perfusion Status of the Tumor

Dynamic contrast–enhanced and dynamic susceptibility contrast MR perfusion are employed routinely in the presurgical evaluation and post-treatment follow-up of the brain tumors. Among all the perfusion parameters, cerebral blood volume (CBV) has been the most extensively studied. Barajas and colleagues[45] studied enhanced and nonenhanced portions of the tumor and correlated them with CBV and peak height values, and decreased percentage of signal recovery and ADC values. They documented that the genes associated with mitosis, angiogenesis, and apoptosis were significantly upregulated in contrast-enhanced regions compared with nonenhanced portion of the tumor (**Fig. 3**).[45,57] In a feasibility study using perfusion CT, Jain and colleagues[58] demonstrated positive correlation between higher perfusion parameters and proangiogenic genes and a negative correlation between these parameters and antiangiogenic genes. Jain and colleagues[59] using dynamic susceptibility contrast–enhanced T2-weighted MR perfusion from TCIA TCGA-GB collection, correlated tumor blood volume with patient survival, and determined its association with molecular subclasses of GB. They measured the mean relative CBV (rCBV) of the contrast-enhanced and nonenhanced regions and correlated with the genomic subclassification. They found that rCBV values had no statistical significance with regard to their molecular classification, but the rCBV max measurements were found to be a strong predictor of overall survival regardless of the molecular subtype.[59] Yamashita and colleagues[51] demonstrated the correlation between IDH1 status and tumor blood flow. Kong and colleagues[60] documented that CBV and cerebral blood flow–related radiomic features were significantly related to up-regulation of PDGF, EGFR, and VEGF pathways and down-regulation of the PTEN pathway.

MR Spectroscopy

Besides MR perfusion, MR spectroscopy has been used commonly in the evaluation of the brain tumor. Mutations of the IDH1 and IDH2 genes result in an over-reduction of the α-ketoglutarate 2-HG metabolite, leading to an accumulation of 2-HG. Choi and colleagues showed the existence of 2-HG and glutamate multiplets in patients with IDH-mutated grade II–III tumors with 100% sensitivity and specificity. A maximum 2-HG peak was identified at approximately 2.25 parts per million (ppm), near the γ-aminobutyric acid peak (2.2–2.4 ppm) and located to the left of the N-acetylaspartate peak, at 2.0 ppm.[61] Similar findings were also seen by Lazovic and colleagues[62] and Pope and colleagues[63] in their studies. In conclusion, documentation of the 2-HG peak is seen with IDH mutation gliomas, and its absence is consistent with IDH wild-type tumors. MR spectroscopy also has been found useful in documenting the treatment response with IDH1/2-mutant inhibitors. Heiland and colleagues[64] explored the relationship between the concentration of metabolites on MR spectroscopy and gene expression pathways. They were able to show spectral differences for different subtypes of GB. The high creatine metabolite was found to be correlated with proneural GB subtype, low creatine was related to mesenchymal subtype; low glutamate and glutamine metabolite was associated with neural subtype, and its high value was related to the classical subtype.[64]

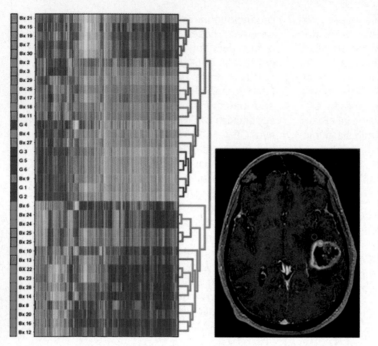

Fig. 3. Presence of contrast enhancement is predictive of GBM genetic expression pattern. (*Right*) Purple and green circles indicate nonenhancing and enhancing biopsy regions, respectively. (*Left*) Genetic expression map of all biopsy samples with hierarchical clustering of the 500 most variant genes shows clustering only by biopsy sample. Purple, nonenhancing samples; blue, gliosis samples; and green, enhancing samples. (*From* Ramon F. Barajas J, Hodgson JG, Chang JS, Vandenberg SR, Yeh R-F, Parsa AT, et al. Glioblastoma Multiforme Regional Genetic and Cellular Expression Patterns: Influence on Anatomic and Physiologic MR Imaging. Radiology. 2010;254(2):564-76.)

MOLECULAR CLASSIFICATION

Verhaak and colleagues[25] described a robust gene expression–based molecular classification of GBs into proneural, neural, classical, and mesenchymal subtypes that integrate multidimensional genomic data to establish patterns of somatic mutations and DNA copy number. Primary GBs represent the classical, mesenchymal, and neural subtypes. The mesenchymal and classical subtypes typically are associated with more aggressive, higher-grade gliomas. The classical subtype demonstrates a greater preponderance of EGFR amplification, decreased rates of *TP53* mutation, and *p16INK4A* and *p14ARF* deletion. One of the earliest studies based on TCGA data set used standardized features sets for image analysis, and associations between imaging features and Verhaak subtypes were assessed. The study found that the proneural subtype was more likely to include a tumor with low levels of contrast enhancement; and the mesenchymal subtype was noted to have lower proportion of nonenhanced T2/FLAIR hyperintense tissue compared with other subtypes.[65] Another study using semantic features found that volume analysis of different tumor regions was able to identify mesenchymal subtype with an area under the curve of 0.93 and *P*<.001. Again, mesenchymal subtypes were associated with lower ratios of nonenhanced T2/FLAIR hyperintensity to contrast enhancement

and necrosis.[66] Jain and colleagues[59] correlated rCBV of the contrast-enhanced and nonenhanced portions of tumors in 50 patients from TCGA set with molecular subclasses and found no significant differences. The study found that rCBV measurements were predictive of overall patient survival independent of molecular classification, although including Verhaak subtypes improved the strength of such association.[59] Overview of studies using radiomic analysis for molecular classification is presented in the next section.

RADIOGENOMIC STUDIES USING RADIOMIC FEATURES

These studies use computer-derived quantitative data derived from clinical imaging, which are not visible to the human eye and not typically measurable in a reading room setting. These features give a detailed overview of the local and global heterogeneity of the tumor environment as seen on clinical images and can be extracted using conventional (human engineered) or deep learning approaches. These data are then analyzed using machine learning or deep learning methods for feature selection and radiogenomic correlation. The entire imaging data set typically is divided into a discovery cohort and a validation cohort. The radiomic features can be derived from clinical sequences, such as T2, FLAIR, T1, and T1 with contrast as well as from advanced imaging techniques, such as diffusion, perfusion, and DTI. Detailed description of radiomic methodology is beyond the scope of this article and is extensively reviewed elsewhere.[67–69]

One of the earliest radiogenomic studies by Itakura and colleagues[70] extracted quantitative features related to shape, texture, and edge sharpness of each lesion and classified the entire cohort into 3 phenotypic clusters, namely premultifocal, spherical, and rim-enhancing. Each cluster was mapped to a unique set of molecular signaling pathways indicating differential molecular activities as well as differential survival probabilities.[70] Kickingereder and colleagues[71] correlated histogram features of anatomic, diffusion, and perfusion imaging with a broad selection of molecular features using machine learning algorithms. Based on MR imaging features, the investigators were able to predict EGFR amplification status and classic subtype with moderate accuracy, although the association strength was not sufficient for generation of a robust model.[71] In a study based on TCGA data set, convolutional neural network was trained to classify IDH1 mutation status, 1p/19q codeletion, and MGMT promoter methylation status based on imaging features. The study demonstrated an accuracy of 94% for IDH1, 92% for 1p/19q, and 83% for MGMT promoter methylations status classification.[72] Several studies have focused on individual molecular characteristics using the radiomic features for imaging phenotypes. For example, using only T2 imaging for texture analysis, Korfiatis and colleagues[73] were able to predict MGMT methylation status with 85% accuracy, whereas Li and colleagues[74] were able to predict the same with 80% accuracy using a multiparametric model using features derived from T1, T1 with contrast, T2, and T2/FLAIR images. In a radiogenomic study based on anatomic and perfusion imaging, the investigators were able to predict EGFRvIII mutation in GBs with 85.3% and 87% accuracy in discovery and validation cohort, respectively.[75] Another study based on perfusion imaging devised a within patient peritumoral heterogeneity index, which compared perfusion parameters of immediate and distant peritumoral edema. Using this index, EGFRvIII mutation was identified with accuracy of 89.9% and specificity of 92%, wherein tumors with this mutation demonstrated a highly infiltrative-migratory phenotype compared with a peritumoral confined vascularization seen in EGFRvIII tumors.[76]

In an attempt to interrogate the hypoxia pathway, Beig and colleagues[77] quantified radiomic texture descriptors of tumor heterogeneity, which were surrogates for tumor hypoxia, and evaluated their role in predicting patient survival. Hu and colleagues[78] used texture analysis techniques to assess genetic heterogeneity in enhancing and nonenhancing regions of GBs and generate predictive models for 6 driver genes. Highest accuracies were observed for PDGFRA (77.1%), EGFR (75%), CDKN2A (87.5%), and RB1 (87.5%), whereas the lowest accuracy was observed in TP53 (37.5%). Higher accuracies were identified using features derived from nonenhanced regions compared with enhancing segments.[78] Dextraze and colleagues[79] identified multiple spatial habitats based on texture features of various tumor regions in a set of 85 GBs from TCGA data set and demonstrated the association of each habitat with unique pathway alterations and association of some of the habitats with overall survival. The phenomenon of angiogenesis and the hypoxia pathway were studied using perfusion imaging in a study by Liu and colleagues.[80] Based on perfusion parameters, a distinct subset of GBs was identified with unique perfusion and molecular characteristics, which pointed to enrichment of angiogenesis and hypoxia pathway markers. This cohort also had poor survival at baseline and had significantly longer survival when treated with antiangiogenic therapy compared with the other subset.[80]

Finally, radiomics-based analysis also has been used for predicting molecular subclasses of GBs. In a study by Macyszyn and colleagues,[81] machine learning techniques were used to analyze radiomic features from multiparametric MR imaging. Using a training data set of 105 and a validation data set of 29 patients, the study demonstrated an accuracy of 76% in classification of GB subtypes.[81] In a subsequent study by Rathore and colleagues,[82] based on radiomic features, 3 distinct subtypes of GB were identified, each with distinct clinical outcome and molecular profile, and relationship between imaging subtypes and molecular subtypes was established (**Fig. 4**).

LIMITATIONS AND FUTURE DIRECTIONS
Reproducibility

Radiogenomics studies, in particular those using radiomic features, are a powerful way to analyze entire tumor environment to identify underlying genomic alterations. Studies so far have demonstrated extremely promising results; however, concerns for generalizability arising from limited radiomic feature robustness remain. These limiting factors can arise at different steps of image acquisition, segmentation, feature extraction, feature selection, and modeling.[83] The imaging community has identified this concern and arrived at a consensus that value of quantitative imaging biomarkers can be improved by reducing variability

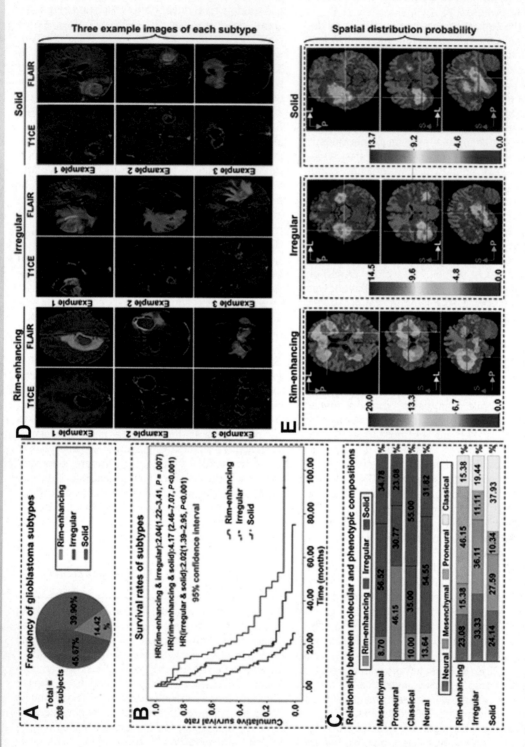

Fig. 4. GB imaging subtypes identified by the clustering process. (A) The frequency of each subtype. (C) Relationship between the molecular composition (neural/mesenchymal/proneural/classical) and imaging subtypes (rim-enhancing/irregular/solid). (D) Three representative subjects of each subtype (closest to the mean of the cluster). (E) Spatial distribution probability of the tumors of each subtype. The color look-up tables show the probability of tumor existence. HR, hazard ratio. (From Rathore S, Akbari H, Rozycki M, Abdullah KG, Nasrallah MP, Binder ZA, et al. Radiomic MRI signature reveals three distinct subtypes of glioblastoma with different clinical and molecular characteristics, offering prognostic value beyond IDH1. Sci Rep. 2018;8(1):5087.)

arising from various steps in analysis (https://www.rsna.org/research/quantitative-imaging-biomarkers-alliance). The Quantitative imaging network (QIN) and Quantitative Imaging Biomarkers Alliance are major collaborative initiatives sponsored by imaging research communities to achieve set goals for biomarker standardization.[84,85] Similarly, efforts are under way to standardize region of interest labeling and segmentation to minimize bias and allow repeatable and reproducible analysis.[86] The Image Biomarker Standardization Initiative has led the effort in validating consensus-based reference values for a set of radiomic features to standardize the feature extraction process.[87] Emerging quantitative techniques, such as MR fingerprinting, with its high reproducibility and repeatability, may have a role to play in ensuring feature robustness in future radiomics studies.[88,89]

Data Size Considerations

Radiomics and radiogenomics studies are highly data intensive. Because the number of features extracted often is large, and sometimes larger than the sample size, overfitting the data always is a risk.[83] Deployment of appropriate feature selection methods can mitigate the problem to a certain degree. Using models that include patient demographics and clinical parameters should be considered so that the results are closer to the ground truth. Given the methodology, having a large, well-curated data set is necessary to achieve robust and reliable results. The QIN with its TCGA initiative has allowed investigators to build a collection of rich imaging, genomic, and clinical data sets. The Radiomics Signatures for Precision Diagnostics consortium on GB is a worldwide collaboration that aims to address the challenges associated with artificial intelligence and machine learning analyses in GBs.[90] Because these are retrospectively collected data sets, however, there is no way to standardize image quality. There is a need for a prospectively generated data repository with rich imaging, clinical, and omics features that will assure image standardization and allow robust analytics.

Translation from Bench to Bedside

A recent systematic review of radiomics applications in neuro-oncology has concluded that the current evidence is not sufficient to support use of radiomics studies in clinical setting.[91] Although the radiomics studies performed well in areas of feature selection and validation, the performance in the areas of protocol quality, reproducibility, biological/clinical validation, and clinical utility was deemed modest, at best. For radiomics and radiogenomics to be adopted successfully in the clinical practice, the steps outlined by National Institutes of Health in the biomarker development process need to be followed.[92] The key areas of technical validation, biological/clinical validation, and cost effectiveness need to be studied rigorously in a prospective approach. In parallel, efforts need to be directed toward conducting hypothesis-driven studies to test the performance of these techniques in a multi-institutional research setting. Until these gaps are bridged, translation of radiomics and radiogenomics from imaging laboratory to reading room remains out of reach.

SUMMARY

Radiogenomics studies offer a powerful way to characterize genomic and molecular characteristics of gliomas noninvasively, using semantic or radiomic features. Although current literature evidence is promising, significant work is needed before application of these techniques in day-to-day clinical practice.

CLINICS CARE POINTS

- Radiogenomics is the study of relationship between imaging features (radiophenotypes) and genetic/molecular profile of disease state, typically neoplasms.

- Current brain tumors research is focused on tumor genomics to identify novel therapeutic targets, devise personalized treatment options, and thereby improve individual patient outcomes.

- The radiomic features derived from clinical sequences, such as T2, FLAIR, T1, and T1 with contrast as well as from advanced imaging techniques, such as diffusion, perfusion, and DTI, can give a detailed overview of the local and global genomic heterogeneity of the tumor environment.

- The key areas of technical validation, biological/clinical validation, and cost effectiveness need to be studied rigorously in a prospective approach. Until these gaps are bridged, translation of radiomics and radiogenomics from imaging laboratory to reading room remains out of reach.

DISCLOSURE

None.

REFERENCES

1. Lander ES, Linton LM, Birren B, et al. Initial sequencing and analysis of the human genome. Nature 2001;409(6822):860–921.
2. Louis DN, Perry A, Reifenberger G, et al. The 2016 world health organization classification of tumors of the central nervous system: a summary. Acta Neuropathol 2016;131(6):803–20.
3. Lim-Fat MJ, Nayak L, Meredith DM. Genomic biomarker assessment in gliomas: impacts of molecular testing on clinical practice and trial design. Surg Pathol Clin 2020;13(2):209–15.
4. Lohmann P, Galldiks N, Kocher M, et al. Radiomics in neuro-oncology: Basics, workflow, and applications. Methods 2020. https://doi.org/10.1016/j.ymeth.2020.06.003.
5. Prior F, Smith K, Sharma A, et al. The public cancer radiology imaging collections of the cancer imaging archive. Sci Data 2017;4(1):170124.
6. Delgado-Lopez P, Corrales-Garcia E, Martino J, et al. Diffuse low-grade glioma: a review on the new molecular classification, natural history and current management strategies. Clin Transl Oncol 2017; 19(8):931–44.
7. Delgado-López PD, Corrales-García EM. Survival in glioblastoma: a review on the impact of treatment modalities. Clin Transl Oncol 2016;18(11):1062–71.
8. Rich JN. Cancer stem cells: understanding tumor hierarchy and heterogeneity. Medicine (Baltimore) 2016;95(1 Suppl 1):S2–7.
9. Ohgaki H, Kleihues P. Genetic pathways to primary and secondary glioblastoma. Am J Pathol 2007; 170(5):1445–53.
10. Mazurowski MA. Radiogenomics: what it is and why it is important. J Am Coll Radiol 2015;12(8):862–6.
11. Yan H, Parsons DW, Jin G, et al. IDH1 and IDH2 mutations in gliomas. N Engl J Med 2009;360(8):765–73.
12. Hartmann C, Hentschel B, Wick W, et al. Patients with IDH1 wild type anaplastic astrocytomas exhibit worse prognosis than IDH1-mutated glioblastomas, and IDH1 mutation status accounts for the unfavorable prognostic effect of higher age: implications for classification of gliomas. Acta Neuropathol 2010;120(6):707–18.
13. Reifenberger J, Reifenberger G, Liu L, et al. Molecular genetic analysis of oligodendroglial tumors shows preferential allelic deletions on 19q and 1p. Am J Pathol 1994;145(5):1175–90.
14. Comprehensive. Integrative genomic analysis of diffuse lower-grade gliomas. N Engl J Med 2015; 372(26):2481–98.
15. Cairncross G, Wang M, Shaw E, et al. Phase III trial of chemoradiotherapy for anaplastic oligodendroglioma: long-term results of RTOG 9402. J Clin Oncol 2013;31(3):337–43.
16. Jenkins RB, Blair H, Ballman KV, et al. A t(1;19)(q10; p10) mediates the combined deletions of 1p and 19q and predicts a better prognosis of patients with oligodendroglioma. Cancer Res 2006;66(20): 9852–61.
17. Griffin CA, Burger P, Morsberger L, et al. Identification of der(1;19)(q10;p10) in five oligodendrogliomas suggests mechanism of concurrent 1p and 19q Loss. J Neuropathol Exp Neurol 2006;65(10):988–94.
18. Eckel-Passow JE, Lachance DH, Molinaro AM, et al. Glioma Groups Based on 1p/19q, IDH, and TERT promoter mutations in tumors. N Engl J Med 2015; 372(26):2499–508.
19. Hegi ME, Diserens A-C, Gorlia T, et al. MGMT gene silencing and benefit from temozolomide in glioblastoma. N Engl J Med 2005;352(10):997–1003.
20. Herrlinger U, Tzaridis T, Mack F, et al. Lomustine-temozolomide combination therapy versus standard temozolomide therapy in patients with newly diagnosed glioblastoma with methylated MGMT promoter (CeTeG/NOA–09): a randomised, open-label, phase 3 trial. Lancet 2019;393(10172):678–88.
21. Gilbert MR, Wang M, Aldape KD, et al. Dose-dense temozolomide for newly diagnosed glioblastoma: a randomized phase III clinical trial. J Clin Oncol 2013;31(32):4085.
22. Leu S, von Felten S, Frank S, et al. IDH/MGMT-driven molecular classification of low-grade glioma is a strong predictor for long-term survival. Neuro Oncol. 2013;15(4):469–79.
23. Kálovits F, Tompa M, Nagy Á, et al. Isocitrate dehydrogenase mutations in defining the biology of and supporting clinical decision making in glioblastoma. Ideggyogy Sz 2018;71(7–08):237–47.
24. Eskilsson E, Røsland GV, Solecki G, et al. EGFR heterogeneity and implications for therapeutic intervention in glioblastoma. Neuro Oncol 2018;20(6): 743–52.
25. Verhaak RG, Hoadley KA, Purdom E, et al. Integrated genomic analysis identifies clinically relevant subtypes of glioblastoma characterized by abnormalities in PDGFRA, IDH1, EGFR, and NF1. Cancer Cell 2010;17(1):98–110.
26. Dunn GP, Rinne ML, Wykosky J, et al. Emerging insights into the molecular and cellular basis of glioblastoma. Genes Dev 2012;26(8):756–84.
27. Brennan CW, Verhaak RG, McKenna A, et al. The somatic genomic landscape of glioblastoma. Cell 2013;155(2):462–77.
28. An Z, Aksoy O, Zheng T, et al. Epidermal growth factor receptor and EGFRvIII in glioblastoma: signaling pathways and targeted therapies. Oncogene 2018; 37(12):1561–75.
29. Zagzag D, Lukyanov Y, Lan L, et al. Hypoxia-inducible factor 1 and VEGF upregulate CXCR4 in glioblastoma: implications for angiogenesis and glioma cell invasion. Lab Invest 2006;86(12):1221–32.

30. Keunen O, Johansson M, Oudin A, et al. Anti-VEGF treatment reduces blood supply and increases tumor cell invasion in glioblastoma. Proc Natl Acad Sci U S A 2011;108(9):3749–54.

31. Young JS, Gogos AJ, Morshed RA, et al. Molecular characteristics of diffuse lower grade gliomas: what neurosurgeons need to know. Acta Neurochir (Wien) 2020;162(8):1929–39.

32. Delgado-López PD, Saiz-López P, Gargini R, et al. A comprehensive overview on the molecular biology of human glioma: what the clinician needs to know. Clin Transl Oncol 2020. https://doi.org/10.1007/s12094-020-02340-8.

33. Park S-H, Won J, Kim S-I, et al. Molecular testing of brain tumor. J Pathol Transl Med 2017;51(3):205–23.

34. Brennan C. Genomic profiles of glioma. Curr Neurol Neurosci Rep 2011;11(3):291–7.

35. Madhavan S, Zenklusen J C, Kotliarov Y, et al. Rembrandt: helping personalized medicine become a reality through integrative translational research. Mol Cancer Res 2009;7(2):157–67.

36. Carrillo JA, Lai A, Nghiemphu PL, et al. Relationship between tumor enhancement, edema, IDH1 mutational status, MGMT promoter methylation, and survival in glioblastoma. AJNR Am J Neuroradiol 2012;33(7):1349–55.

37. Metellus P, Coulibaly B, Colin C, et al. Absence of IDH mutation identifies a novel radiologic and molecular subtype of WHO grade II gliomas with dismal prognosis. Acta Neuropathol 2010;120(6):719–29.

38. Paldor I, Pearce FC, Drummond KJ, et al. Frontal glioblastoma multiforme may be biologically distinct from non-frontal and multilobar tumors. J Clin Neurosci 2016;34:128–32.

39. Sonoda Y, Shibahara I, Kawaguchi T, et al. Association between molecular alterations and tumor location and MRI characteristics in anaplastic gliomas. Brain Tumor Pathol 2015;32(2):99–104.

40. Qi S, Yu L, Li H, et al. Isocitrate dehydrogenase mutation is associated with tumor location and magnetic resonance imaging characteristics in astrocytic neoplasms. Oncol Lett 2014;7(6):1895–902.

41. Hong EK, Choi SH, Shin DJ, et al. Radiogenomics correlation between MR imaging features and major genetic profiles in glioblastoma. Eur Radiol 2018;28(10):4350–61.

42. Ellingson BM, Lai A, Harris RJ, et al. Probabilistic radiographic atlas of glioblastoma phenotypes. AJNR Am J Neuroradiol 2013;34(3):533–40.

43. Zinn PO, Sathyan P, Mahajan B, et al. A novel volume-age-KPS (VAK) glioblastoma classification identifies a prognostic cognate microRNA-gene signature. PLoS One 2012;7(8):e41522.

44. Pope WB, Chen JH, Dong J, et al. Relationship between gene expression and enhancement in glioblastoma multiforme: exploratory DNA microarray analysis. Radiology 2008;249(1):268–77.

45. Barajas RF Jr, Phillips JJ, Parvataneni R, et al. Regional variation in histopathologic features of tumor specimens from treatment-naive glioblastoma correlates with anatomic and physiologic MR Imaging. Neuro Oncol 2012;14(7):942–54.

46. Zinn PO, Mahajan B, Sathyan P, et al. Radiogenomic mapping of edema/cellular invasion MRI-phenotypes in glioblastoma multiforme. PLoS One 2011;6(10): e25451.

47. Barker FG, Davis RL, Chang SM, et al. Necrosis as a prognostic factor in glioblastoma multiforme. Cancer 1996;77(6):1161–6.

48. Pope WB, Sayre J, Perlina A, et al. MR imaging correlates of survival in patients with high-grade gliomas. AJNR Am J Neuroradiol 2005;26(10): 2466–74.

49. Colen RR, Wang J, Singh SK, et al. Glioblastoma: imaging genomic mapping reveals sex-specific oncogenic associations of cell death. Radiology 2015;275(1):215–27.

50. Van Meter T, Dumur C, Hafez N, et al. Microarray analysis of MRI-defined tissue samples in glioblastoma reveals differences in regional expression of therapeutic targets. Diagn Mol Pathol 2006;15(4): 195–205.

51. Yamashita K, Hiwatashi A, Togao O, et al. MR imaging–based analysis of glioblastoma multiforme: estimation of idh1 mutation status. AJNR Am J Neuroradiol 2016;37(1):58–65.

52. Zinn PO, Hatami M, Youssef E, et al. Diffusion weighted magnetic resonance imaging radiophenotypes and associated molecular pathways in glioblastoma. Neurosurgery 2016;63(CN_suppl_1):127–35.

53. Cui Y, Ren S, Tha KK, et al. Volume of high-risk intratumoral subregions at multi-parametric MR imaging predicts overall survival and complements molecular analysis of glioblastoma. Eur Radiol 2017;27(9): 3583–92.

54. Han Y, Yan LF, Wang XB, et al. Structural and advanced imaging in predicting MGMT promoter methylation of primary glioblastoma: a region of interest based analysis. BMC Cancer 2018;18(1):215.

55. Rundle-Thiele D, Day B, Stringer B, et al. Using the apparent diffusion coefficient to identifying MGMT promoter methylation status early in glioblastoma: importance of analytical method. J Med Radiat Sci 2015;62(2):92–8.

56. Heiland DH, Simon-Gabriel CP, Demerath T, et al. Integrative diffusion-weighted imaging and radiogenomic network analysis of glioblastoma multiforme. Sci Rep 2017;7:43523.

57. Ramon F, Barajas J, Hodgson JG, et al. Glioblastoma multiforme regional genetic and cellular expression patterns: influence on anatomic and physiologic MR imaging. Radiology 2010;254(2):564–76.

58. Jain R, Poisson L, Narang J, et al. Correlation of perfusion parameters with genes related to

angiogenesis regulation in glioblastoma: a feasibility study. AJNR Am J Neuroradiol 2012;33(7):1343–8.

59. Jain R, Poisson L, Narang J, et al. Genomic mapping and survival prediction in glioblastoma: molecular subclassification strengthened by hemodynamic imaging biomarkers. Radiology 2013;267(1):212–20.

60. Kong D-S, Kim J, Ryu G, et al. Quantitative radiomic profiling of glioblastoma represents transcriptomic expression. Oncotarget 2018;9(5):6336.

61. Choi C, Ganji S, DeBerardinis R, et al. 2-hydroxy-glutarate detection by magnetic resonance spectroscopy in IDH-mutated patients with gliomas. Nat Med 2012;18(4):624–9.

62. Lazovic J, Soto H, Piccioni D, et al. Detection of 2-hydroxyglutaric acid in vivo by proton magnetic resonance spectroscopy in U87 glioma cells overexpressing isocitrate dehydrogenase–1 mutation. Neuro Oncol 2012;14(12):1465–72.

63. Pope WB, Prins RM, Thomas MA, et al. Non-invasive detection of 2-hydroxyglutarate and other metabolites in IDH1 mutant glioma patients using magnetic resonance spectroscopy. J Neurooncol 2012;107(1):197–205.

64. Heiland DH, Wörner J, Haaker JG, et al. The integrative metabolomic-transcriptomic landscape of glioblastome multiforme. Oncotarget 2017;8(30):49178.

65. Gutman DA, Cooper LA, Hwang SN, et al. MR imaging predictors of molecular profile and survival: multi-institutional study of the TCGA glioblastoma data set. Radiology 2013;267(2):560–9.

66. Naeini KM, Pope WB, Cloughesy TF, et al. Identifying the mesenchymal molecular subtype of glioblastoma using quantitative volumetric analysis of anatomic magnetic resonance images. Neuro Oncol. 2013;15(5):626–34.

67. Lambin P, Leijenaar RTH, Deist TM, et al. Radiomics: the bridge between medical imaging and personalized medicine. Nat Rev Clin Oncol 2017;14(12):749–62.

68. Gore S, Chougule T, Jagtap J, et al. A review of radiomics and deep predictive modeling in glioma characterization. Acad Radiol 2020. https://doi.org/10.1016/j.acra.2020.06.016.

69. Soni N, Priya S, Bathla G. Texture analysis in cerebral gliomas: a review of the literature. AJNR Am J Neuroradiol 2019;40(6):928–34.

70. Itakura H, Achrol AS, Mitchell LA, et al. Magnetic resonance image features identify glioblastoma phenotypic subtypes with distinct molecular pathway activities. Sci Transl Med 2015;7(303):303ra138.

71. Kickingereder P, Bonekamp D, Nowosielski M, et al. Radiogenomics of glioblastoma: machine learning–based classification of molecular characteristics by using multiparametric and multiregional MR imaging features. Radiology 2016;281(3):907–18.

72. Chang P, Grinband J, Weinberg BD, et al. Deep-learning convolutional neural networks accurately classify genetic mutations in gliomas. AJNR Am J Neuroradiol 2018. https://doi.org/10.3174/ajnr.A5667.

73. Korfiatis P, Kline TL, Coufalova L, et al. MRI texture features as biomarkers to predict MGMT methylation status in glioblastomas. Med Phys 2016;43(6Part1):2835–44.

74. Li Z-C, Bai H, Sun Q, et al. Multiregional radiomics features from multiparametric MRI for prediction of MGMT methylation status in glioblastoma multiforme: a multicentre study. Eur Radiol 2018;28(9):3640–50.

75. Akbari H, Bakas S, Pisapia JM, et al. In vivo evaluation of EGFRvIII mutation in primary glioblastoma patients via complex multiparametric MRI signature. Neuro Oncol 2018;20(8):1068–79.

76. Bakas S, Akbari H, Pisapia J, et al. In vivo detection of EGFRvIII in glioblastoma via perfusion magnetic resonance imaging signature consistent with deep peritumoral infiltration: the φ-index. Clin Cancer Res 2017;23(16):4724–34.

77. Beig N, Patel J, Prasanna P, et al. Radiogenomic analysis of hypoxia pathway is predictive of overall survival in Glioblastoma. Sci Rep 2018;8(1):7.

78. Hu LS, Ning S, Eschbacher JM, et al. Radiogenomics to characterize regional genetic heterogeneity in glioblastoma. Neuro Oncol. 2017;19(1):128–37.

79. Dextraze K, Saha A, Kim D, et al. Spatial habitats from multiparametric MR imaging are associated with signaling pathway activities and survival in glioblastoma. Oncotarget 2017;8(68):112992.

80. Liu TT, Achrol AS, Mitchell LA, et al. Magnetic resonance perfusion image features uncover an angiogenic subgroup of glioblastoma patients with poor survival and better response to antiangiogenic treatment. Neuro Oncol 2017;19(7):997–1007.

81. Macyszyn L, Akbari H, Pisapia JM, et al. Imaging patterns predict patient survival and molecular subtype in glioblastoma via machine learning techniques. Neuro Oncol 2015;18(3):417–25.

82. Rathore S, Akbari H, Rozycki M, et al. Radiomic MRI signature reveals three distinct subtypes of glioblastoma with different clinical and molecular characteristics, offering prognostic value beyond IDH1. Sci Rep 2018;8(1):5087.

83. Gillies RJ, Kinahan PE, Hricak H. Radiomics: images are more than pictures, they are data. Radiology 2016;278(2):563–77.

84. Sullivan DC, Obuchowski NA, Kessler LG, et al. Metrology standards for quantitative imaging biomarkers. Radiology 2015;277(3):813–25.

85. Farahani K, Tata D, Nordstrom RJ. QIN benchmarks for clinical translation of quantitative imaging tools. Tomography 2019;5(1):1–6.

86. Bakas S, Akbari H, Sotiras A, et al. Advancing the cancer genome atlas glioma MRI collections with

expert segmentation labels and radiomic features. Sci Data 2017;4:170117.

87. Zwanenburg A, Vallières M, Abdalah MA, et al. The image biomarker standardization initiative: standardized quantitative radiomics for high-throughput image-based phenotyping. Radiology 2020;295(2):328–38.

88. Körzdörfer G, Kirsch R, Liu K, et al. Reproducibility and repeatability of MR fingerprinting relaxometry in the human brain. Radiology 2019;292(2):429–37.

89. Dastmalchian S, Kilinc O, Onyewadume L, et al. Radiomic analysis of magnetic resonance fingerprinting in adult brain tumors. Eur J Nucl Med Mol Imaging 2020. https://doi.org/10.1007/s00259-020-05037-w.

90. Davatzikos C, Barnholtz-Sloan JS, Bakas S, et al. AI-based prognostic imaging biomarkers for precision neuro-oncology: the ReSPOND consortium. Neuro Oncol 2020;22(6):886–8.

91. Park JE, Kim HS, Kim D, et al. A systematic review reporting quality of radiomics research in neuro-oncology: toward clinical utility and quality improvement using high-dimensional imaging features. BMC Cancer 2020;20(1):29.

92. O'Connor JP, Aboagye EO, Adams JE, et al. Imaging biomarker roadmap for cancer studies. Nat Rev Clin Oncol 2017;14(3):169–86.

Imaging Mimics of Brain Tumors

Joseph H. Donahue, MD[a], Sohil H. Patel, MD[a], Camilo E. Fadul, MD[b],
Sugoto Mukherjee, MD[a],*

KEYWORDS

- Brain tumor • Central nervous system neoplasm • Tumor mimic • Tumefactive demyelination

KEY POINTS

- Tumor mimics may account for 4% to 13% of referrals to a neuro-oncology service, so consideration of nonneoplastic processes is critical during initial evaluation of CNS neoplasia.
- Leveraging specific imaging signs and advanced imaging techniques detailed herein may add diagnostic confidence when considering various autoimmune, infectious, and vascular tumor mimics.
- Variability in ancillary laboratory diagnostics, including serologic and various immunohistochemical tests, may confer sufficiently low negative predictive values such that tumor mimics may still be considered on a clinical and imaging basis despite an unrevealing laboratory evaluation.

INTRODUCTION

Although most patients referred to neuro-oncology with the suspicion of brain tumor by imaging harbor a neoplasm, in some cases the abnormality has a nonneoplastic cause. A wide variety of nonneoplastic entities may closely resemble the imaging findings of primary or metastatic intracranial neoplasia, posing diagnostic challenges for the referring provider and the radiologist. Autoimmune, infectious, and vascular diseases have particular potential for misdiagnosis as brain tumors given the often nonspecific neurologic symptoms and ambiguous imaging features.[1–3] These "tumor mimics" may account for 4% to 13% of patient referrals to neuro-oncology; and when imaging is ordered by neuro-oncologists with the presumptive diagnosis of "brain tumor," it may foster a framing bias that leads the radiologist to misinterpretation of the examination.[4,5] Advances in neuroimaging quality and availability, which have increased the detection of "incidentalomas" (approximately 3% of MR imaging brain scans), potentiates the possibility for such referrals to neuro-oncologists or neurosurgeons.[6–8] The consequences of an incorrect imaging diagnosis of intracranial neoplasia are obvious, with unnecessary surgical procedures and misdirected medical therapies yielding a likelihood of patient harm and legal liability.

In this article, we provide a framework for the radiologist to identify "brain tumor mimics" by highlighting imaging and laboratory pearls and pitfalls, and illustrating unique and frequently encountered lesions. Because the initial imaging in most patients with these lesions follows a generic brain MR imaging protocol dictated by institutional practice, we describe features of the various tumor mimics on common MR imaging brain sequences that are applicable to routine clinical imaging studies.

IMAGING FINDINGS
Demyelinating and Inflammatory Disorders

Although multiple sclerosis typically displays small multifocal perivenular demyelinating plaques with a propensity for the call ososeptal interface that disseminate in space and time, larger tumefactive lesions may occasionally constitute the imaging

[a] Department of Radiology and Medical Imaging, University of Virginia Health System, PO Box 800170, Charlottesville, VA 22908-0170, USA; [b] Department of Neurology, University of Virginia Health System, PO Box 800432, Charlottesville, VA 22908-0170, USA
* Corresponding author.
E-mail address: sm5qd@virginia.edu

Radiol Clin N Am 59 (2021) 457–470
https://doi.org/10.1016/j.rcl.2021.02.003

presentation. In such cases, almost one-third of the larger tumefactive lesions can be the only lesion, potentially leading to misdiagnosis as neoplasia. Solitary and/or tumefactive lesions are more likely to occur in the uncommon multiple sclerosis variants of Marburg and Schilder diseases.[9]

The tumefactive demyelinating lesions can have local mass effect and edema (although disproportionally less when compared with tumors of the same size), centered within the deep white matter in the supratentorial cortex. Other imaging features include computed tomography (CT) hypoattenuation and T2 hypointense rim.[10] When these demonstrate enhancement, it is classically in the form of an incomplete ring, with the incomplete segment of the ring facing the cortex.[11] The enhancing segment represents the leading edge of demyelination, facing the white matter side of the lesion. Dilated veins have been seen within the central part of these lesions, and may be well demonstrated on susceptibility-weighted imaging (SWI). Usually these lesions demonstrate increased diffusivity, with decreased perfusion and nonspecific MR spectroscopy findings (with elevated choline, decreased N-acetylaspartate (NAA), and high lactate) when compared with lymphomas.[12] A rapid response to steroid helps in narrowing the diagnosis.

Acute disseminated encephalomyelitis (ADEM) is a unique autoimmune-mediated demyelinating disease, initiated by an infection (or immunization), which leads to myelin antibodies. Imaging usually reveals multifocal subcortical and periventricular lesions, with involvement of the basal ganglia, posterior fossa, and cranial nerves. Many of the white matter lesions have ill-defined "cotton-ball" like appearance on T2 and FLAIR series with a varied enhancing appearance ranging from linear, punctate, to partial/incomplete ring like enhancement for some of the larger lesions.[13] Larger "tumefactive" lesions when present appear similar to those seen in multiple sclerosis (**Fig. 1**). In cases of acute hemorrhagic leukoencephalitis, microhemorrhages or macrohemorrhages are most evident on SWI sequences,[14] occasionally resembling hemorrhagic neoplasms.

Neuromyelitis optica and neuromyelitis optica spectrum disorder (NMOSD) are autoimmune-mediated demyelinating disorders because of antibodies against aquaporin-4. Neuromyelitis optica–IgG is a specific biomarker that is present in most of these patients. The brain lesions in NMOSD involve the brainstem, hypothalamus, and other periventricular areas, and unlike tumefactive demyelinating lesions, it is unlikely for them to be mistaken for tumors.[15] In rare cases, tumefactive demyelinating lesions is seen in neuromyelitis optica or NMOSD, with similar imaging features as discussed previously. It is more likely for the long segment cord lesions to be mistaken for a spinal cord tumor if there is lack of intracranial or optic nerve involvement.

Myelin oligodendrocyte glycoprotein (MOG) is a cellular adhesion molecule expressed on the cell surface of oligodendrocytes and myelin sheaths within the central nervous system (CNS). Clinical presentation is strongly influenced by age and correlates generally with imaging phenotypes. The usual imaging patterns of presentation include a leukodystrophy-like pattern, an ADEM-like pattern, and an NMOSD-like pattern. However, they can rarely present on imaging as a demyelinating pseudotumor with imaging findings similar to a tumefactive demyelinating lesion detailed previously.[16]

Neurosarcoid

Sarcoidosis is a complex multisystem granulomatous disease that is believed to have an autoimmune origin.[17] Although the most commonly involved organ is the lung, extrapulmonary sarcoidosis frequently occurs, with CNS involvement present in 10% to 20% of patients. Many patients with neurosarcoidosis remain asymptomatic, with only 5% demonstrating significant imaging findings, including possible involvement of the brain, blood vessels, spinal cord, dura, optic nerves, bones, and the adjacent soft tissues in the head and neck.

Neurosarcoidosis can mimic brain tumors in multiple different ways.[18] Large dural-based masses can mimic meningiomas, whereas nodular enhancing lesions along cranial nerves is characterized as schwannomas or neurofibromas. Involvement of choroid plexuses can mimic enhancing intraventricular tumors. Although the parenchymal involvement in neurosarcoidosis is frequently along perivascular spaces, causing a vasculitic-like picture, larger coalescing granulomas within the brain can present as expansile tumefactive lesions with local mass effect and edema (**Fig. 2**).[19] Unless the neuroradiologist is cognizant of this entity, these lesions are misdiagnosed as lymphoma or idiopathic inflammatory pseudotumor. Rarely, there is need for a biopsy to demonstrate the noncaseating granulomas, multinucleated giant cells, epithelioid histiocytes, and benign lymphocytes and plasma cells characteristic of this entity.

Autoimmune Encephalitis

Autoimmune encephalitis represents a challenging set of diagnoses with varied clinical presentations.

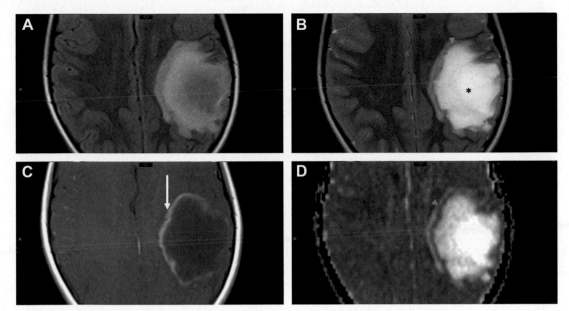

Fig. 1. Tumefactive demyelinating lesion in ADEM. Axial FLAIR (*A*), axial T2-weighted (*B*), axial postcontrast T1-weighted (*C*), and axial apparent diffusion coefficient (ADC) map (*D*) MR images in an 8 year old with complaints of foot numbness and progressive clumsiness determined to have ADEM. The leading edge of demyelination is characterized by the incomplete rim enhancement (*white arrow* in *C*) with corresponding thin linear T2 and ADC hypointensity (*blue arrowheads* in *B* and *D*, respectively). The T2 images show a characteristic "zoned" appearance with the central lesion showing marked hyperintensity (*asterisk* in *B*), which is marginated by the leading edge of demyelination (*blue arrowhead* in *B*) that separates the central lesion from a rim of perilesional edema (*red arrowhead* in *B*).

In most cases, specific antibodies directed against CNS cells are found in peripheral blood or cerebrospinal fluid (CSF). Although autoimmune encephalitis has been grouped according to the antibodies recognized epitope (intracellular vs cellular surface) and if the antibodies are mechanistically responsible for the disease or an epiphenomenon, the MR imaging findings are indistinguishable between these two groups. The most common imaging appearance is the involvement of the limbic system, which manifests as either unilateral or bilateral involvement of mesial temporal lobes and thalami/basal ganglia with patchy enhancement.[20] Nevertheless, the imaging abnormalities may occur in other cerebral lobes. Rarely, these lesions exhibit swelling and edema that can mimic infiltrative gliomas.

TREX1-Associated Retinal Vasculopathy with Cerebral Leukodystrophy

TREX1 gene–related mutations causing retinal vasculopathy and cerebral leukodystrophy are rare autosomal-dominant disorders secondary to underlying frameshift mutations that encode for major DNA exonucleases.[21] The mutations result in accumulation of abnormal DNA and RNA within cells, which are then mistakenly targeted by the

host immune cells with devastating consequences. Most of these patients are middle aged, present with vision and neurologic symptoms, and have a positive family history.

The most common imaging findings include hyperintense white matter lesions on T2/FLAIR with near complete sparing of the gray matter. Lesions, which are usually supratentorial, may demonstrate nodular enhancement with restricted diffusion or larger mass-like lesions with irregular rim enhancement and extensive surrounding edema (**Fig. 3**). After immunosuppressive treatment, the lesions can transiently decrease in size with newer lesions appearing at different sites, giving the appearance of a migratory tumefactive process.[22]

Central Nervous System Infection Tumor Mimics

Pyogenic infections

Cerebral abscesses are occasionally difficult to distinguish from neoplasm, particularly metastatic disease, because both may appear as disseminated ring-enhancing lesions localizing to the gray-white matter interface. In a series of 221 ring-enhancing lesions, Schwartz and colleagues[23] found that although neoplasia (primary

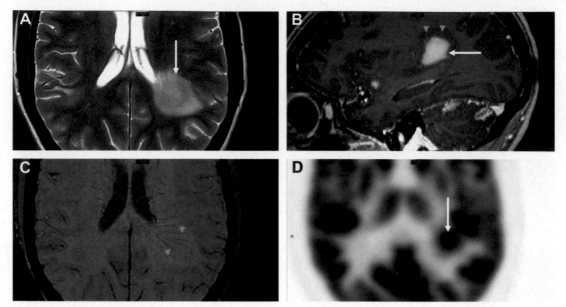

Fig. 2. Neurosarcoidosis. Axial T2-weighted MR image (*A*), sagittal T1-weighted postcontrast MR image (*B*), axial SWI MR image (*C*), and axial fluorodeoxyglucose PET image (*D*) in a 23 year old presenting with multiple subacute focal neurologic deficits. A mass-like area of left periatrial signal abnormality demonstrates slightly mixed intermediate/high T2 signal (*white arrow* in *A*) with corresponding homogeneous enhancement (*white arrow* in *B*). Note that the medullary veins maintain a straight course through the lesion and demonstrate slight engorgement on SWI and postcontrast series (*blue arrowheads* in *B* and *C*). Additional areas of cerebellar folia parenchymal and leptomeningeal enhancement are present (*red arrowheads* in *B*). Fluorodeoxyglucose PET images show radiotracer accumulation within the periatrial lesion (*white arrow* in *D*), measuring an average and maximum standardized uptake value of 9.2 and 12.9, respectively.

and metastatic) accounted for 72% of cases, pyogenic abscess and atypical infections accounted for 8% and 4%, respectively. In a similar investigation by Kim and colleagues,[24] concordant findings were reported, with 4% pyogenic abscess and 2.6% atypical infections.

Although metastasis are the more common underlying cause of ring-enhancing lesions, some imaging features should prompt consideration of an infectious tumor mimic. The SWI dual rim sign displays a hypointense outer rim posited to represent the fibrocollagenous abscess capsule surrounding a hyperintense inner rim thought to correspond to a zone of granulation tissue between the necrotic core and the capsule. In a study of 32 brain masses, the dual rim sign was present in 9 of 12 abscesses and 0 of 20 glioblastomas, conferring a sensitivity of 75% and a specificity of 100%.[25]

Restricted diffusion of cavity contents, one of the best known imaging features of pyogenic abscesses, is caused by the highly viscous nature of the proteinaceous exudate admixed with viable bacteria, inflammatory cells, and debris (**Fig. 4**). A meta-analysis of 11 studies found a pooled sensitivity and specificity of 95% and 94%, respectively, for the use of diffusion-weighted images

(DWI) to distinguish abscess from other cerebral ring-enhancing lesions.[26] However, some pyogenic abscesses (~4%), atypical infections, or pyogenic abscesses imaged after initiation of antibiotic therapy or in an immunocompromised host may not show diffusion restriction.[27,28]

Atypical Infections

Toxoplasmosis
Toxoplasma gondii is a ubiquitous protozoan parasite prone to cause opportunistic cerebral infection, typically reactivation of latent infection, in the setting of severe immunosuppression (CD4 <100 cells/μL). Differentiating cerebral toxoplasmosis from primary CNS lymphoma (PCNSL) is often challenging on a clinical, laboratory, and imaging basis. Although there is considerable overlap of imaging, PCNSL is statistically the more likely cause in immunocompromised patients with a solitary parenchymal mass, particularly one demonstrating subependymal spread of disease, whereas toxoplasmosis is more likely multifocal with basal ganglia predilection. Both "eccentric" and "concentric" target signs favor toxoplasmosis. The eccentric target sign, present in less than 30% of cases, is recognized on postcontrast MR imaging series as a ring-enhancing lesion

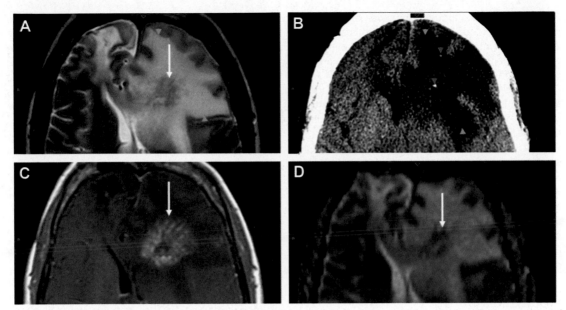

Fig. 3. TREX1-associated retinal vasculopathy with cerebral leukodystrophy. Axial T2-weighted MR image, axial noncontrast CT scan, axial postcontrast T1-weighted image, and axial ADC map MR image in a 45 year old presenting with headache and weakness. Extensive left frontal vasogenic edema (*blue arrowheads* in *A* and *B*) surrounds an irregular mass-like area of periventricular enhancement (*white arrow* in *C*) with corresponding intermediate signal on T2 and ADC series (*white arrows* in *A* and *D*, respectively). A few punctate foci of calcification are displayed on CT images (*red arrowheads* in *B*). A nearly identical lesion was previously present in the right frontal lobe (not shown) with biopsy revealing subacute infarction with extensive gliosis and nonspecific vasculopathy.

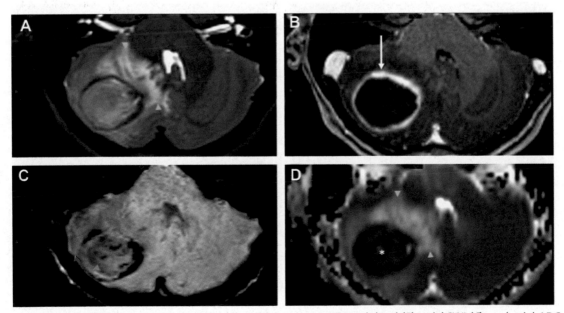

Fig. 4. Pyogenic abscess. Axial T2-weighted (*A*), axial postcontrast T1-weighted (*B*), axial SWI (*C*), and axial ADC map (*D*) MR images in a 10 year old presenting with headache. Vasogenic edema (*green arrowheads* in *A* and *D*) surrounds the smoothly rim-enhancing right cerebellar mass (*white arrow* in *B*). A partial dual rim sign is displayed on SWI as an inner hyperintense rim and an outer hypointense rim (*blue* and *red arrowheads* in *C*, respectively). The central abscess cavity shows nearly homogeneous diffusion restriction as low signal intensity on ADC (*asterisk* in *D*).

with a small nodular focus of enhancement along the lesion wall. The concentric target sign is shown on T2-weighted images as alternating zones of hypointensity/hyperintensity and is believed to be a more specific imaging feature (**Fig. 5**).[29]

Cerebral toxoplasmosis may demonstrate lower perfusion indices (regional cerebral blood volume <1.3–1.5 × normal white matter) and higher diffusion coefficient (apparent diffusion coefficient >1.6 normal white matter) than PCNSL.[30–32] By MR spectroscopy, cerebral toxoplasmosis and PCSNL may both demonstrate lipid/lactate peaks, with toxoplasmosis generally showing a suppression of other metabolite peaks and PCNSL potentially showing a prominent choline peak. The specificity of MR spectroscopy for differentiating PCNSL from other diagnoses in immunocompromised patients ranges from 27% to 83%.[33]

Neurocysticercosis

The cestode *Taenia solium* (pork tapeworm) causes cysticercosis, a globally common parasitic infection in which humans act as the intermediate dead-end host. The parasitic embryos disseminate hematogenously and commonly deposit within skeletal muscle, the globes, and neural tissues, where the cysticerci then evolve through four stages of disease: vesicular, colloidal vesicular, granular nodular, and nodular calcified.

Neurocysticercosis may occasionally masquerade as CNS neoplasia, particularly in the colloidal vesicular or granular nodular stages of intraparenchymal disease when rim enhancement and perilesional edema may be present. The racemose disease form, infection of the subarachnoid space, may also mimic intraventricular or suprasellar neoplasia, such as craniopharyngioma.

If present, larvae in various life stages or of varying compartmental distribution are an important feature in recognizing neurocysticercosis. For instance, the co-occurrence of parenchymal ringenhancing lesions with calcified parenchymal or craniofacial soft tissue foci may be present. Identification of the parasitic scolex in the vesicular and colloidal vesicular stages adds certainty to the diagnosis. Typically, the scolex appears as a DWI and/or T1 hyperintense eccentric nodule or comma-shaped structure within the larger cyst (**Fig. 6**). DWI hyperintensity of the cysts may occur during evolution to the granular nodular phase when the fluid contents becomes more viscous.

Imaging Features Suggesting a Vascular Tumor Mimic

Aneurysm

Most intracranial aneurysms are acquired "true" aneurysms that arise at the branch points of major intracranial arteries, and are caused by

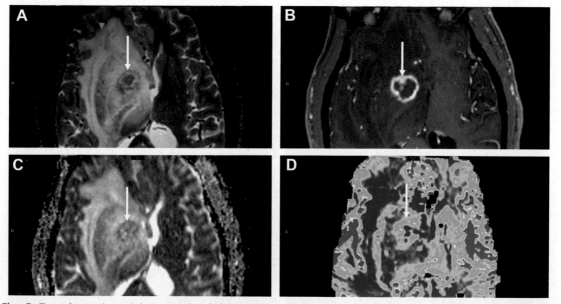

Fig. 5. Toxoplasmosis. Axial T2-weighted (*A*), axial postcontrast T1-weighted (*B*), ADC map (*C*), and axial perfusion-weighted (PWI) cerebral blood volume map (*D*) MR images in a 47-year-old immunocompromised patient presenting with headache. Right basal ganglia lesion shows the "concentric target sign" on T2-weighted images as alternating zones of hypointensity/hyperintensity (*white arrow* in *A*) and substantial perilesional vasogenic edema (*blue arrowheads* in *A*). T1-weighted images show the "eccentric target sign" as a small nodular focus of enhancement along the lesion wall (*white arrow* in *B*). The lesion shows predominantly intralesional T2 shine through on ADC map (*white arrow* in *C*) and mild capsular hyperperfusion on PWI (*white arrow* in *D*).

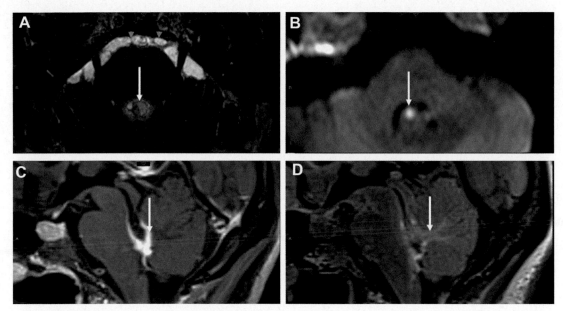

Fig. 6. Neurocysticercosis. Axial heavily T2-weighted (*A*), axial diffusion-weighted (*B*), sagittal T1-weighted post-contrast (*C*), and sagittal FLAIR (*D*) MR imaging in a 30-year-old patient with headache. The scolex is identifiable as a cystic intraventricular focus with corresponding diffusion restriction (*white arrows* in *A* and *B*). Inflammatory ependymal enhancement (*white arrow* in *C*) and periventricular edema (*white arrow D*) contribute to obstruction of the fourth ventricular outflow foramina and hydrocephalus (not shown). Additional racemose disease is appreciable in the prepontine cistern on heavily T2-weighted images (*blue arrowheads* in *A*).

hemodynamic stresses that are potentiated by various environmental (smoking, hypertension, alcohol abuse) and genetic factors.[34] "False" aneurysms, or pseudoaneurysms, involve complete arterial wall disruption with a specific cause, such as trauma or infection, and are variably contained by hemorrhage, clot, and fibrin, and are therefore at high risk of rupture.

On angiographic examinations (CT angiography, MR angiography), most intracranial aneurysms are easily diagnosed, appearing as rounded/saccular outpouchings that arise from branch points of the major cerebral arteries. However, aneurysms can have atypical appearances or be initially detected on nonangiographic studies, which can create diagnostic uncertainty. In particular, giant intracranial aneurysms (>2.5 cm) frequently contain mural thrombus of variable and heterogeneous signal intensity on T1- and T2-weighted imaging, an appearance that might mimic a complex, hemorrhagic neoplasm.[35] Giant aneurysms may cause local brain parenchymal mass effect and edema, similar to extra-axial neoplasms. The contrast enhancement of an aneurysm lumen can be mistaken for the avid contrast enhancement of a vascularized neoplasm. Furthermore, the location of an aneurysm may cause diagnostic confusion depending on the context. Cavernous internal carotid

aneurysms might be mistaken for cavernous sinus neoplasms (eg, schwannoma, meningioma, pituitary macroadenoma). Fusiform aneurysms of the petrous internal carotid artery might be mistaken for petrous apex masses, such as cholesterol granuloma, mucocele, dermoid, or epidermoid.[36]

Several diagnostic clues may aid in the accurate identification of an intracranial aneurysm that mimics a neoplasm. On CT, aneurysms appear as rounded masses with attenuation values similar to neighboring vessels. Peripheral calcification may be present. On MR imaging, T2-weighted imaging frequently shows marked hypointense signal ("flow void") in the aneurysm lumen, although the signal intensity may vary depending on flow turbulence. Pulsation artifact in the phase encoding direction is an extremely useful sign, but not always present. Aneurysm wall thrombus commonly demonstrates "blooming" on T2*/SWI; T1 shortening; and a concentric, lamellated pattern. Contrast-enhanced three-dimensional gradient echo T1-weighted sequences (eg, MPRAGE, VIBE, BRAVO) are particularly useful for visualizing the artery from which the aneurysms arises. On such sequences, the degree of contrast enhancement of the aneurysm lumen usually matches that of the surrounding vasculature (**Fig. 7**). When aneurysm is suspected, CT angiography and MR angiography should be pursued for confirmation, with

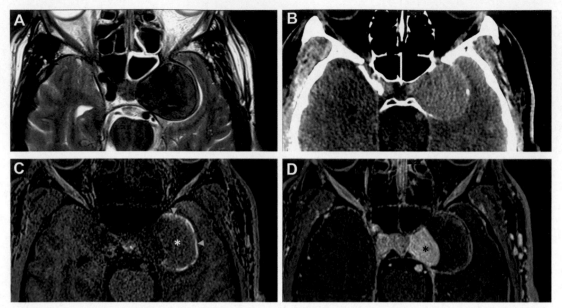

Fig. 7. Giant aneurysm. Axial T2-weighted MR image (*A*), axial noncontrast CT (*B*), axial noncontrast T1-weighted MR image (*C*), and axial postcontrast T1-weighted MR image (*D*) in a 63 year old presenting with left cranial nerve III palsy. The left cavernous carotid artery aneurysm wall demonstrates smooth low signal intensity on T2-weighted images (*blue arrowheads* in *A*) and peripheral calcification (*red arrowhead* in *B*). The patent portion of the aneurysm sac shows avid contrast enhancement, which approximates that of other vascular structures (*asterisk* in *D*). The nonenhancing mural thrombus within the aneurysm sac shows variable signal, with discontinuous peripheral hyperintensity (*green arrowheads* in *C*) and vague central hypointensity (*asterisk* in *C*) on T1-weighted images.

the authors generally preferring high-quality CT angiography for this purpose. On time-of-flight MR angiography, the hyperintense signal of mural thrombus caused by T1-shortening can mimic flow-related signal. Conversely, turbulent or slow blood flow through the aneurysm lumen may result in reduced flow-related signal.[37]

Subacute arterial infarction
Subacute arterial cerebral infarctions (generally considered 2 days to 2 weeks following the ischemic event) mimic many of the imaging features of neoplasm. Mass effect from edema and heightened risk for hemorrhage occur during the subacute phase. DWI is variable at this stage, reflecting a combination of cytotoxic and vasogenic edema. Subacute infarctions often show contrast enhancement, reflecting endothelial damage and ingrowth of vessels with "leaky" blood-brain barriers. "Luxury" perfusion, representing infarct-bed hyperemia after arterial recanalization, shows increased cerebral blood flow on perfusion-weighted imaging.[38]

Nonetheless, there are several clues to the diagnosis of a subacute infarction. A history of acute symptom onset suggests ischemic stroke. Parenchymal injury is often restricted to a single arterial

territory. The pattern of contrast enhancement is usually gyriform for cortical infarctions, or may isolate to the deep gray structures. Angiographic imaging can identify an occluded artery in the territory of the infarction. MR spectroscopy shows reduction in NAA from neuronal damage, a lactate peak, and lack of significant Cho elevation.[39] Short-term follow-up neuroimaging usually clarifies the diagnosis.

Venous infarction
Venous infarctions result from venous sinus or cortical vein thrombosis. Predisposing conditions include various hypercoagulable diseases, oral contraceptive use, pregnancy, dehydration, underlying infection, neoplasm, and trauma. The clinical presentation of venous infarctions is more variable than for arterial infarctions, with symptoms that include headache, seizure, nausea and vomiting, focal neurologic deficits, and altered mental status.

Neuroimaging features include parenchymal hemorrhage, mixed vasogenic and cytotoxic edema, and mass effect.[40] The appearance of hemorrhage is variable, but may show a lobar or petechial gyriform pattern. The location of venous infarctions is an important clue to their cause because they follow the territory drained by the thrombosed vein. For instance, thrombosis of the internal cerebral veins can cause bilateral thalamic venous ischemia.

An important step in confirming a diagnosis of venous infarction is identifying the thrombosed venous sinus or cortical vein, best displayed on MR or CT venography. Note that lack of flow void on T2 and FLAIR-weighted imaging should be interpreted with caution, and can result from turbulent and slow flow in a patient venous structure.[41]

Low-flow cerebral vascular malformations

Cerebral cavernous malformations (CCMs) are slow-flow venous malformations composed of clustered thin-walled capillaries and thin fibrous adventitia, surrounded by hemosiderin and gliosis. Although most are sporadic and solitary, familial CCM syndrome or prior radiation therapy may result in multiple intracranial CCMs.[42] Although most are asymptomatic, hemorrhage into a CCM can result in headache, seizures, or focal neurologic deficit. On CT, CCMs are typically hyperdense and some show calcification. MR imaging shows a characteristic "popcorn" morphology, with regions of hypointense/hyperintense signal on T1- and T2-weighted imaging, often with a hypointense rim. T2*/SWI shows marked

susceptibility blooming (**Fig. 8**). There is mild or no contrast enhancement. Recent hemorrhage of a cavernous malformation associates with acute/subacute blood products, blood-fluid levels, and adjacent brain edema. CCMs may mimic neoplasms if they are large and/or recently hemorrhaged. An important clue is the presence of a neighboring developmental venous anomaly, which frequently co-occur with CCMs.[43] In familial CCM syndrome, the presence of multiple CCMs may suggest a differential diagnosis of metastases. In this situation, most of the CCMs should neither enhance nor cause local edema, allowing for differentiation from metastasis.

Capillary telangiectasias are benign low-flow malformations composed of dilated capillaries with normal intervening brain parenchyma, usually discovered incidentally on neuroimaging. Most occur in the pons, with a minority occurring in the cerebellum and basal ganglia.[44] Capillary telangiectasias are asymptomatic lesions discovered incidentally on neuroimaging. They show subtle if any signal alteration on T1- and T2-weighted imaging. T2*/SWI shows low signal "blooming" from slow-flowing deoxyhemoglobin (**Fig. 9**). They show contrast enhancement, which, in our experience, most frequency causes a diagnostic dilemma when a patient is undergoing MR imaging to evaluate for brain metastases. Lack of edema

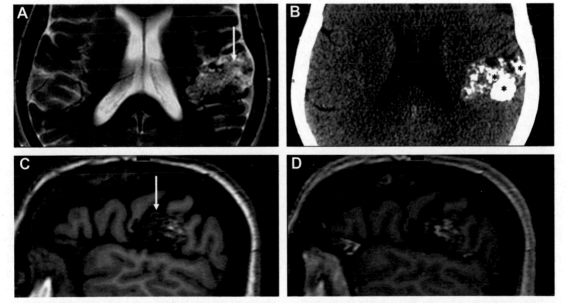

Fig. 8. Giant CCM. Axial T2-weighted MR image, axial noncontrast CT, and sagittal precontrast and postcontrast T1-weighted MR images in a 66 year old with focal epilepsy. The giant CCM demonstrates markedly heterogeneous hypointense/hyperintense signal on T2 and T1 images (*white arrows* in *A* and *C*, respectively) with surrounding chronic hemosiderin deposition noted as linear low T2 signal (*red arrowheads* in *A*). Faint contrast enhancement is present at the posterior lesion margin (*blue arrowhead* in *D*). The large intralesional calcific foci present in this case (*asterisks* in *B*) may be more dense and conspicuous than in other cases.

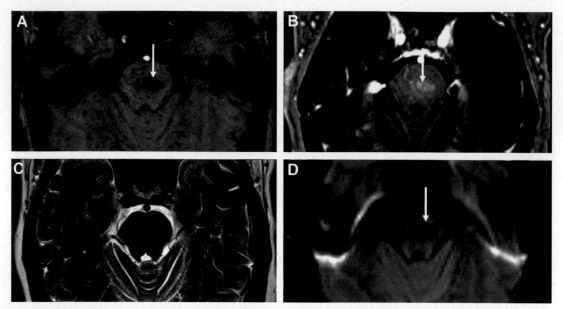

Fig. 9. Capillary telangiectasia. Axial SWI (*A*), axial postcontrast T1-weighted (*B*), axial T2-weighted (*C*), and axial DWI (*D*) MR images in a 72-year-old patient with lung carcinoma undergoing cerebral metastasis screening. The central pontine capillary telangiectasia is most conspicuous as a low signal intensity focus on SWI (*arrow* in *A*) with corresponding amorphous faint contrast enhancement (*arrow* in *B*). The capillary telangiectasia is nearly imperceptible on T2-weighted images and demonstrates T2 blackout effect (low signal intensity) on DWI series (*arrow* in *D*).

and mass effect, and an associated branching vein are helpful clues to the diagnosis. Stability on follow-up imaging helps confirm the diagnosis.

Cerebral amyloid angiopathy

Cerebral amyloid angiopathy (CAA) results from abnormal accumulation of amyloid-β protein in cerebral cortical and leptomeningeal vessels, which predisposes to vessel rupture and hemorrhage, typically in a lobar distribution. CAA is most commonly sporadic and occurs in elderly patients. The most important neuroimaging features are sequela of prior lobar hemorrhage, including cortical/subcortical microhemorrhages and superficial siderosis, with relative sparing of the deep gray nuclei and pons. Hemorrhages are best visualized with SWI.[45] Most patients with CAA also exhibit changes of small vessel ischemia on T2-weighted imaging.

Manifestations of CAA that can mimic neoplasms are CAA-related inflammation and cerebral amyloidoma. Patients with CAA-related inflammation present with headache, rapid cognitive decline, seizure, and focal neurologic deficits. CAA-related inflammation shows large confluent regions of white matter edema with leptomeningeal contrast enhancement and local mass effect. This disease can often be identified by appreciating coexistent lobar microhemorrhages on

hemosiderin-sensitive sequences (**Fig. 10**). Cerebral amyloidoma is a rare mass-like lesion that occurs in middle age patients. On imaging, it appears as a solidly enhancing white matter mass with local edema, which is difficult to prospectively distinguish from neoplasm.[46]

LABORATORY TEST PEARLS AND PITFALLS

When confronted by imaging with a brain tumor mimic, the clinical history is crucial to guide the need for laboratory studies that may help in the diagnosis. For instance, imaging characteristics in the context of a history of immunosuppression or epidemiologic exposure raises the suspicion of an infectious cause. Thus, a detailed medical history increases the utility of ordering serologic and CSF tests. Unfortunately, for most circumstances there are no studies that determine the sensitivity and specificity of integrating the imaging characteristics and laboratory studies for a diagnosis. A pitfall of serologic diagnosis of CNS infections is the variability in sensitivity and specificity of assays and delayed antibody response after symptom onset.[47]

When a brain-enhancing lesion appears in an immunosuppressed patient, the differential diagnosis is usually between toxoplasmosis and lymphoma. Most patients with cerebral toxoplasmosis

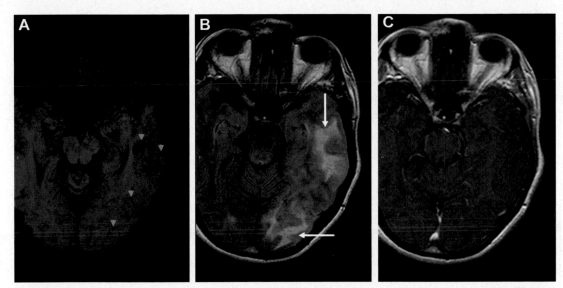

Fig. 10. CAA-related inflammation. Axial SWI (*A*), axial FLAIR (*B*), and axial postcontrast T1-weighted (*C*) MR images in a 66 year old with altered mental status. SWI demonstrates numerous parenchymal microhemorrhages as low signal intensity foci in a peripheral lobar distribution (*blue arrowheads* in *A*), which corresponds to the large area of temporo-occipital vasogenic edema noted on FLAIR images (*white arrows* in *B*). Minimal if any regional leptomeningeal enhancement is present on postcontrast imaging.

have high titers of antibodies against *T gondii* in blood, but a negative serologic result does not exclude the diagnosis.[48] If able to perform a lumbar puncture without risk of herniation, doing polymerase chain reaction in the CSF for *Toxoplasma* and Epstein-Barr virus may help in the diagnosis without need for a biopsy.[49] Although the specificity of CSF *Toxoplasma* polymerase chain reaction is 100%, the sensitivity is approximately 86%.[50] Therefore, a negative polymerase chain reaction does not rule out the diagnosis of CNS toxoplasmosis.

Neurocysticercosis will be in the differential diagnosis, when a brain tumor mimic is seen in an individual coming from or living in an endemic area, but there are rare cases without a clear exposure history to *T solium*. The utility of immunologic testing varies depending if the neurocysticercosis is parenchymal, extraparenchymal, or both, and the stage of the disease (viable, degenerating, or nonviable). The complement fixation test and the enzyme-linked immunosorbent assay have poor sensitivity and specificity.[51] The enzyme-linked immunoelectrotransfer blot assay in serum, which has a higher sensitivity than in CSF, is the preferred immunologic diagnostic method. Its sensitivity, however, varies from very high when there are multiple parenchymal and extraparenchymal lesions to low when there is a single parenchymal calcified lesion. Another caveat is that there may be false-positive results because of prior infection with the parasite, but without neurocysticercosis.

In the absence of systemic involvement, the diagnosis of neurosarcoidosis may be challenging. Determination of angiotensin-converting enzyme concentration is a valuable biomarker for systemic sarcoidosis. Both serum and CSF angiotensin-converting enzyme concentration, however, carry low sensitivity and specificity in neurosarcoidosis and have no predictive value in the differential diagnosis of a brain tumor mimic on MR imaging.[52]

When clinically isolated syndrome is the initial presentation of multiple sclerosis, the presence of IgG oligoclonal bands in CSF may support the diagnosis. Qualitative analysis using isoelectric focusing with immunofixation in CSF and parallel serum is the recommended methodology.[53] In two studies with long-term follow-up of patients with isolated tumefactive lesions, CSF oligoclonal bands were present in about half of the cases.[54,55] Therefore, the sensitivity for patients with multiple sclerosis presenting with a tumefactive lesion seems to be low, whereas the specificity is unknown. The anti-MOG antibody should be requested in all patients with ADEM or atypical demyelinating disease because it is a marker that in addition to imaging finding may help establish the diagnosis of MOG-associated antibody disease. The presence of anti-aquaporin-4 antibody in blood is a specific biomarker for NMOSD in the appropriate clinical and imaging settings.

SUMMARY

Prospective identification of brain tumor mimics is an opportunity for the interpreting radiologist to add value to patient care by decreasing time to diagnosis and avoiding unnecessary surgical procedures and medical therapies, but requires familiarity with mimic entities and an appropriately high degree of suspicion.

CLINICS CARE POINTS

- Tumor mimics may account for 4% to 13% of referrals to a neuro-oncology service, so consideration of nonneoplastic processes is critical during initial evaluation of CNS neoplasia.

- Leveraging specific imaging signs and advanced imaging techniques detailed herein may add diagnostic confidence when considering various autoimmune, infectious, and vascular tumor mimics.

- Variability in ancillary laboratory diagnostics, including serologic and various immunohistochemical tests, may confer sufficiently low negative predictive values such that tumor mimics may still be considered on a clinical and imaging basis despite an unrevealing laboratory evaluation.

DISCLOSURE

The authors have nothing to disclose.

REFERENCES

1. Go JL, Acharya J, Rajamohan AG. Is it or is it not? Brain tumor mimics. Semin Roentgenol 2018;53(1): 62–76.

2. Leclercq D, Trunet S, Bertrand A, et al. Cerebral tumor or pseudotumor? Diagn Interv Imaging 2014; 95(10):906–16.

3. Bradley D, Rees J. Brain tumour mimics and chameleons. Pract Neurol 2013;359–71. https://doi.org/10. 1136/practneurol-2013-000652.

4. Starkey J, Li Y, Tihan T, et al. Clinical series: five simple MR imaging features to identify tumor mimics. Neurographics 2016;6(4):229–36.

5. Maldonado MD, Batchala P, Ornan D, et al. Features of diffuse gliomas that are misdiagnosed on initial neuroimaging: a case control study. J Neurooncol 2018;140(1):107–13.

6. Bos D, Poels MMF, Adams HHH, et al. Prevalence, clinical management, and natural course of incidental findings on brain MR images: the population-based Rotterdam Scan Study. Radiology 2016;281(2):507–15.

7. Morris Z, Whiteley WN, Longstreth WT Jr, et al. Incidental findings on brain magnetic resonance imaging: systematic review and meta-analysis. BMJ 2009;339:b3016.

8. Niessen WJ, Breteler MMB, Van Der Lugt A. Incidental findings on brain MRI in the general population. N Engl J Med 2007;357:1821–8.

9. Sarbu N, Shih RY, Jones RV, et al. White matter diseases with radiologic-pathologic correlation. Radiographics 2016;36(5):1426–47.

10. Kim E. Distinguishing tumefactive demyelinating lesions from glioma or central nervous system lymphoma: added value of unenhanced CT. Radiology 2009;251(2):467–75.

11. Given CA 2nd, Stevens BS, Lee C. The MRI appearance of tumefactive demyelinating lesions. AJR Am J Roentgenol 2004;182(1):195–9.

12. Suh CH, Kim HS, Jung SC, et al. MRI findings in tumefactive demyelinating lesions: a systematic review and meta-analysis. AJNR Am J Neuroradiol 2018;39(9):1643–9.

13. Khurana DS, Melvin JJ, Kothare SV, et al. Acute disseminated encephalomyelitis in children: discordant neurologic and neuroimaging abnormalities and response to plasmapheresis. Pediatrics 2005; 116(2):431–6.

14. Kao H-W, Alexandru D, Kim R, et al. Value of susceptibility-weighted imaging in acute hemorrhagic leukoencephalitis. J Clin Neurosci 2012;19(12):1740–1.

15. Wingerchuk DM, Banwell B, Bennett JL, et al. International consensus diagnostic criteria for neuromyelitis optica spectrum disorders. Neurology 2015; 85(2):177–89.

16. Shu Y, Long Y, Wang S, et al. Brain histopathological study and prognosis in MOG antibody-associated demyelinating pseudotumor. Ann Clin Transl Neurol 2019;6(2):392–6.

17. Starshinova AA, Malkova AM, Basantsova NY, et al. Sarcoidosis as an autoimmune disease. Front Immunol 2019;10:2933.

18. Bathla G, Singh AK, Policeni B, et al. Imaging of neurosarcoidosis: common, uncommon, and rare. Clin Radiol 2016;71(1):96–106.

19. Smith JK, Matheus MG, Castillo M. Imaging manifestations of neurosarcoidosis. AJR Am J Roentgenol 2004;182(2):289–95.

20. Kelley BP, Patel SC, Marin HL, et al. Autoimmune encephalitis: pathophysiology and imaging review of an overlooked diagnosis. AJNR Am J Neuroradiol 2017;38(6):1070–8.

21. Richards A, van den Maagdenberg AMJM, Jen JC, et al. C-terminal truncations in human 3'-5' DNA exonuclease TREX1 cause autosomal dominant retinal vasculopathy with cerebral leukodystrophy. Nat Genet 2007;39(9):1068–70.

22. Mateen FJ, Krecke K, Younge BR, et al. Evolution of a tumor-like lesion in cerebroretinal vasculopathy and TREX1 mutation. Neurology 2010;75(13): 1211–3.

23. Schwartz KM, Erickson BJ, Lucchinetti C. Pattern of T2 hypointensity associated with ring-enhancing brain lesions can help to differentiate pathology. Neuroradiology 2006;48(3):143–9.

24. Kim JE, Kim DG, Paek SH, et al. Stereotactic biopsy for intracranial lesions: reliability and its impact on the planning of treatment. Acta Neurochir (Wien) 2003;145(7):547–55.

25. Toh CH, Wei K-C, Chang C-N, et al. Differentiation of pyogenic brain abscesses from necrotic glioblastomas with use of susceptibility-weighted imaging. AJNR Am J Neuroradiol 2012;33(8):1534–8.

26. Xu X-X, Li B, Yang H-F, et al. Can diffusion-weighted imaging be used to differentiate brain abscess from other ring-enhancing brain lesions? A meta-analysis. Clin Radiol 2014;69(9):909–15.

27. Reddy JS, Mishra AM, Behari S, et al. The role of diffusion-weighted imaging in the differential diagnosis of intracranial cystic mass lesions: a report of 147 lesions. Surg Neurol 2006;66(3):246–50.

28. Kim JH, Park SP, Moon BG, et al. Brain abscess showing a lack of restricted diffusion and successfully treated with linezolid. Brain Tumor Res Treat 2018;6(2):92–6.

29. Mahadevan A, Ramalingaiah AH, Parthasarathy S, et al. Neuropathological correlate of the "concentric target sign" in MRI of HIV-associated cerebral toxoplasmosis. J Magn Reson Imaging 2013;38(2): 488–95.

30. Dibble EH, Boxerman JL, Baird GL, et al. Toxoplasmosis versus lymphoma: cerebral lesion characterization using DSC-MRI revisited. Clin Neurol Neurosurg 2017;152:84–9.

31. Floriano VH, Torres US, Spotti AR, et al. The role of dynamic susceptibility contrast-enhanced perfusion MR imaging in differentiating between infectious and neoplastic focal brain lesions: results from a cohort of 100 consecutive patients. PLoS One 2013;8(12): e81509.

32. Camacho DLA, Smith JK, Castillo M. Differentiation of toxoplasmosis and lymphoma in AIDS patients by using apparent diffusion coefficients. AJNR Am J Neuroradiol 2003;24(4):633–7.

33. Yang M, Sun J, Bai HX, et al. Diagnostic accuracy of SPECT, PET, and MRS for primary central nervous system lymphoma in HIV patients. Medicine (Baltimore) 2017;96(19):1–6.

34. Kulcsár Z, Ugron Á, Marosfoi M, et al. Hemodynamics of cerebral aneurysm initiation: the role of wall shear stress and spatial wall shear stress gradient. AJNR Am J Neuroradiol 2011;32(3):587–94.

35. Martin AJ, Hetts SW, Dillon WP, et al. MR imaging of partially thrombosed cerebral aneurysms: characteristics and evolution. AJNR Am J Neuroradiol 2011;32(2):346–51.

36. Liu JK, Gottfried ON, Amini A, et al. Aneurysms of the petrous internal carotid artery: anatomy, origins, and treatment. Neurosurg Focus 2004;17(5):1–9.

37. De Jesús O, Rifkinson N. Magnetic resonance angiography of giant aneurysms. Pitfalls and surgical implications. P R Health Sci J 1997;16(2):131–5.

38. Lev MH. Perfusion imaging of acute stroke: its role in current and future clinical practice. Radiology 2013; 266(1):22–7.

39. Mathews P, Barker PB, Chatham JC, et al. Cerebral metabolites in patients with acute and subacute strokes: by quantitative proton. AJR Am J Roentgenol 1995;165:633–8.

40. Gaskill-shipley MF. Imaging of cerebral venous thrombosis: current techniques, spectrum of findings, and diagnostic pitfalls. RadioGraphics 2006; 26(suppl_1):19–42.

41. Chang Y, Porbandarwala N, Rojas R. Unilateral nonvisualization of a transverse dural sinus on phasecontrast MRV: frequency and differentiation from sinus thrombosis on noncontrast MRI. AJNR Am J Neuroradiol 2019;41(1):115–21.

42. Brunereau L, Labauge P, Tournier-Lasserve E, et al. Familial form of intracranial cavernous angioma: MR imaging findings in 51 families. French Society of Neurosurgery. Radiology 2000;214(1):209–16.

43. Wang KY, Idowu OR, Lin DDM. Chapter 24 - Radiology and imaging for cavernous malformations. In: Spetzler RF, Moon K, Almefty RO, editors. Handbook of clinical neurology, vol. 143. The Netherlands: Elsevier; 2017. p. 249–66. https://doi.org/10.1016/B978-0-444-63640-9.00024-2.

44. Castillo M, Morrison T, Shaw JA, et al. MR imaging and histologic features of capillary telangiectasia of the basal ganglia. AJNR Am J Neuroradiol 2001; 22(8):1553–5. Available at: http://www.ajnr.org/content/22/8/1553.abstract.

45. Haacke EM, DelProposto ZS, Chaturvedi S, et al. Imaging cerebral amyloid angiopathy with susceptibility-weighted imaging. AJNR Am J Neuroradiol 2007;28(2):316–7. Available at: http://www.ajnr.org/content/28/2/316.abstract.

46. Miller-Thomas MM, Sipe AL, Benzinger TLS, et al. Multimodality review of amyloid-related diseases of the central nervous system. RadioGraphics 2016; 36(4):1147–63.

47. He T, Kaplan S, Kamboj M, et al. Laboratory diagnosis of central nervous system infection. Curr Infect Dis Rep 2016;18(11):35.

48. Colombo FA, Vidal JE, Penalva de Oliveira AC, et al. Diagnosis of cerebral toxoplasmosis in AIDS patients in Brazil: importance of molecular and immunological methods using peripheral blood samples. J Clin Microbiol 2005;43(10):5044–7.

49. Antinori A, Ammassari A, De Luca A, et al. Diagnosis of AIDS-related focal brain lesions: a decision-making analysis based on clinical and neuroradiologic characteristics combined with polymerase chain reaction assays in CSF. Neurology 1997; 48(3):687–94.

50. Anselmo LMP, Vilar FC, Lima JE, et al. Usefulness and limitations of polymerase chain reaction in the etiologic diagnosis of neurotoxoplasmosis in immunocompromised patients. J Neurol Sci 2014;346(1–2):231–4.

51. Del Brutto OH. Neurocysticercosis. Handb Clin Neurol 2014;121:1445–59.

52. Bridel C, Courvoisier DS, Vuilleumier N, et al. Cerebrospinal fluid angiotensin-converting enzyme for diagnosis of neurosarcoidosis. J Neuroimmunol 2015;285:1–3.

53. Freedman MS, Thompson EJ, Deisenhammer F, et al. Recommended standard of cerebrospinal fluid analysis in the diagnosis of multiple sclerosis: a consensus statement. Arch Neurol 2005;62(6): 865–70.

54. Altintas A, Petek B, Isik N, et al. Clinical and radiological characteristics of tumefactive demyelinating lesions: follow-up study. Mult Scler 2012;18(10): 1448–53.

55. Siri A, Carra-Dalliere C, Ayrignac X, et al. Isolated tumefactive demyelinating lesions: diagnosis and long-term evolution of 16 patients in a multicentric study. J Neurol 2015;262(7):1637–45.

Imaging of Tumor Syndromes

Prem P. Batchala, MD, Thomas J. Eluvathingal Muttikkal, MD, Sugoto Mukherjee, MD*

KEYWORDS

- Cancer syndromes • Neurofibromatosis type 1 • Neurofibromatosis type 2 • Ataxia telangiectasia
- Tuberous sclerosis complex • von Hippel-Lindau syndrome • Basal cell nevus syndrome
- Li-Fraumeni syndrome

KEY POINTS

- Cancer predisposition syndromes affecting the central nervous system represent a diverse subgroup of lesions, including intra-axial malignant brain tumors, extra-axial nerve sheath tumors, spinal cord tumors, vascular masses, pituitary tumors, and various hamartomas, with markedly different phenotypes both within and outside the neural axis.
- Advances in knowledge of the underlying genomics and cancer pathways has enhanced understanding of the tumor behavior, resulting in improved diagnostics, better imaging screening, and better surveillance strategies.
- Imaging serves a critical role in early diagnosis, screening, and long-term follow-up of these patients, requiring specialized whole-body protocols and surveillance techniques for optimal management.

INTRODUCTION

The tumor syndromes covered here include both inheritable and noninheritable cancer syndromes. These syndromes are more appropriately referred to as cancer predisposition syndromes, because of their complex cancer pathways, and how it is passed on from one generation to the next. Well-identified genetic mutations, which often characterize these syndromes, predispose to phenotypically distinct tumors throughout the body. The syndromes present a unique challenge to oncologists and radiologists owing to multiorgan involvement, aggressive nature of the tumors, and associated endocrine abnormalities. Recent genomic characterization of these syndromes has led to revision and reclassification of the established syndromes as well as development of targeted therapies.

Screening and diagnosis for these syndromes require a plethora of advanced laboratory tests, which include comprehensive genetic testing. Multimodality, multiorgan imaging plays a quintessential role in the screening, early diagnosis, surveillance, and management of these syndromes.

Whole-Body Imaging

In addition to targeted organ-specific protocols, dedicated whole-body imaging is becoming an indispensable tool in evaluating cancer syndromes. Occasionally, whole-body imaging refers to a combination of different modalities including ultrasonography (US), computed tomography (CT), and magnetic resonance (MR) imaging, done separately. Another emerging approach is single-modality whole-body scanning to evaluate local multiorgan tumors as well as distant metastatic disease. In this scenario, whole-body MR imaging has taken precedence over whole-body CT or PET/CT, because of lack of ionizing radiation (given that many of these patients are in the

Department of Radiology and Medical Imaging, University of Virginia Health System, 1215 Lee Street, Charlottesville, VA 22903, USA
* Corresponding author. PO Box 800170, 1215 Lee Street, Charlottesville, VA 22908-0170.
E-mail address: SM5QD@hscmail.mcc.virginia.edu

Radiol Clin N Am 59 (2021) 471–500
https://doi.org/10.1016/j.rcl.2021.01.009

pediatric age group and need repeated follow-up scans), excellent soft tissue contrast, and bone marrow evaluation.[1] Single-modality imaging also has the advantage of 1-time sedation or general anesthesia when required.

MR imaging has limitations, which include cost, decreased specificity, artifacts related to patient hardware and motion, repeated gadolinium dosage and accumulation, as well as technical issues with older scanners. However, recent advances have allowed many of the limitations to be overcome, which include rolling table platforms, multiple phased array coils, parallel imaging techniques, and wider field of view (FOV). These advances have led to improvement in resolution, decreased artifacts and scan time, with reduction in the need for repeated gadolinium administration. The principles of whole-body MR scans include using series of images at multiple stations (targeting specific body parts based on the FOV and patient size), in multiple planes (usually axial and coronal planes with sagittal plane used for spine), while using a combination of sequences tailored for specific disorders. The stations include combinations such as the chest-abdomen-pelvis station, neck-chest-abdomen-pelvis station, or brain–head and neck–spine station. Typically a combination of diffusion and fluid-sensitive sequences are used, with respiratory gating for chest and antiperistaltic drugs for abdomen. Use of gadolinium is reserved for specific syndromes and clinical situations.

CANCER PREDISPOSITION SYNDROMES
Neurofibromatosis

Neurofibromatosis is a group of hereditary syndromes with tumors involving the central and peripheral nervous systems, including neurofibromatosis type 1 (NF1), neurofibromatosis type 2 (NF2), and schwannomatosis.

Neurofibromatosis Type 1

NF1, also known as peripheral neurofibromatosis and von Recklinghausen disease, is an autosomal dominant (AD) syndrome, with high penetrance and variable expressivity, with an incidence of 1 in 3000. The mutation affects the neurofibromin tumor suppressor gene located in the long arm of chromosome 17 (17q11.2). About half are inherited and the rest result from sporadic mutations. The segmental form with a limited distribution of lesions can be seen with mosaicism.[2,3] Familial spinal neurofibromatosis is a rare form, with neurofibromas affecting nerve roots bilaterally at all spinal levels, with most patients lacking the cutaneous and ocular lesions of NF.[4] The diagnostic criteria for NF1 are summarized in **Box 1**.

Neurofibromas

Neurofibromas, which are nerve sheath tumors, are the most common tumors in NF1, and can involve both superficial and deep soft tissues, including the nerve roots in the spinal canal and neural foramen. Morphologic subtypes include localized neurofibroma, plexiform neurofibroma (PNF), and diffuse neurofibroma.[5]

Localized cutaneous neurofibroma is the most common form, presenting as nodular or polypoid lesion often with epidermal hyperpigmentation. Localized intraneural neurofibroma causes fusiform enlargement of the affected nerve.[5] The lesions appear hypodense with minimal enhancement in CT scans, well defined and hyperintense on T2-weighted imaging (T2WI), with intermediate to low signal intensity on T1-weighted imaging (T1WI), with homogeneous, slightly heterogeneous, or central enhancement (**Figs. 1 and 2**). The lesions may show target sign with low central signal with peripheral high signal in T2WI (see **Fig. 2**), and a central dense area on CT. Target sign can sometimes also be seen with schwannoma and malignant peripheral nerve tumors. Neurofibroma is challenging to differentiate from schwannoma by imaging. T2 hyperintense rim and intratumoral cysts are more common with schwannoma than with neurofibroma.[3,6]

PNF is virtually pathognomonic of NF1, and appears as lobulated, tortuous thickening of nerves with a bag-of-worms appearance (**Fig. 3**). The lesion appears as an infiltrative multispatial soft tissue density lesion in CT (**Fig. 4**). Target sign is commonly seen (see **Fig. 4**). The lesion has intermediate signal intensity in T1-weighted images, with central dotlike or diffuse heterogeneous enhancement (see **Figs. 3 and 4**).[3,5]

Box 1
National Institutes of Health Consensus criteria for neurofibromatosis type 1 diagnosis

Diagnostic criteria of NF1: 2 or more of the following criteria should be met:

1. At least 6 café-au-lait macules (diameter>5 mm in prepubertal individuals and >15 mm in postpubertal individuals)

2. Freckling in axillary or inguinal regions

3. Optic glioma

4. At least 2 Lisch nodules (iris hamartomas)

5. At least 2 neurofibromas of any type, or 1 plexiform neurofibroma

6. A distinctive osseous lesion (sphenoid dysplasia or tibial pseudarthrosis)

7. A first-degree relative with NF1

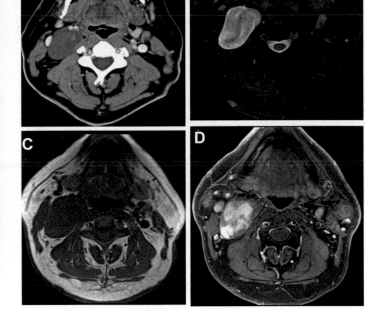

Fig. 1. Sympathetic trunk neurofibroma in a 47-year-old male patient with NF1. (A) Contrast-enhanced CT shows a well-defined low-density mass in the right carotid space with minimal enhancement. (B, C) On axial fat-suppressed T2WI and T1WI, the mass is hyperintense and isointense compared with muscle. (D) Contrast-enhanced fat-suppressed axial T1WI shows heterogeneous enhancement in the mass.

Diffuse neurofibromas most commonly occur in children and young adults as plaquelike or infiltrative, poorly defined, reticulated lesions in skin and subcutaneous fat.[3]

Malignant peripheral nerve sheath tumor
Malignant peripheral nerve sheath tumors (MPNSTs) usually arise from plexiform neurofibromas, and less commonly from localized neurofibromas. Malignant transformation of neurofibroma is often associated with rapid growth and worsening pain. Infiltrative margin, heterogeneous enhancement with necrotic areas, peripheral edema, and osseous destruction are features suggestive of malignant transformation (**Fig. 5**). MPNST shows high ^{18}F-fluorodeoxyglucose

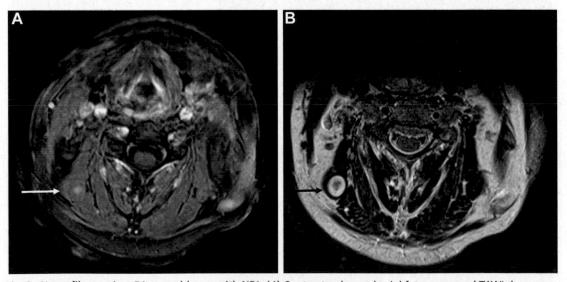

Fig. 2. Neurofibroma in a 54-year-old man with NF1. (A) Contrast-enhanced axial fat-suppressed T1WI shows central enhancement in an intramuscular neurofibroma (*white arrow*). (B) Axial T2WI shows target sign with central T2 hypointensity (*black arrow*).

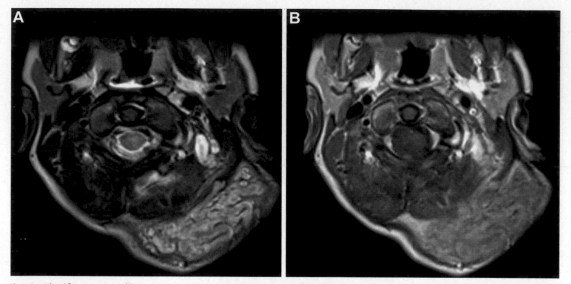

Fig. 3. Plexiform neurofibroma in a 12-year-old female patient with NF1. (*A*) Axial T2WI shows bag-of-worms appearance in the left suboccipital region. (*B*) Contrast-enhanced axial T1-weighted image shows diffuse heterogeneous enhancement.

(FDG) uptake on PET scans. About half of the MPNSTs occur in patients with NF1, and about 5% of patients with NF1 develop MPNST.[2,3]

Optic pathway gliomas

NF1-associated optic pathway glioma (OPG) typically presents in young children. OPGs usually are low-grade pilocytic astrocytomas.[2] Less than half of the cases are symptomatic. OPG in patients with NF1 commonly involves the optic nerve, followed by the chiasm, unlike OPG in patients without NF1. Hypothalamic involvement can present with premature or delayed puberty.[7]

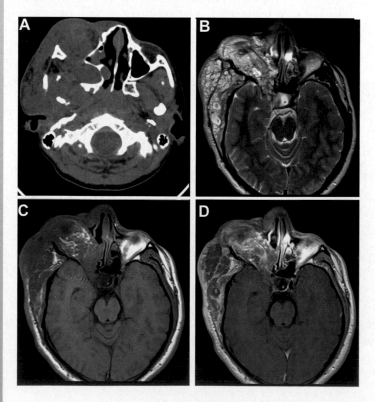

Fig. 4. Plexiform neurofibroma in a 17-year-old male patient with NF1. (*A*) Axial CT scan shows an infiltrative multispatial soft tissue density mass in right side of the face and temporal fossa. (*B*) Axial T2WI shows multiple target sign within the plexiform neurofibroma. (*C*) Axial T1WI and (*D*) postcontrast T1WI show intermediate signal lesion with heterogeneous enhancement.

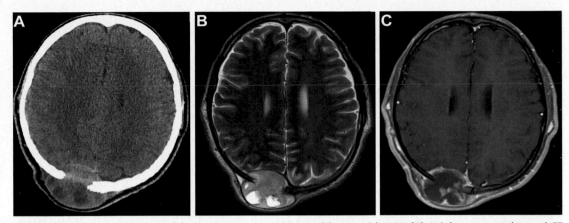

Fig. 5. Rapidly growing right parietal scalp mass in a 28-year-old man with NF1. (*A*) Axial contrast-enhanced CT, (*B*) axial T2WI, and (*C*) postcontrast T1WI show heterogeneously enhancing mass with cysts and necrosis. There is also calvarial destruction by the mass.

OPG appears as fusiform enlargement of the nerve that is isodense to slightly hypodense on CT scans. The optic canal may appear enlarged. Calcification is rare, which helps to differentiate OPG from optic sheath meningioma. OPG appears hyperintense on T2WI, and shows variable contrast enhancement (**Fig. 6**). Cysts are uncommon in OPG associated with NF1.[7,8]

Other central nervous system and extra–central nervous system tumors

Brainstem gliomas are the second most common intracranial tumors in NF1 (**Fig. 7**), frequently pilocytic astrocytomas with few transforming into aggressive gliomas (**Figs. 8 and 9**). There is increased risk of rhabdomyosarcomas, gastrointestinal stromal tumors, endocrine tumors of gastrointestinal tract, pheochromocytomas, breast cancer, and hematopoietic malignancies.[2]

Other neuroimaging findings

An unusual but characteristic imaging finding, known as focal abnormal signal intensity (FASI), can be seen in basal ganglia, thalamus, pons, midbrain, cerebellar peduncles, cerebellar white matter, dentate nuclei, and less commonly supratentorial white matter, likely from myelin vacuolization (**Fig. 10**). These findings are usually hyperintense on T2WI, isointense on T1WI, with a few appearing mildly hyperintense on T1 in basal

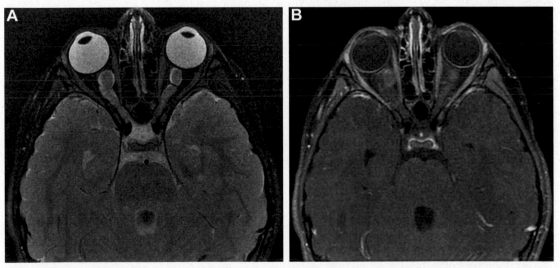

Fig. 6. Bilateral optic glioma in a 5-year-old female patient with NF1. (*A*) Axial fat-suppressed T2WI shows fusiform enlargement of bilateral optic nerves. (*B*) Contrast-enhanced axial fat-suppressed T1WI showing mild enhancement of enlarged optic nerves.

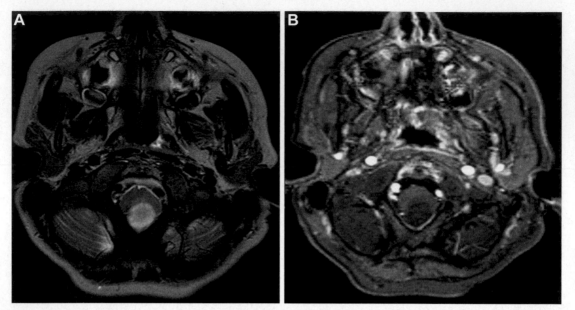

Fig. 7. Exophytic brainstem glioma in an 8-year-old boy with NF1. (*A*) Axial T2WI shows a well-defined hyperintense exophytic dorsal brainstem. (*B*) Contrast-enhanced magnetization prepared rapid gradient echo (MPRAGE) T1WI shows no enhancement in the mass.

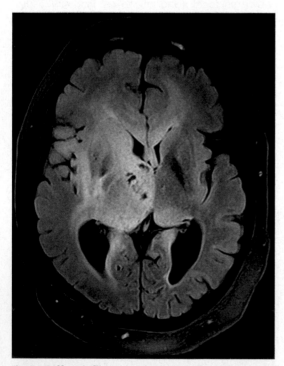

Fig. 8. Diffuse infiltrative astrocytoma in a 21-year-old man with NF1. Axial fluid-attenuated inversion recovery (FLAIR) image shows a diffuse infiltrative tumor involving the right basal ganglia, right thalamus, left thalamic pulvinar, right insular cortex, corpus callosum, and periventricular white matter.

ganglia, likely because of microcalcifications. Although they typically have no associated mass effect or enhancement, rarely they show mild mass effect in basal ganglia. FASI can become bigger in early childhood before they regress.[9,10] Cerebrovascular dysplasia including stenosis, hypoplasia, moyamoya pattern (**Fig. 11**), and aneurysms can occur.[11]

Neurofibromatosis Type 2

Just like NF1, NF2 is also an AD genetic syndrome, with high penetrance and variable expressivity. However, it is rarer, with an incidence of 1 in 25,000. NF2 results from a mutation of the NF2 gene, which codes for the cytoskeletal protein schwannomin (merlin) located on chromosome 22 (22q12.2), which acts as a tumor suppressor protein. About half of the cases have de novo mutation, with somatic mosaicism in about one-third of these cases.[2]

The diagnostic criteria for NF2 are summarized in **Box 2**. The 1987 National Institute of Health (NIH) criteria were modified to include patients with multiple schwannomas and or meningiomas with no family history and who have not yet developed bilateral eighth nerve tumors. These criteria include the Manchester criteria, National Neurofibromatosis Foundation (NNFF) criteria, and Baser criteria[12] (**Box 3**). Young patients (<18 years old) with apparently isolated meningioma or vestibular schwannoma have a 20% and 10% likelihood,

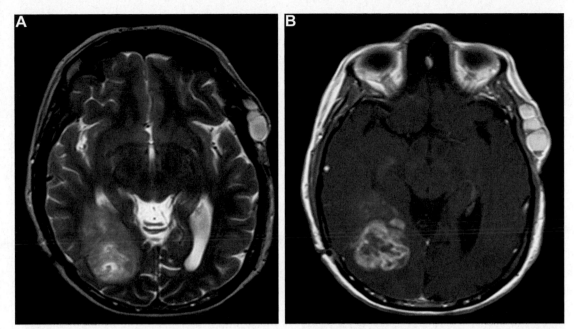

Fig. 9. High-grade glial tumor in a 42-year-old woman with NF1. (*A*) Axial T2WI and (*B*) postcontrast T1WI show a heterogeneously enhancing right posterior temporo-occipital lobe tumor.

respectively, of developing NF2. After 20 years, likelihood decreases, and NF2 becomes very unlikely after 30 years.[13] In contrast, 50% of patients more than 70 years of age with bilateral vestibular schwannoma without other features of NF2 represent a chance occurrence rather than underlying mosaic or constitutional NF2 mutation.[14]

Schwannomas

In addition to bilateral vestibular schwannomas (**Fig. 12**A, B) usually occurring by 30 years of age in about 90% to 95% of patients, schwannomas of other cranial nerves are present in up to about half of the patients (**Fig. 12**C). Unilateral hearing loss and tinnitus are the presenting symptoms in

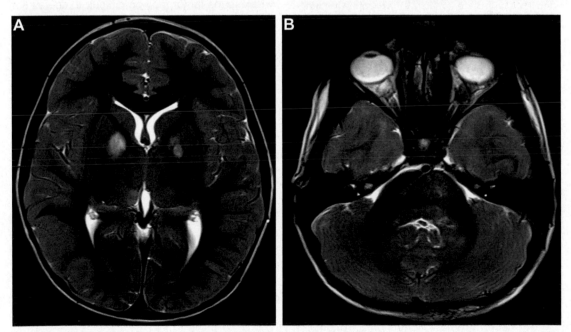

Fig. 10. FASI in a 7-year-old boy with NF1. Axial T2WI at the level of (*A*) basal ganglia and (*B*) pons show hyperintense foci in bilateral globus pallidi, dorsomedial thalami, pons, cerebellar peduncles, cerebellar white matter, and dentate nuclei.

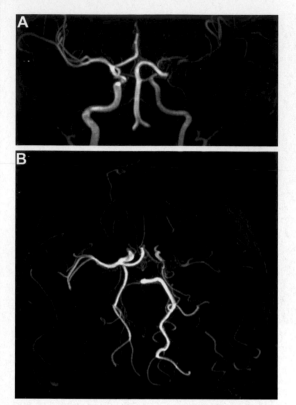

Fig. 11. Moyamoya pattern in a 9-year-old girl with NF1. (*A*) Coronal and (*B*) axial maximum intensity projections of three-dimensional (3D) time-of-flight MR angiography (MRA) head show occlusion of left intracranial internal carotid artery with prominent left sided lenticulostriate collaterals (moyamoya or puff-of-smoke pattern).

more than half of the adults and about a quarter of the children.[15] Schwannomas can also affect spinal (**Fig. 13**) and peripheral nerves. Vestibular schwannomas appear as enhancing masses that are ovoid when small, and ice cream cone–shaped when large enough to extend in to the cerebellopontine angle from the internal auditory canal (IAC). These lesions show up as filling defects

---

Box 2
National Institutes of Health criteria for neurofibromatosis type 2 diagnosis

A patient who meets either condition A or B has NF2.

A. Bilateral vestibular schwannomas

B. First-degree family relative with NF2 and unilateral vestibular schwannoma or any 2 of neurofibroma, meningioma, glioma, schwannoma, or juvenile posterior subcapsular lenticular opacity

---

Box 3
Revised Manchester criteria for neurofibromatosis type 2

A patient who meets any 1 of the following criteria has NF2:

1. Bilateral vestibular schwannomas if less than 70 years of age.

2. First-degree relative with family history of NF2 (excluding siblings with clearly unaffected parents) and unilateral vestibular schwannoma if less than 70 years of age.

3. First-degree relative with family history of NF2 or unilateral vestibular schwannoma and 2 of the following lesions: meningioma, ependymoma, schwannoma, cataract, cerebral calcification. LZTR1 (leucine-zipperlike transcription regulator 1) test has to be negative, if unilateral vestibular schwannoma plus ≥ 2 nonintradermal schwannomas.

4. Multiple meningiomas (2 or more) and 2 of unilateral vestibular schwannoma, schwannoma, cataract, cerebral calcification.

5. Constitutional pathogenic NF2 gene variant in blood or identical in 2 tumors.

---

within the cerebrospinal fluid (CSF) on high-resolution heavily T2-weighted sequences (see **Fig. 12**). CT scan shows widening of the IAC, whereas the tumor may be difficult to see on soft tissue windows.

Meningiomas
Intracranial meningiomas are present in about half of the patients, and spinal meningiomas are present in about 20%. Although many of these lesions remain asymptomatic, larger lesions, as well as smaller lesions within the spinal canal, optic canal, or skull base, can be symptomatic.[15] They appear as extra-axial masses, usually with intense contrast enhancement (see **Fig. 12**; **Fig. 14**), similar to sporadic meningiomas.

Ependymomas
Ependymomas are present in up to about half of patients, mostly within the upper cervical canal or at the craniocervical junction. On imaging, these look similar to their sporadic counterparts, including showing hemosiderin cap and homogeneous enhancement (see **Fig. 14**).[15]

Other central nervous system tumors
Intramedullary astrocytomas and schwannomas of the spinal cord and meningioangiomatosis have also been reported in NF2.[15,16]

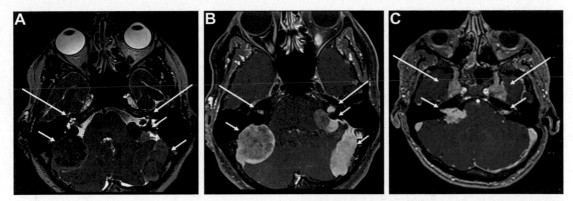

Fig. 12. NF2. (*A*) Axial high resolution heavily weighted T2 and (*B*) contrast-enhanced fat-suppressed axial T1WI at the level of internal auditory canals in a 60-year-old man with NF2 show T2-hypointense enhancing bilateral vestibular schwannomas (*long arrows*) and multiple posterior fossa meningiomas (*short arrows*). The low T2 signal in the meningiomas reflects calcification. (*C*) Contrast-enhanced axial MPRAGE image in a 42-year-old woman with NF2 shows bilateral vestibular (*short arrows*) and trigeminal schwannomas (*long arrows*).

Schwannomatosis

Schwannomatosis is the third major form of neurofibromatosis, with an incidence of 1 in 60,000 to 70,000, characterized by multiple schwannomas without evidence of bilateral vestibular schwannomas. Inheritance is AD, with a sporadic predominance. The tumor suppressor genes identified are SMARCB1 (SWI/SNF-Related Matrix-associated Actin-dependent Regulator of Chromatin Subfamily B Member 1) and *LZTR1* (leucine-zipperlike transcription regulator 1), located in the long arm of chromosome 22.[17] The diagnostic criteria for schwannomatosis are summarized in **Box 4**.[17] The overlap in presentation and phenotype of schwannomatosis and NF2 makes the clinical differentiation difficult. On imaging, the schwannomas look identical to those in NF2. Spinal ependymomas are not present in schwannomatosis, which helps in differentiating from NF2.

von Hippel-Lindau Syndrome

von Hippel-Lindau (VHL) is an AD syndrome arising from mutations in the VHL tumor suppressor gene located in chromosome 3 (3p25-26). The mutation causes overexpression of hypoxia-inducible messenger RNAs, including vascular endothelial growth factor, which results in angiogenesis, and proliferation of endothelial cells and pericytes that are characteristic of VHL-related tumors. Hemangioblastoma (HB) and endolymphatic sac tumor (ELST) are the most common central nervous system (CNS) tumors in VHL, with rare reports of choroid plexus papilloma. The average age of presentation of VHL-related tumors is the third to fourth decade.[18] Tumor combinations in VHL often overlap with other syndromes, such as NF1 and multiple endocrine neoplasia (MEN) and pose a diagnostic challenge.[18] The recommended diagnostic criteria by the Danish VHL coordination group are summarized in **Box 5**.[18] The recommended NIH screening guidelines for VHL tumors are summarized in **Table 1**.[19]

Central nervous system hemangioblastoma

CNS hemangioblastomas (HBs) are World Health Organization (WHO) grade I tumors that present at a younger age in VHL compared with their sporadic counterparts. Their frequency varies along the craniospinal axis, with cerebellar being most common (44%–72%), followed by brainstem (10%–25%), spinal cord (13%–50%), cauda equina (<1%), and supratentorial compartment (<1%).[20] HBs vary in size at the time of presentation. Early symptomatic HBs tend to have larger cystic components and often present with headache, cerebellar signs, cranial nerve palsies, or cord compression. Wanebo and colleagues[21] in their series of 160 patients reported more frequent association of cysts in symptomatic cerebellar HB than in asymptomatic cases (72% vs 13%, *P*<.0001). In close to 80% of VHL cases, HBs are multifocal.[21]

HBs are best evaluated by MR imaging and present as cyst with a mural nodule (most common type) or a solid nodule without or with internal cystic change (**Fig. 15A**).[22,23] Pure cystic morphology is very rare. The nodule shows intense postcontrast enhancement with characteristic superficial or pial location, and predilection to the posterior aspects of cerebellum, brainstem, and spinal cord. The nodule is isointense to

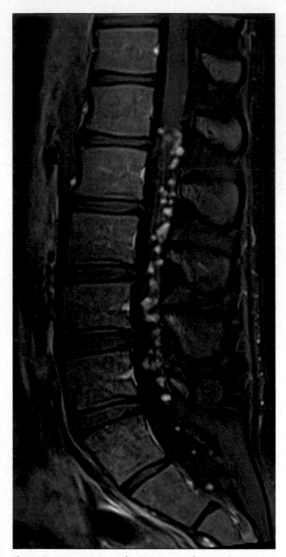

Fig. 13. Numerous enhancing cauda equina nerve root schwannomas seen in this sagittal fat-suppressed postcontrast T1WI of the lumbar spine in a 21-year-old man with NF2.

hypointense on T1WI and hyperintense on T2WI. The cystic component is usually hyperintense to CSF on T1WI and fluid-attenuated inversion recovery (FLAIR). Vasogenic edema may be seen around the HB (**Fig. 15**B). Flow voids or prominent vessels around the HB indicates its vascular nature (**Fig. 16**). Catheter angiography is not required for the diagnosis and can also display intense prolonged contrast staining of the nodules with arteriovenous shunting (**Fig. 15**C). Spinal cord HBs also show similar imaging features. In addition, a syrinx may be seen.[23] In patients with VHL, renal cell carcinoma (RCC) CNS metastasis should always be considered in the differential diagnosis.

RCC metastasis can mimic HB on histopathology and also on imaging.

Retinal hemangioblastomas
Retinal HBs are seen in 52% to 84% of VHL cases and can be the only presentation in as many as 11%.[18,20,24,25] In 50%, they are multifocal and bilateral. Most are asymptomatic with a limited role for imaging. If seen on MR imaging, HBs are mildly hyperintense on T1WI relative to vitreous with intense postcontrast enhancement (**Fig. 17**).

Endolymphatic sac tumor
ELST is seen in 11% of VHL cases, and the average age of presentation is 22 years.[20] It is a locally aggressive, slow-growing neoplasm arising from endolymphatic sac housed in the posterior aspect of the petrous bone and has low metastatic potential. Akin to vestibular schwannoma in NF2, bilateral ELST is pathognomonic of VHL. Bilateral tumors are seen in 30% of patients with VHL.[26] The presenting symptoms vary between hearing loss, tinnitus, imbalance, and facial nerve palsy.

Contrast-enhanced MR imaging and/or CT are typically used for diagnosing ELST. Small lesions may not be readily apparent on CT (**Fig. 18**). Larger lesions typically show a moth-eaten type of osteolysis with spiculated tumor matrix calcification.[23] Intense enhancement can be seen in the soft tissue component. On MR imaging, the soft tissue shows heterogeneous signal, mildly hyperintense on T1WI (because of hemorrhage) and hyperintense on T2WI and FLAIR sequences. Stippled or paint-brush pattern of enhancement has also been described on MR imaging[27] (**Fig. 19**). In the setting of VHL, it is important to remember that paraganglioma or metastatic carcinoma can also appear similar on imaging.

Tuberous Sclerosis

Tuberous sclerosis (TS) is an AD syndrome linked to mutations in TS complex (TSC) 1 and TSC2 genes in chromosomes 9q34 and 16p13.3 respectively.[28] TSC1 and TSC2 genes code for hamartin and tuberin proteins respectively, which together form a heterodimer that inhibits mammalian target of rapamycin (mTOR) pathway. Mutations activate the mTOR pathway, which causes unregulated cellular growth and formation of CNS and extra-CNS hamartomas. The classic TS clinical triad is epilepsy, mental retardation, and facial angiofibromas. Other CNS-related symptoms include cognitive dysfunction, neuropsychiatric abnormalities, or increased intracranial pressure caused by obstructive hydrocephalus from subependymal giant cell astrocytoma (SGCA). The diagnostic criteria recommended by the 2012 International

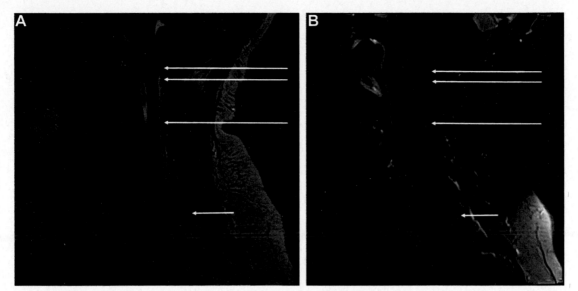

Fig. 14. Spinal ependymoma and meningioma in a 32-year-old patient with NF2. (*A*) Sagittal T2WI and (*B*) fat-suppressed postcontrast T1WI show intramedullary T2-hyperintense enhancing ependymomas (*long arrows*) and extramedullary intradural T2 intermediate signal enhancing meningiomas (*short arrow*).

Tuberous Sclerosis Complex Consensus Group are summarized in **Table 2**.[29] CNS manifestations of TS include cortical/subcortical tubers, radial migration lines, subependymal nodules (SENs), and SGCA, and each constitutes a major feature in the diagnostic criteria.

Cortical/subcortical tubers, radial migration lines

Tubers are hamartomas that arise from abnormal neuronal migration, differentiation, and organization and are seen in 95% of patients with TS.[30] Tubers are cortical/subcortical in location with supratentorial and frontal lobe predominance. Cerebellar tubers have been reported in 12% to 30% of cases.[30,31] Number and size of the tubers vary in individual patients. Tubers typically expand the affected gyri with mushroomlike or wartlike protrusions.

Imaging appearance and conspicuity of tubers are partly influenced by the degree of myelination.

Box 4
Diagnostic criteria for schwannomatosis

A patient should meet the following criteria for a diagnosis of schwannomatosis:

1. Anatomically distinct 2 nonintradermal schwannomas, 1 of which has to be histologically confirmed.

2. No evidence of bilateral vestibular schwannomas on imaging or NF2 mutation.

3. Presence of 1 pathologically confirmed schwannoma, unilateral vestibular schwannoma, or intracranial meningioma and schwannomatosis in a first-degree relative.

Box 5
Danish diagnostic criteria for von Hippel-Lindau

VHL diagnostic criteria: positive if individual satisfies criteria 1 or 2 or both

Criterion 1	At least 2 manifestations stated below
Criterion 2	At least 1 manifestation stated below plus pathogenic mutation of VHL (or) at least 1 first-degree relative with VHL

VHL manifestations that satisfy criteria

Retina	Hemangioblastoma
CNS	Hemangioblastoma of cerebellum, medulla oblongata, and/or spinal cord
Temporal bone	Endolymphatic sac tumor
Kidney	Renal cell carcinoma
Pancreas	Neuroendocrine tumor and/or multiple cysts
Adrenal gland/ sympathetic chain	Pheochromocytoma, paraganglioma, and/or glomus tumor

Table 1
Screening recommendations for central nervous system tumors of von Hippel-Lindau

Tumor	Screening Recommendation
CNS hemangioblastoma	MR imaging of brain and spine every 2 y starting from 11 y of age
Retinal hemangioblastoma	Annual ophthalmoscopy starting from infancy
Endolymphatic sac tumor	Annual audiometry starting from 5 y of age and, if abnormal, dedicated temporal bone MR imaging/CT

In general, the thickened peripheral cortex is isointense to gray matter on T1WI and T2WI. The inner core of the tuber is hypointense on T1WI and hyperintense on T2WI/FLAIR, and sometimes appears cystic[32](**Fig. 20**A, B). In infants less than 6 months old, because of the lack of myelination, the tuber can appear hyperintense on T1WI and hypointense on T2WI. Postcontrast enhancement is a rare feature seen in less than 5% of tubers.[30] Tubers show facilitated diffusion, and the ones with higher apparent diffusion coefficient (ADC) values can be epileptogenic. On CT, the subcortical components of the tubers are seen as hypodense areas, which can become isodense over

time. Altman and colleagues[33] reported tuber calcifications in 54% of cases on CT.

Cerebellar tubers differ from supratentorial lesions in their imaging appearance.[31] The lesions appear dystrophic rather than dysplastic, and show wedge-shaped morphology like infarcts. Folial retraction can be present, and calcifications and enhancement are more frequent (**Fig. 21**). Cerebellar lesions have been linked to TSC2 mutations. Cerebellar lesions are most frequent in the posterior lobe.

Radial migration lines are wedge-shaped, straight, or curvilinear lines extending from periventricular white matter toward the cortex, often toward the tuber like a comet tail (**Fig. 20**C). These lines represent heterotopic glial and neuronal cells along the migratory pathway. On MR imaging, the lines are isointense to hypointense on T1WI and hyperintense on T2WI/FLAIR.

Subependymal nodules and subependymal giant cell astrocytoma

SENs are also hamartomas, located along the ependyma, and are seen in 95% of patients with TS.[30] There is a strong predilection to caudate nucleus and caudothalamic groove, but they can be found at other locations, including the third and fourth ventricles. SENs measure 1 to 12 mm and show no growth in longitudinal studies. On MR, SENs appear mildly hyperintense on T1WI and isointense to hyperintense on T2WI/FLAIR sequences. Calcification is seen in 88% as low signal on susceptibility-weighted imaging (SWI). Enhancement is present in 30% to 80% and is not a sign for transformation into SGCA (**Fig. 22**).

SENs larger than 13 mm or that continue to grow are considered as imaging criteria for

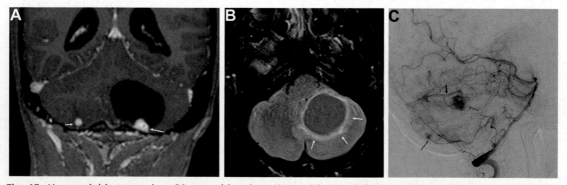

Fig. 15. Hemangioblastomas in a 20-year-old male patient with VHL. (*A*) Postcontrast T1WI showing cerebellar HBs. Cyst with a mural nodule morphology in left cerebellum (*long arrow*) and solid morphology in right cerebellum (*short arrow*). Nodules show intense postcontrast enhancement with superficial/pial location. (*B*) Vasogenic edema around the nontumor cystic component of the left cerebellar HB (*arrows*). (*C*) Catheter angiography after vertebral artery injection shows cerebellar HBs (*red arrows*) as focal intense staining with venous shunting (*black arrow*).

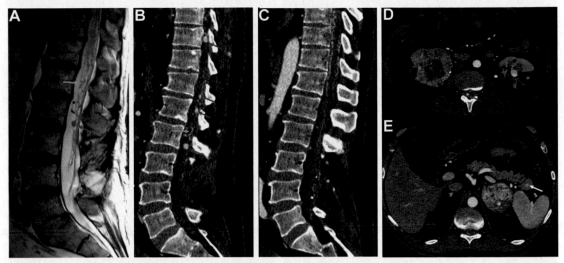

Fig. 16. A 55-year-old man with a known diagnosis of VHL. (*A*) Sagittal T2WI. (*B, C*) Sagittal reformations of post-contrast abdominal CT show multiple HBs (*red arrows*) along the conus and cauda equine roots. Flow voids on T2WI (*blue arrows*) and corresponding enhancing tortuous vessels on CT are also present. (*D, E*) Axial postcontrast abdomen CT show multiple renal cysts (*blue asterisk*), right renal cell carcinoma (*red asterisk*), left pheochromo-cytoma (*yellow asterisk*), and pancreatic tail neuroendocrine tumor (*white arrow*).

SGCA. SGCA is the most common CNS tumor (WHO grade I) in patients with TS, seen in 10% to 15%.[34] SGCAs are most commonly detected during early childhood (5–10 years), and are presumed to arise from a preexisting SEN.[35] They are typically found along the lateral ventricular wall, near the foramen of Monro, can be unilateral or bilateral, and can cause obstructive hydrocephalus. SGCAs show heterogeneous signal on MR. They are predominantly hypointense to white matter on T1WI and hyperintense on T2WI (**Fig. 23**).[35] Flow voids can be seen in the tumor with bright postcontrast enhancement indicating vascularity. Rarely, intraventricular hemorrhage arises from SGCA.[36] Sener[37] reported ADC values in SGCA to be similar to normal white matter (0.89×10^{-3} mm^2/s). Like other brain neoplasms, SGCA can show high choline/creatine ratio and low N-acetyl aspartate (NAA)/creatine ratio on MR spectroscopy (**Fig. 24**).[38] Symptomatic SGCAs are managed by surgical resection. mTOR pathway inhibitors (eg, everolimus) are used in nonsurgical candidates.

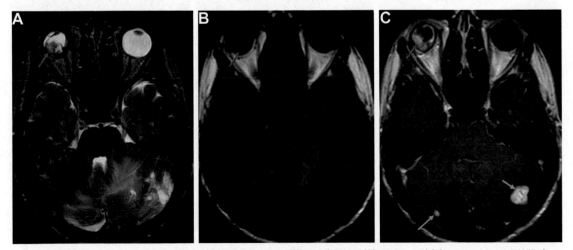

Fig. 17. A 39-year-old man with VHL and blind right eye. (*A*) Axial T2WI, (*B*) T1WI, and (*C*) postcontrast T1WI show retinal HB in right globe (*red arrow*). The mass shows T1 shortening and intense postcontrast enhancement. Cerebellar HBs are also seen (*blue arrows*), consistent with VHL.

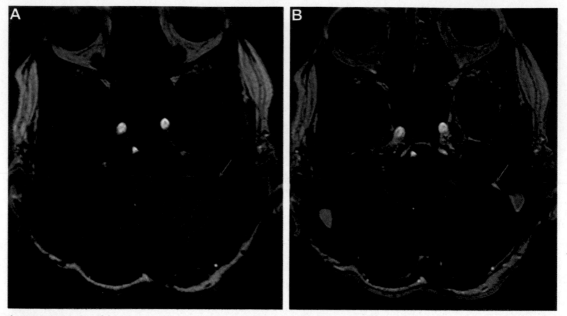

Fig. 18. A 69-year-old woman with VHL. (*A*) Axial T1WI and (*B*) postcontrast T1WI show focal enhancement in left endolymphatic sac compatible with early endolymphatic sac tumor (*red arrows*).

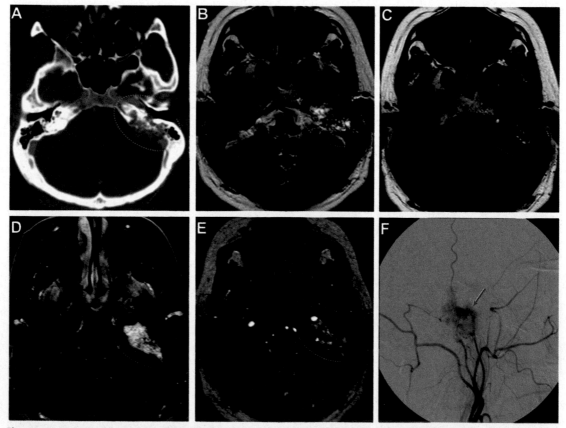

Fig. 19. A 59-year-old woman with endolymphatic sac tumor (*dotted ellipse*) in left temporal bone. (*A*) Axial CT shows moth-eaten type of osteolysis. (*B*) Axial T2WI, (*C*)T1WI, and (*D*) postcontrast T1WI show left temporal bone mass with areas of T1 shortening and intense postcontrast enhancement. (*E*) Axial 3D time-of-flight MRA and (*F*) catheter angiography (left external carotid artery injection) show tumor vascularity (*red arrow*).

Table 2
2012 International Tuberous Sclerosis Complex Consensus Conference diagnostic criteria

1. Genetic diagnostic criteria
   Identification of either TSC1 or TSC2 pathogenic mutation in DNA from normal tissue is sufficient to make a definite diagnosis of TSC. A pathogenic mutation is defined as a mutation that clearly inactivates the function of the TSC1 or TSC2 proteins. Note: 10%–25% of patients with TSC have no mutation identified by conventional genetic testing, and a normal result does not exclude TSC or have any effect on the use of clinical diagnostic criteria to diagnose TSC
2. Clinical diagnostic criteria
   Definitive diagnosis: 2 major features or 1 major plus ≥2 minor features
   Possible diagnosis: 1 major feature or ≥2 minor features

Major feature	Cutaneous
	• Hypomelanotic macules: ≥3 of at least 5 mm diameter
	• Angiofibromas (≥3) or fibrous cephalic plaque
	• Ungual fibromas (≥2)
	• Shagreen patch
	Retinal
	• Multiple retinal hamartomas
	CNS
	• Cortical tubers or radial migration lines
	• Subependymal nodules
	• SGCA
	Chest
	• Cardiac rhabdomyoma
	• Lymphangioleiomyomatosis
	Renal
	• Angiomyolipomas (≥2)
Minor feature	Cutaneous
	• Confetti skin lesions
	Orodental
	• Dental enamel pits (>3)
	• Intraoral fibromas (≥2)
	Retinal
	• Retinal achromic patch
	Renal
	• Multiple renal cysts
	• Nonrenal hamartomas

Ataxia Telangiectasia

Ataxia telangiectasia (AT) is an autosomal recessive condition resulting from a mutation in the *ATM* gene in chromosome 11q22-23. The gene product is involved in DNA repair and apoptosis.

Affected individuals present with cerebellar ataxia, immunodeficiency, repeated sinopulmonary infections, increased alpha-fetoprotein level, and telangiectasias in eye and brain. AT is also characterized by radiosensitivity. Lymphoreticular cancers are the most common malignancies in AT. CNS tumors reported in AT are glioma, pilocytic astrocytoma, medulloblastoma, and meningiomas.[19] The imaging features of these tumors are similar to those outside of AT.

Cerebellar volume loss is the hallmark of AT (**Fig. 25**). In particular, superior vermis and lateral cerebellum show the earliest changes.[39] The other reported neuroimaging features are punctate susceptibility low signal foci in the cerebral white matter resulting from microbleeds and capillary telangiectasia, enhancement related to capillary telangiectasias, and white matter FLAIR hyperintense signal changes possibly related to gliosis.[39–42]

Basal Cell Nevus Syndrome (Gorlin Syndrome)

Basal cell nevus syndrome (BCNS) is an AD disorder characterized by mutation in the *PTCH1* tumor suppressor gene in chromosome 9q22.3-31. Multiple basal cell carcinomas (particularly in adolescence) and multiple odontogenic keratocysts (OKCs) are the hallmarks of this syndrome.

Medulloblastoma (MB), especially the desmoplastic subtype, is the most common CNS malignancy reported in BCNS.[43] Imaging findings are similar to the sporadic medulloblastoma tumors. Other reported CNS tumors include oligodendroglioma and craniopharyngioma.[19,43] Meningiomas have also been reported in BCNS, with many of them possibly secondary to cranial radiation. Important neuroimaging clues that point toward Gorlin syndrome are dural calcifications (bilamellar calcifications involving falx and tentorium), OKC in the jaw bones, mandibular coronoid process hyperplasia, scoliosis, frontal bossing, hypertelorism, and cleft lip/palate abnormalities (**Fig. 26**).[19,43,44] The diagnostic criteria recommended by the international colloquium on BCNS is laid out in **Table 3**.[45] The recommendation for neuroimaging surveillance in BCNS is summarized in **Table 4**. Of course, whole-spine imaging should be done in patients with evidence of MB.

Gastrointestinal Polyposis-Related Tumor Syndromes

Cowden syndrome

Cowden syndrome, a phosphatase and tensin homolog (PTEN) hamartoma tumor syndrome, is a group of disorders caused by a mutation in the PTEN gene, located on chromosome 10q23.

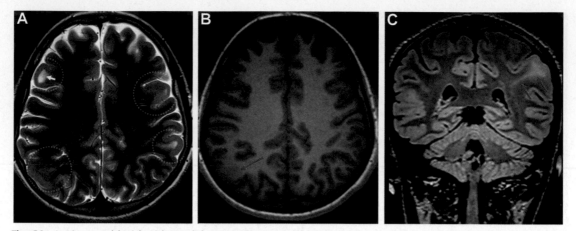

Fig. 20. A 13-year-old girl with TS. (*A*) Axial T2WI and (*B*) T1WI show multiple cortical/subcortical mushroom-shaped tubers (*dotted circles*) with gray-white matter blur in right parietal tuber (*red arrow*). The right frontal subcortical tuber shows cystic change (*yellow arrow*). (*C*) Coronal FLAIR image shows wedge-shaped radial migration line (*red arrows*) extending from tuber to ventricular surface.

These patients have increased risk of breast, endometrial, thyroid, kidney, and colon cancers.[46]

The characteristic CNS lesion in this syndrome is dysplastic cerebellar gangliocytoma (DCG), a hamartomatous tumor, the presence of which in an adult is highly suggestive of Cowden syndrome.[47] DCG appears as a hypodense mass on CT (**Fig. 27**A) with occasional calcification. On MR, DCG has a characteristic striated appearance with thickened folia. The tumor is hypointense on T1WI, hyperintense on T2WI, without postcontrast enhancement, and with facilitated diffusion (**Fig. 27**B–E; **Fig. 28**). On MR spectroscopy, DCG shows decreased NAA and choline levels, with increased lactate level (**Fig. 27**G–I). On FDG-PET/CT, the tumor is hypermetabolic (**Fig. 27**F).[47,48]

Turcot syndrome

Turcot syndrome, also referred to as brain-tumor polyposis syndrome, has 2 subtypes, types 1 and 2. Type 1 is associated with hereditary nonpolyposis colorectal cancer, secondary to germline mutations in mismatch repair genes, and predisposes patients to colorectal, endometrial, gastric, pancreaticobiliary, and genitourinary cancers along with malignant astrocytomas. Type 2 is associated with familial adenomatous polyposis, secondary to mutations in the APC gene, and these patients present with colorectal cancers and skin/osseous lesions along with medulloblastomas.[49–51] On imaging, these tumors look similar to their sporadic counterparts, except that the median age of these patients is less than 20 years.

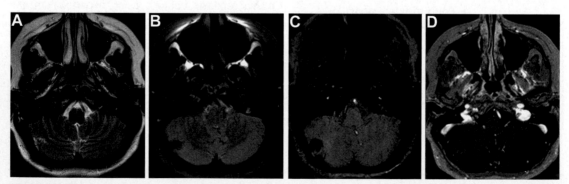

Fig. 21. A 46-year-old woman with TSC2 mutation mosaicism. (*A*) Axial T2WI, (*B*) FLAIR, (*C*) susceptibility-weighted imaging, and (*D*) postcontrast T1WI showing a typical right cerebellar tuber, a wedge-shaped lesion in right cerebellum with susceptibility low signal caused by calcification and heterogeneous postcontrast enhancement.

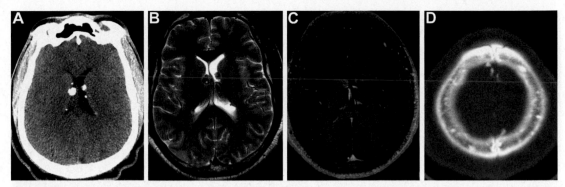

Fig. 22. A 34-year-old patient with TS. (*A*) Axial CT, (*B*) T2WI, and (*C*) postcontrast T1WI show calcified multiple SENs with low T2 signal and postcontrast enhancement. (*D*) Axial CT bone window shows multiple sclerotic foci in the calvarium.

Li-Fraumeni Syndrome

Li-Fraumeni syndrome (LFS) is an AD cancer predisposition disorder, resulting in cancers arising in children and younger adults. This disorder is usually secondary to mutation of tumor suppressor gene TP53, located in the short arm of chromosome17 (17p13.1). Cancers seen in LFS include soft tissue sarcomas, osteosarcomas, premenopausal breast cancers, brain tumors, adrenal cortical carcinomas, leukemias, and lung cancers. Classic LFS diagnosis is based on a combination of clinical presentation and family history, which includes any sarcoma diagnosed before age 45 years, and a first-degree relative with any cancer diagnosed before age 45 years and another first-degree or second-degree relative with any cancer diagnosed before age 45 years or a sarcoma diagnosed at any age. The modified Chompret criteria from 2009 have been developed to identify affected families beyond the classic criteria listed earlier.[52] Lastly, there's an additional set of criteria for Li-Fraumeni–like syndrome.

The CNS tumors seen in LFS include astrocytomas (diffusely infiltrating fibrillary type; WHO grades II–IV) and gliosarcomas, choroid plexus

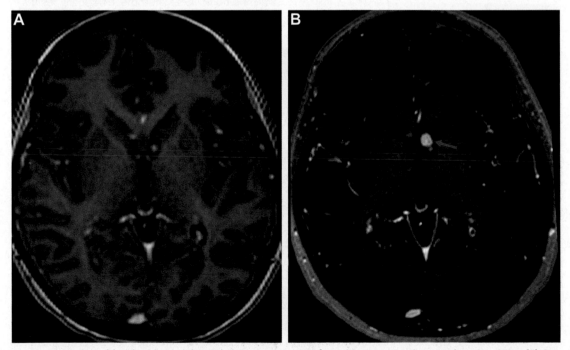

Fig. 23. A 15-year-old girl with TS. (*A*) Axial postcontrast T1WI from 10 years ago shows enhancing SENs. (*B*) One of the SENs (*red arrow*) shows interval enlargement, suggesting transformation into SGCA.

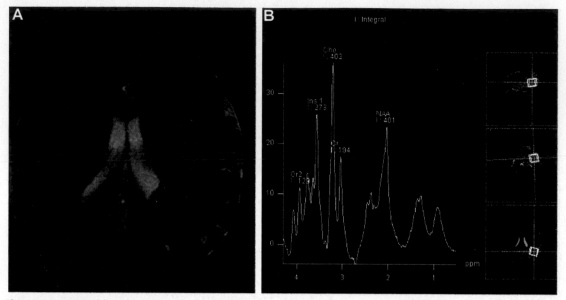

Fig. 24. A 5-year-old patient with non-TS SGCA. (*A*) Axial T2*WI showing a partially calcified left parietal region mass lesion, which was resected and found to be SGCA on histopathology. (*B*) MR spectroscopy revealed increased choline level and decreased N-acetyl aspartate level in the tumor like other neoplasms.

carcinoma, medulloblastoma, and supratentorial primitive neuroectodermal tumors.[53] Imaging findings are similar to sporadic counterparts. Imaging is also an essential part of screening and surveillance of these patents given that almost half of these patients develop an invasive cancer by age 30 years. Both whole-body MR imaging and brain MR imaging scans are recommended annually in addition to clinical and laboratory evaluations.

Multiple Endocrine Neoplasia Type 1

MEN type 1 (MEN1), also referred to commonly by the mnemonic 3Ps syndrome, classically results in

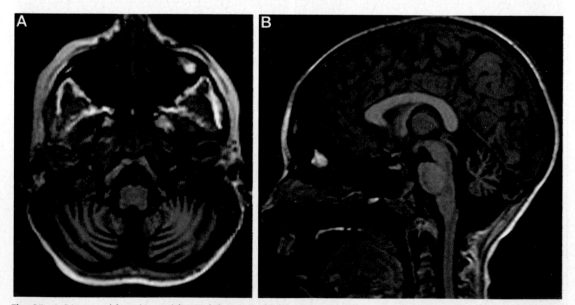

Fig. 25. A 21-year-old patient with AT. (*A*) Axial and (*B*) sagittal T1WI show significant cerebellar parenchymal volume loss, including vermis (*arrows*) with atrophic folia and prominent sulci. The supratentorial parenchyma is spared.

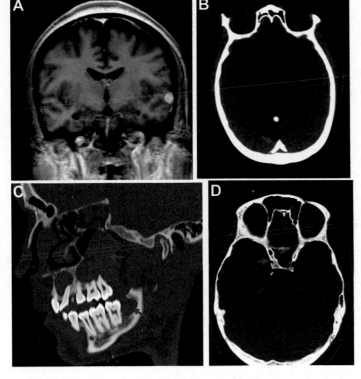

Fig. 26. BCNS. (*A*) Coronal postcontrast T1WI shows a meningioma in left temporal convexity (*arrow*) in a 30-year-old patient with BCNS. (*B*) Axial CT head shows dural calcifications (*arrow*) in the same patient. (*C*) Sagittal oblique reformat of CT face of a 26-year-old patient with BCNS shows multiple OKCs in maxilla and mandible (*arrows*). (*D*) Axial head CT in the same patient shows sellar bridging (*arrow*).

tumors of the parathyroid glands, anterior pituitary, and pancreatic islet cells. It is a high-penetrance AD heritable cancer syndrome, with a prevalence of approximately 2 per 100,000. The basis of oncogenesis in this syndrome is assumed to be the underlying mutation involving the MEN1 gene located on chromosome 11q13, which encodes for the protein menin, thought to be a tumor suppressor gene. Knudson's 2-hit hypothesis is thought to be the underlying mechanism

Table 3	
Diagnostic criteria for basal cell nevus syndrome based on the consensus statement from the First International Colloquium (May 2005)	
Diagnostic criteria: 2 major criteria (or) 1 major plus 2 minor criteria (or) 1 major criteria plus molecular confirmation	
Major criteria	• Multiple (>2) basal cell carcinomas or 1 before 20 y of age • Odontogenic keratocysts of the jaws before 20 y of age • Palmar or plantar pits • Calcification of the falx cerebri • Medulloblastoma, typically desmoplastic • First-degree relatives with BCNS
Minor criteria	• Rib anomalies (bifid, fused, or markedly splayed ribs) • Cleft lip or palate • Other specific skeletal malformations and radiologic changes (vertebral anomalies, kyphoscoliosis, short fourth metacarpals, postaxial polydactyly) • Macrocephaly • Ovarian/cardiac fibroma • Lymphomesenteric cysts • Ocular abnormalities (ie, strabismus, hypertelorism, congenital cataracts, glaucoma, coloboma)

Table 4 Neuroimaging screening recommendations in Gorlin syndrome	
Tumor/Abnormality	**Screening Recommendation**
Medulloblastoma	Baseline MR imaging brain with contrast followed by annual examination until 8 y
Odontogenic keratocyst	Baseline panorex followed by annual examination until the detection of a jaw cyst. From then, every 6 mo until no jaw cysts for 2 y or until 21 y of age
Scoliosis	Baseline at age 1 y or at time of diagnosis; repeat if symptomatic; if abnormal, repeat every 6 mo

combining the effects of the inherited gene followed by a somatic mutation.[54]

MEN1 diagnosis can be made clinically or on family history, as well as solely from a mutation without any obvious clinical/biochemical manifestations, as summarized in **Table 5**. The most common components of MEN1 are multiple parathyroid tumors causing primary hyperparathyroidism, followed by gastrinomas and pituitary adenomas (**Fig. 29**). However, patients with MEN1 can have multiple tumors other than those in the parathyroid and pituitary, and pancreatic islet cells, the discussion of which is outside the scope of this review.

Neuroradiologists can encounter patients with MEN1 in different settings of both neuro-oncology and neuroendocrine consults secondary to the involvement of parathyroid glands, pituitary, as well as the rare associations with meningiomas and cord ependymomas. MEN1 lesions relevant to neuroradiologists and their prevalence are summarized in **Table 6**.[55]

Pituitary adenomas associated with MEN1 are similar in imaging appearance to sporadic adenomas and can present as both microadenomas ($\leq$10 mm in maximal dimension) and macroadenomas ($\geq$10 mm in maximal dimension). However, adenomas associated with MEN1 are typically larger (more likely to be macroadenomas), more invasive, and difficult to resect surgically.[56] Imaging varies depending on the size of the lesion. The larger macroadenomas are usually isointense to the gray matter on T1/T2 sequences, unless they have calcification, hemorrhage, or cystic changes. On contrast-enhanced sequences, macroadenomas show robust heterogeneous enhancement. In contrast, microadenomas are inconspicuous on nonenhanced sequences and appear slightly hypointense relative to the normal pituitary gland on postcontrast sequences. Also, given that these enhance slowly compared with the pituitary gland, dynamic contrast-enhanced sequences are more sensitive in identifying these lesions.

Primary hyperparathyroidism in MEN1 is usually caused by multiglandular disease. The treatment is usually surgical, which requires the surgeon to do a 4-gland exploration. This requirement limits the role of routine preoperative screening. However, many surgeons prefer to get imaging in patients with atypical clinical presentation/biochemical profiles as well as to evaluate for ectopic glands. US is usually the first-line imaging, with nuclear scintigraphy and multiphase CT being second-line studies. On US, parathyroid adenomas appear as a well-defined, oval, hypoechoic masses adjacent to the thyroid gland, when in eutopic locations. Frequently, an enlarged/prominent vessel referred to as a polar vessel can be seen adjacent to the lesion. However, US is limited in evaluating ectopic locations. (99m)Tc-methoxyisobutylisonitrile (MIBI) planar and single-photon emission CT scintigraphy images of the neck and mediastinum are sensitive for picking up small and ectopic adenomas. In addition, multiphasic CT (also referred to as 4DCT), which involves noncontrast CT and arterial and delayed venous phase acquisitions, is another tool for evaluating these patients, and is preferred by many surgeons because of the excellent anatomic localization, particularly for ectopic adenomas as well as to differentiate from other mimics. In this technique, a parathyroid adenoma is identified by a combination of its shape, location, and enhancement characteristics with early arterial enhancement and washout.

Screening for MEN1-associated tumors is usually done using serum calcium, parathyroid hormone assays, and prolactin measurements annually. Although there is no universal consensus regarding the role of imaging in screening, some experts suggest screening individuals at high risk (such as MEN1 mutant gene carriers) at baseline and every 1 to 3 years using pituitary and abdominal imaging (eg, MR imaging or CT).[55]

Miscellaneous Syndromes

Other CNS-related cancer predisposition syndromes include neurocutaneous melanosis (NCM)[57] (**Fig. 30**), meningioangiomatosis (MA)[58]

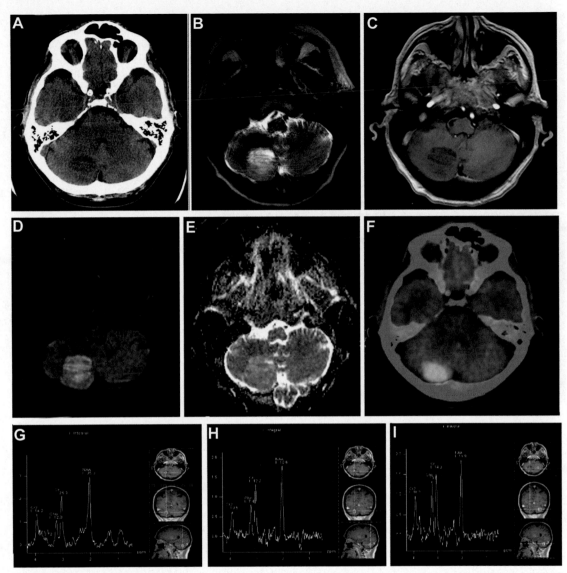

Fig. 27. Dysplastic cerebellar gangliocytoma in a 53-year-old man with Cowden syndrome. (*A*) Axial CT, (*B*) T2WI, (*C*) postcontrast T1WI, (*D*) diffusion-weighted imaging (DWI), and (*E*) ADC images show a CT hypodense, nonenhancing, T2 hyperintense mass in the right cerebellum without restricted diffusion, with striated morphology. (*F*) Fused axial FDG-PET/CT shows hypermetabolic activity of the right cerebellar lesion. MR spectroscopy of the cerebellar mass with (*G*) low and (*H*) intermediate echo time (TE) shows lactate doublet peak inverting in the intermediate TE sequence. (*I*) MR spectroscopy with intermediate TE from contralateral side shown for comparison with normal metabolite peaks.

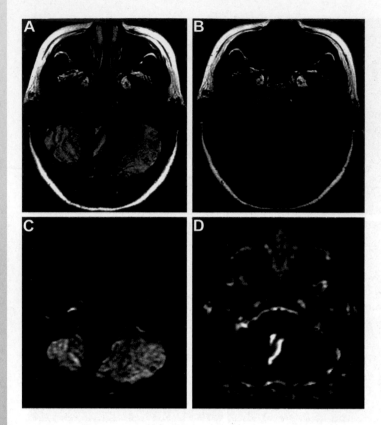

Fig. 28. Bilateral dysplastic cerebellar gangliocytoma in a 40-year-old woman with Cowden syndrome. (A) Axial T2WI and (B) T1WI shows bilateral T2 hyperintense and T1 hypointense masses with striated appearance on T2WI. (C) Axial DWI and (D) ADC images show mild restricted diffusion in the cerebellar masses.

Table 5
Diagnostic criteria for multiple endocrine neoplasia type 1

Clinical	A patient with 2 or more MEN1-associated tumors
Familial	A patient with 1 MEN1-associated tumor and a first-degree relative with MEN1
Genetic	An individual with MEN1 mutation who does not have clinical/biochemical manifestations of MEN1

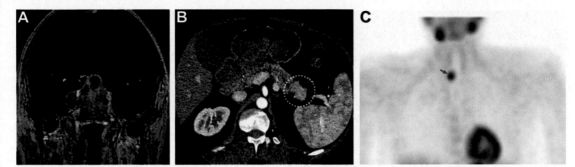

Fig. 29. MEN1. (*A*) Coronal post-T1WI of the brain shows an invasive pituitary macroadenoma with right cavernous sinus invasion in a 40-year-old patient with MEN1. (*B*) Axial CT abdomen in the same patient shows a surgically proven neuroendocrine tumor in the tail of pancreas (*circle*). (*C*) Maximum intensity projection of a delayed (90 minute) ^{99m}Tc-sestamibi scan shows a right inferior parathyroid adenoma (*arrow*) in 49-year-old patient with MEN1.

Table 6
Multiple endocrine neoplasia type 1 lesions relevant to neuroradiologists and their prevalence

Endocrine Lesions	Nonendocrine Lesions
Parathyroid adenomas (90%)	Lipomas (30%)
Anterior pituitary adenomas (30%–40%)	Facial angiofibromas (85%)
Prolactinoma (20%)	Spinal ependymomas (1%)
Prolactinoma plus growth hormone, growth hormone, nonfunctioning (5%)	Meningiomas (8%)
Adrenocorticotropin stimulating (2%)	
Thyroid-stimulating hormone–secreting adenomas (rare)	

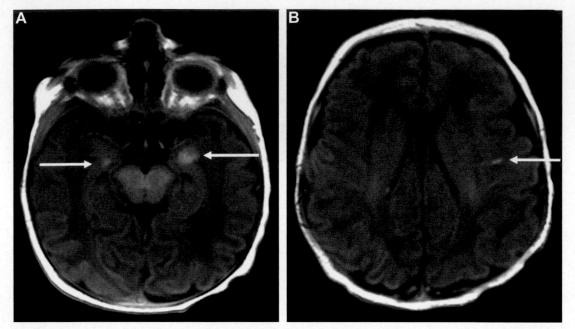

Fig. 30. Parenchymal melanosis in a 2-day-old neonate with neurocutaneous melanosis. Axial T1WI at the level of (*A*) temporal and (*B*) frontal lobes shows T1 hyperintense signal in bilateral amygdala and in left frontal deep white matter corresponding with perivascular melanocytes (*arrows*).

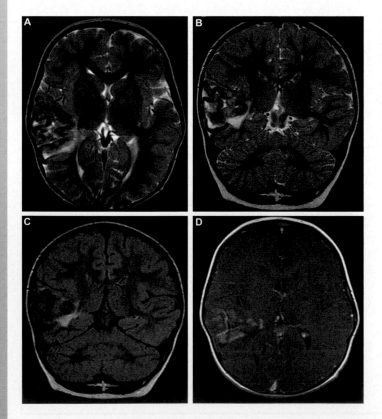

Fig. 31. Meningioangiomatosis in a 3-year-old patient. (*A*) Axial and (*B*) coronal T2WI show thickened dysmorphic right temporal lobe cortex with hypointense T2 signal caused by calcification. (*C*) Coronal FLAIR shows the adjacent white matter edema. (*D*) Axial postcontrast T1WI showing heterogeneous enhancement in the meningioangiomatosis.

Table 7
Miscellaneous central nervous system–related cancer predisposition syndromes

Syndrome	Mutations	Clinical	Tumors	Imaging
NCM	Somatic, NRAS, chromosome 1p13.2	Large (>20 cm) or multiple (>3) congenital nevi Seizure, hydrocephalus with associated clinical features Poor prognosis for both leptomeningeal melanocytosis and leptomeningeal melanomatosis	CNS: parenchymal and leptomeningeal melanoma Leptomeningeal melanomatosis Skin: malignant melanoma	Ideally MR imaging done before 6 mo of age in suspected infants, with follow-up surveillance scans Can be normal Meningeal Leptomeningeal focal melanocytic neoplasms: T1 shortening Leptomeningeal melanocytosis: T1 shortening with or without diffuse enhancement Leptomeningeal melanomatosis: T1 shortening with diffuse enhancement FLAIR sequence may show diffuse sulcal hyperintensity in leptomeningeal melanocytosis and melanomatosis Parenchymal Parenchymal melanosis: T1 shortening without enhancement, amygdala and cerebellum are most common sites

(continued on next page)

Table 7
(continued)

Syndrome	Mutations	Clinical	Tumors	Imaging
				Malignant melanoma: T1 shortening, enhancement can be heterogeneous
MA	Some are associated with NF2	Seizure	Benign hamartomatous malformation	Cortical/subcortical lesion, often shows calcification. Variable enhancement of the leptomeninges and the cortical component. There can be edema in the subjacent white matter
RTPS	*RTPS1 SMARCB1* *RTPS2: SMARCA4*	Typically present at very young age	Brain: atypical teratoid/rhabdoid tumor Rhabdoid tumor of the kidney and other organs Schwannoma	Heterogeneous in T1WI and T2WI, may show hemorrhage and cysts. Restricted diffusion, heterogeneous enhancement
MAS	Germline, *CDKN2A* tumor suppressor gene, chromosome 9p21	Seizure, cutaneous lesions from melanoma	Melanoma, astrocytoma, occasionally meningiomas, schwannoma, and neurofibroma	Imaging features are similar to the tumors seen in nonsyndromic patients
CC	*PRKAR1A*, chromosome 17q22–24 Chromosome 2p16	Pigmented lesions of the skin and mucosa, cardiac myxoma: stroke, cardiac failure, sudden death, acromegaly,	Cardiac myxoma, cutaneous and other soft tissue myxomas. Endocrine tumors: pituitary, adrenocortical, thyroid. Testicular,	Imaging features of pituitary adenomas are similar to the tumors seen in nonsyndromic patients

			Cushing, precocious puberty	ovarian and breast tumors. Pancreatic tumors, and so forth	
RTS	CREBBP, EP300	Mental retardation, behavioral problems, growth retardation, and multiple congenital anomalies, especially of the face and distal limbs, keloids		Meningioma, pilomatrixoma	Imaging features are similar to the tumors seen in nonsyndromic patients

Abbreviations: CC, Carney complex; *CDKN2A*, cyclin-dependent kinase inhibitor 2A; *CREBBP*, CREB-binding protein; *EP*, E1A-binding protein p300; MA, meningioangiomatosis; *NRAS*, N-Ras proto-oncogene; *PRKAR1A*, protein kinase cAMP-dependent type I regulatory subunit alpha; *SMARCA4/B1*, SWI/SNF-related, matrix-associated, actin-dependent regulator of chromatin.

(**Fig. 31**), rhabdoid tumor predisposition syndromes (RTPS),[59] melanoma-astrocytoma syndrome (MAS),[60] Carney complex,[61] and Rubinstein-Taybi syndrome (RTS).[62] The significant characteristics of these syndromes are summarized in **Table 7**.

CLINICS CARE POINTS

- Heritable and non-heritable cancer syndromes affecting the central nervous system have distinctive underlying mutations and molecular pathways, resulting in a myriad of both tumors, and non-tumorous lesions, with unique histopathological and imaging features.

- Recent advances in radiogenomics and understanding of cancer pathways, have led to renewed emphasis on screening and early diagnosis, targeting for innovating therapies, optimizing surveillance for monitoring therapies and follow up with imaging playing a central role in many of the above.

- Both organ specific and whole body protocols using multimodality imaging represent a crucial tool in optimizing imaging for both lesions involving the brain and spinal cord, as well as lesions outside the central nervous system, which requires leveraging the advancements in scanners and optimizing protocols.

- In addition to their expertise in imaging findings, radiologists need to have familiarity with radiogenomics and molecular cancer pathways to better serve both patients and clinicians.

DISCLOSURE

None.

REFERENCES

1. Greer MLC, Voss SD, States LJ. Pediatric cancer predisposition imaging: focus on whole-body MRI. Clin Cancer Res 2017;23(11):e6–13.

2. Kresak J, Walsh M. Neurofibromatosis: a review of NF1, NF2, and schwannomatosis. J Pediatr Genet 2016;05(02):098–104.

3. Lin J, Martel W. Cross-sectional imaging of peripheral nerve sheath tumors. Am J Roentgenol 2001; 176(1):75–82.

4. Pascual-Castroviejo I, Pascual-Pascual SI, Velazquez-Fragua R, et al. Familial spinal neurofibromatosis. Neuropediatrics 2007;38(2):105–8.

5. Woodruff J. Pathology of tumors of the peripheral nerve sheath. Am J Med Genet 1999;89(1):23–30.

6. Jee W-H, Oh S-N, McCauley T, et al. Extraaxial neurofibromas versus neurilemmomas: discrimination with MRI. Am J Roentgenol 2004;183(3):629–33.

7. Kornreich L, Blaser S, Schwarz M, et al. Optic Pathway glioma: correlation of imaging findings with the presence of neurofibromatosis. AJNR Am J Neuroradiol 2001;22(10):1963–9.

8. Binning MJ, Liu JK, Kestle JRW, et al. Optic pathway gliomas: A review. Neurosurg Focus 2007;23(5):1–8.

9. DiPaolo DP, Zimmerman RA, Rorke LB, et al. Neurofibromatosis type 1: Pathologic substrate of high-signal-intensity foci in the brain. Radiology 1995; 195(3):721–4.

10. Itoh T, Magnaldi S, White RM, et al. Neurofibromatosis type 1: The evolution of deep gray and white matter MR abnormalities. AJNR Am J Neuroradiol 1994;15(8):1513–9.

11. Cairns AG, North KN. Cerebrovascular dysplasia in neurofibromatosis type 1. J Neurol Neurosurg Psychiatry 2008;79(10):1165–70.

12. Baser ME, Friedman JM, Joe H, et al. Empirical development of improved diagnostic criteria for neurofibromatosis 2. Genet Med 2011;13(6):576–81.

13. Evans DGR. Neurofibromatosis type 2 (NF2): A clinical and molecular review. Orphanet J Rare Dis 2009;4(1):1–11.

14. Evans DG, King AT, Bowers NL, et al. Identifying the deficiencies of current diagnostic criteria for neurofibromatosis 2 using databases of 2777 individuals with molecular testing. Genet Med 2019;21(7):1525–33.

15. Asthagiri AR, Parry DM, Butman JA, et al. Neurofibromatosis type 2. Lancet 2009;373(9679):1974–86.

16. Coy S, Rashid R, Stemmer-Rachamimov A, et al. An update on the CNS manifestations of neurofibromatosis type 2. Acta Neuropathol 2020;139(4):643–65.

17. Evans DG, Bowers NL, Tobi S, et al. Schwannomatosis: A genetic and epidemiological study. J Neurol Neurosurg Psychiatry 2018;1215–9. https://doi.org/10.1136/jnnp-2018-318538.

18. Binderup MLM, Bisgaard ML, Harbud V, et al. Von Hippel-Lindau disease (vHL). National clinical guideline for diagnosis and surveillance in Denmark. 3rd edition. Dan Med J 2013;60(12):B4763.

19. Vijapura C, Saad Aldin E, Capizzano AA, et al. Genetic syndromes associated with central nervous system tumors. Radiographics 2017;37(1):258–80.

20. Lonser RR, Glenn GM, Walther M, et al. von Hippel-Lindau disease. Lancet 2003;361(9374):2059–67.

21. Wanebo JE, Lonser RR, Glenn GM, et al. The natural history of hemangioblastomas of the central nervous

system in patients with von Hippel-Lindau disease. J Neurosurg 2003;98(1):82–94.

22. Lee SR, Sanches J, Mark AS, et al. Posterior fossa hemangioblastomas: MR imaging. Radiology 1989; 171(2):463–8.

23. Leung RS, Biswas SV, Duncan M, et al. Imaging features of von Hippel-Lindau disease. Radiographics 2010;28(1):65–79 [quiz: 323].

24. Binderup MLM, Stendell A-S, Galanakis M, et al. Retinal hemangioblastoma: prevalence, incidence and frequency of underlying von Hippel-Lindau disease. Br J Ophthalmol 2018;102(7):942–7.

25. Wiley HE, Krivosic V, Gaudric A, et al. MANAGEMENT OF RETINAL HEMANGIOBLASTOMA IN VON HIPPEL-LINDAU DISEASE. Retina 2019; 39(12):2254–63.

26. Lonser RR, Kim HJ, Butman JA, et al. Tumors of the endolymphatic sac in von Hippel-Lindau disease. N Engl J Med 2004;350(24):2481–6.

27. Shanbhogue KP, Hoch M, Fatterpaker G, et al. von Hippel-Lindau disease: review of genetics and imaging. Radiol Clin North Am 2016;54(3):409–22.

28. Melean G, Sestini R, Ammannati F, et al. Genetic insights into familial tumors of the nervous system. Am J Med Genet C Semin Med Genet 2004;129C(1): 74–84.

29. Northrup H, Krueger DA. International Tuberous Sclerosis Complex Consensus Group. Tuberous sclerosis complex diagnostic criteria update: recommendations of the 2012 International Tuberous Sclerosis Complex Consensus Conference. Pediatr Neurol 2013;49(4):243–54.

30. Braffman BH, Bilaniuk LT, Naidich TP, et al. MR imaging of tuberous sclerosis: pathogenesis of this phakomatosis, use of gadopentetate dimeglumine, and literature review. Radiology 1992;183(1):227–38.

31. Manara R, Bugin S, Pelizza MF, et al. Genetic and imaging features of cerebellar abnormalities in tuberous sclerosis complex: more insights into their pathogenesis. Dev Med Child Neurol 2018;60(7): 724–5.

32. Manoukian SB, Kowal DJ. Comprehensive imaging manifestations of tuberous sclerosis. AJR Am J Roentgenol 2015;204(5):933–43.

33. Altman NR, Purser RK, Post MJD. Tuberous sclerosis: characteristics at CT and MR imaging. Radiology 1988;167(2):527–32.

34. DiMario FJ. Brain abnormalities in tuberous sclerosis complex. J Child Neurol 2004;19(9):650–7.

35. Inoue Y, Nemoto Y, Murata R, et al. CT and MR imaging of cerebral tuberous sclerosis. Brain Dev 1998; 20(4):209–21.

36. Waga S, Yamamoto Y, Kojima T, et al. Massive hemorrhage in tumor of tuberous sclerosis. Surg Neurol 1977;8(2):99–101.

37. Sener RN. Tuberous sclerosis: diffusion MRI findings in the brain. Eur Radiol 2002;12(1):138–43.

38. de Carvalho Neto A, Gasparetto EL, Bruck I. Subependymal giant cell astrocytoma with high choline/creatine ratio on proton MR spectroscopy. Arq Neuropsiquiatr 2006;64(3B):877–80.

39. Tavani F, Zimmerman RA, Berry GT, et al. Ataxia-telangiectasia: The pattern of cerebellar atrophy on MRI. Neuroradiology 2003;45(5):315–9.

40. Sardanelli F, Parodi RC, Ottonello C, et al. Cranial MRI in ataxia-telangiectasia. Neuroradiology 1995; 37(1):77–82.

41. Sahama I, Sinclair K, Pannek K, et al. Radiological imaging in ataxia telangiectasia: A review. Cerebellum 2014;13(4):521–30.

42. Lin DDM, Barker PB, Lederman HM, et al. Cerebral abnormalities in adults with ataxia-telangiectasia. AJNR Am J Neuroradiol 2014;35(1):119–23.

43. Thalakoti S, Geller T. 1st edition. Basal cell nevus syndrome or Gorlin syndrome, vol. 132. The Netherlands: Elsevier B.V.; 2015.

44. Leonardi R, Caltabiano M, Lo Muzio L, et al. Bilateral hyperplasia of the mandibular coronoid processes in patients with nevoid basal cell carcinoma syndrome: An undescribed sign [4]. Am J Med Genet 2002;110(4):400–3.

45. Bree AF, Shah MR. Consensus statement from the first international colloquium on basal cell nevus syndrome (BCNS). Am J Med Genet A 2011;155(9): 2091–7.

46. Pilarski R, Burt R, Kohlman W, et al. Cowden syndrome and the PTEN hamartoma tumor syndrome: Systematic review and revised diagnostic criteria. J Natl Cancer Inst 2013;105(21):1607–16.

47. Klisch J, Juengling F, Spreer J, et al. Lhermitte-Duclos disease: Assessment with MR imaging, positron emission tomography, single-photon emission CT, and MR spectroscopy. AJNR Am J Neuroradiol 2001;22(5):824–30.

48. Awwad EE, Levy E, Martin DS, et al. Atypical MR appearance of Lhermitte-Duclos disease with contrast enhancement. AJNR Am J Neuroradiol 1995;16(8):1719–20.

49. Bronner MP. Gastrointestinal inherited polyposis syndromes. Mod Pathol 2003;16(4):359–65.

50. Lebrun C, Olschwang S, Jeannin S, et al. Turcot syndrome confirmed with molecular analysis. Eur J Neurol 2007;14(4):470–2.

51. Mullins KJ, Rubio A, Myers SP, et al. Malignant ependymomas in a patient with Turcot's Syndrome: Case report and management guidelines. Surg Neurol 1998;49(3):290–4.

52. Malkin D. Li-fraumeni syndrome. Genes and Cancer 2011;2(4):475–84.

53. Orr BA, Clay MR, Pinto EM, et al. An update on the central nervous system manifestations of Li–Fraumeni syndrome. Acta Neuropathol 2020; 139(4):669–87.

54. Lemos MC, Thakker RV. Multiple endocrine neoplasia type 1 (MEN1): analysis of 1336 mutations reported in the first decade following identification of the gene. Hum Mutat 2008;29(1):22–32.

55. Thakker RV, Newey PJ, Walls GV, et al. Clinical practice guidelines for multiple endocrine neoplasia type 1 (MEN1). J Clin Endocrinol Metab 2012;97(9): 2990–3011.

56. Burgess JR, Shepherd JJ, Parameswaran V, et al. Spectrum of pituitary disease in multiple endocrine neoplasia type 1 (MEN 1): clinical, biochemical, and radiological features of pituitary disease in a large MEN 1 kindred. J Clin Endocrinol Metab 1996;81(7):2642–6.

57. Ramaswamy V, Delaney H, Haque S, et al. Spectrum of central nervous system abnormalities in neurocutaneous melanocytosis. Dev Med Child Neurol 2012; 54(6):563–8.

58. Aizpuru RN, Quencer RM, Norenberg M, et al. Meningioangiomatosis: clinical, radiologic, and histopathologic correlation. Radiology 1991;179(3): 819–21.

59. Sredni ST, Tomita T. Rhabdoid tumor predisposition syndrome. Pediatr Dev Pathol 2015;18(1):49–58.

60. Chan AK, Han SJ, Choy W, et al. Familial melanoma-astrocytoma syndrome: Synchronous diffuse astrocytoma and pleomorphic xanthoastrocytoma in a patient with germline CDKN2A/B deletion and a significant family history. Clin Neuropathol 2017;36(5): 213–21.

61. Correa R, Salpea P, Stratakis CA. Carney complex: an update. Eur J Endocrinol 2015;173(4):M85–97.

62. Boot MV, van Belzen MJ, Overbeek LI, et al. Benign and malignant tumors in Rubinstein–Taybi syndrome. Am J Med Genet A 2018;176(3):597–608.

Moving?

Make sure your subscription moves with you!

To notify us of your new address, find your **Clinics Account Number** (located on your mailing label above your name), and contact customer service at:

Email: journalscustomerservice-usa@elsevier.com

800-654-2452 (subscribers in the U.S. & Canada)
314-447-8871 (subscribers outside of the U.S. & Canada)

Fax number: 314-447-8029

Elsevier Health Sciences Division
Subscription Customer Service
3251 Riverport Lane
Maryland Heights, MO 63043

*To ensure uninterrupted delivery of your subscription, please notify us at least 4 weeks in advance of move.